T0257954

Encyclopedia of Tuberculosis: Diagnostic Approaches

Volume III

Encyclopedia of Tuberculosis: Diagnostic Approaches
Volume III

Edited by **Morris Beckler**

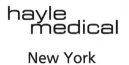

New York

Published by Hayle Medical,
30 West, 37th Street, Suite 612,
New York, NY 10018, USA
www.haylemedical.com

Encyclopedia of Tuberculosis: Diagnostic Approaches
Volume III
Edited by Morris Beckler

© 2015 Hayle Medical

International Standard Book Number: 978-1-63241-204-1 (Hardback)

Contents

Preface

Mycobacterium tuberculosis is a highly infectious disease and it is suspected that close to one-third of the world's human population has already been affected by it. Nearly, one-tenth of the infected individuals stand the chance of developing the disease, which makes its eradication a serious challenge. It is an airborne disease and easily spreads through aerosols. However, the most worrisome fact is that most affected people are absolutely unaware of their condition because the responsible bacterium causes no specific symptoms. Nevertheless, the infected cannot spread the infection any further. At the stage of development, the disease becomes dangerously contagious and the symptoms make rapid advances. Hence, detection and differentiation between infection and disease has become a serious problem. This book presents the experiences of global experts on the detection and treatment of this disease.

All of the data presented henceforth, was collaborated in the wake of recent advancements in the field. The aim of this book is to present the diversified developments from across the globe in a comprehensible manner. The opinions expressed in each chapter belong solely to the contributing authors. Their interpretations of the topics are the integral part of this book, which I have carefully compiled for a better understanding of the readers.

At the end, I would like to thank all those who dedicated their time and efforts for the successful completion of this book. I also wish to convey my gratitude towards my friends and family who supported me at every step.

Editor

Experience on Laboratory Diagnosis Around the World

1

Laboratory Diagnosis of Latent and Active Tuberculosis Infections in Trinidad & Tobago and Determination of Drug Susceptibility Profile of Tuberculosis Isolates in the Caribbean

Patrick Eberechi Akpaka and Shirematee Baboolal
Unit of Microbiology & Pathology, Department of Para Clinical Sciences,
Faculty of Medical Sciences, The University of the West Indies, St. Augustine
Trinidad & Tobago

1. Introduction

Tuberculosis (TB) is a life-threatening, infectious disease caused by the bacteria *Mycobacterium tuberculosis*. The disease has plagued human beings for many centuries as signs of tubercular damage have been found in Egyptian mummies and bones dating back at least 5,000 years ago [1]. Today, despite advances in diagnosis and treatment, TB is still a global pandemic, fueled by the spread of the Human Immunodeficiency Virus (HIV), the Acquired Immunodeficiency Syndrome (AIDS), poverty and a lack of proper health services in many developing countries [2]. As a developing nation, many of the Caribbean countries face serious challenges in the diagnosis, treatment, care and management of patients with TB. Some of these challenges include TB/HIV co-infection, drug resistance, inadequate laboratory services, growth of inequity stemming from rising poverty and the presence of weak health systems in many countries [3]. A major challenge that affects the Caribbean is the lack of proper facilities for laboratory diagnosis of TB; and there is a dire shortage of laboratory facilities and capability for culture and drug susceptibility testing. Because of this, many cases of TB with low bacillary load may be missed by smear microscopy if culture is not routinely performed. This is even more so in HIV/AIDS patients where smear microscopy may be negative due to the small numbers of bacilli being produced as a result of reduced pulmonary cavity formation [4].

Weak laboratory service is one of the major obstacles to reducing the global burden of TB. The clinical mycobacteriology laboratory plays a major role in the prevention strategies and control measures of TB [5]. A wide spectrum of laboratory techniques has been developed to confirm the diagnosis of active and latent TB infection. No single laboratory test method is perfect, and unfortunately, some of the methods of diagnosis on which clinicians still rely on were developed more than a century ago.

It was based on these challenges that the aims of this study were conceived - to compare the available screening and investigative methods for detection of latent TB in Trinidad and Tobago; and also to evaluate methods for detection of drug resistance to *Mycobacterium tuberculosis* isolates recovered from clinical and cultured specimens from several Caribbean countries.

2. Materials and methods

Study setting and Site: The overall study design and methods have been described previously [6, 7]. Briefly, this prospective observational cross sectional population and laboratory based study was carried out at the Mycobacteriology laboratory at the Caribbean Epidemiology Centre (CAREC) in Trinidad and Tobago. The materials used for the study included individuals and clinical specimens from patients managed for TB infection in Trinidad and Tobago collected over a twelve month period as well as convenient clinical specimens and *M. tuberculosis* isolates from several countries in the Caribbean that were referred to CAREC for culture, identification and drug susceptibility testing over a twenty four month period.

Specimen collection: The specimens used included sputum and other clinical specimens from several Caribbean countries including Antigua, Belize, Dominica, Jamaica, Montserrat, St. Kitts, Nevis, St. Lucia, St. Vincent and the Grenadines, Trinidad and Tobago and Turks and Caicos Islands. While sputum and clinical specimens were referred from countries that did not perform culture or was not performing culture for TB during the study, cultures on Lowestein Jensen (LJ) slants were referred from countries that had the capability to perform culture for mycobacteria but were unable to perform identification and drug susceptibility testing. These countries included The Bahamas, Barbados, Trinidad and Tobago, Suriname and Guyana. For specimens coming from Trinidad and Tobago, both clinical specimens and cultures on LJ were included in the study. Diagnosis of latent TB infection was performed using the Quantiferon Gold Assay. For this test blood samples were collected in heparinized tubes. Individuals for this assay included contacts of confirmed tuberculosis patients, health care workers from the Caura Chest Hospital and the Chest Clinic at the Eric Williams Medical Sciences Complex, inmates of the maximum security prison (where a case of TB was identified) and HIV positive patients attending routine care and treatment clinic.

All specimens referred to CAREC over a two year period (September 2006 – August 2008) from the CAREC Member Countries except Trinidad and Tobago were included in the study. Only specimens from Trinidad and Tobago referred to CAREC over a one year period (September 2006 to October 2007) were included in the study. Clinical specimens were collected from hospitalized patients, chest clinics and sometimes from patients attending the offices of their private physicians and sent to the hospital laboratory or public health laboratory in each country for acid fast bacilli. For culture and drug susceptibility testing (DST), a portion of the specimen was referred, while for laboratories that are able to culture for mycobacteria, clinical specimens were processed using the N-acetyl-L-cysteine-sodium hydroxide (NALC-NaOH) method, inoculated and incubated until visible growth was seen on the LJ slants. Slants showing positive growth were then referred for identification and DST. Patients from Trinidad and Tobago in addition to giving blood specimens placed in heparin and transported at room temperature to the laboratory for detection of latent TB also had tuberculin skin tests (Mantoux test) administered on their forearm. Results of the reaction were was read after 72 hours.

Inclusion and exclusion criteria: (a) Only specimens showing positive growth on LJ or BACTEC 460 TB system were further analysed. (b) Repeat specimens or culture were not included. (c) Specimens without basic demographic data were excluded. (d) Cultures that showed growth of contaminating organisms were also not included in the study.

Data collection: For specimens originating from Trinidad & Tobago, a standardized questionnaire was used to obtain additional information of the test subjects. The questionnaire was divided into several sections including demographics, clinical information, medical history, laboratory investigation, radiographic findings, risk factors and treatment. Several methods were used to collate data, including going through the patient's file at the hospital and speaking to the County and the Public Health Nurses. Information (usually age, gender, type of specimen, HIV status and nationality) of specimens from other countries was taken from the patient's form that accompanied the specimens when they were received at the laboratory for culture, identification and DST. Information obtained was then entered into Excel spreadsheet for analysis.

Digestion and Decontamination of the specimens: All clinical specimens were processed in a Biological Safety Cabinet (BSC) using the NALC-NaOH method as previously described in literature [8]. Specimens on LJ slants were also processed in a BSC observing all safety precautions that are applicable when working with live tuberculosis cultures as has been described [9]. From the LJ slants colonies of growth were removed with a sterile disposable loop and placed in tubes containing glass beads and 0.5ml sterile distilled water. The tubes were vortexed for approximately 10 seconds to break up the large clumps of mycobacteria and then left undisturbed for 5-10 minutes. Following this, 0.1 ml portions of the supernatant were used to inoculate into BACTEC 12B vials only.

Processing of blood sample for latent TB detection: Blood specimens in heparin tubes were incubated overnight with antigens according to the manufacturer's (Cellestis Inc., USA) instructions. To do this the blood was mixed at least 20 times by gently inverting the tube, then in a 24 well culture plate 1.0ml of blood was placed in each of 4 wells. To each well 3 drops of the respective reagent was added; saline (NIL), early secretory antigen target-6 (ESAT-6), culture filtrate protein-10 (CFP-10) and phytohemaglutinin (Mitogen control), mixed thoroughly into the blood using a plate shaker for 1-2 minutes and then incubated overnight at 37°C. After overnight incubation, the plasma was removed from each well, placed in labeled tubes and stored at 4°C after which the enzyme linked immunosorbent assay (ELISA) test for the detection of IFN-γ was performed.

Culture of clinical specimens: Clinical specimens were cultured using two types of media, the LJ media and 12B media using the BACTEC 460 TB system (Becton Dickenson). For this 0.1 ml of sediments were added aseptically into each of these two media using a tuberculin syringe and needle. Supernatant from LJ cultures were only inoculated on 12B media as above. Both LJ slants and 12B vials were incubated at 37°C. 12B vials were read twice weekly for the first 2 weeks and then once a week for the next 6 weeks for the presence of growth while LJ slants were read weekly for up to 8 weeks. 12B cultures showing positive growth (between 50 to 100 growth units) or LJ slants showing colonies of mycobacteria were removed and identified using the NAP (p-nitro-α-acetylamino-β-hydroxyl-propiophenone) test. Cultures that showed growth of contaminating organisms were discarded. The supernatant was reprocessed and reinoculated. If the cultures were still contaminated, they were discarded.

Identification of mycobacteria using the NAP test: When mycobacterial growth was detected from either the 12B growth media or the LJ slants, each isolate was further identified using the NAP test. This test was performed by adding 1.0 ml of positive culture media to a vial containing p-nitro-α-acetylamino β-hydroxyl-propiophenone. This vial together with the original culture vial was incubated at 37⁰C and read daily for 4 consecutive days. The culture was identified as *M. tuberculosis* Complex (MTBC) if the tube containing NAP did not allow growth of the mycobacteria while the original tube continued to grow. If growth was detected in both tubes, then the culture was identified as non-tuberculous mycobacteria (NTM); and these were further identified to species level using the Common Mycobacteria (CM) genotyping line probe assay from Hain Lifesciences (Germany). For quality control, a Clinical and Laboratory Standards Institute (CLSI) strain of *M. tuberculosis*, H37Rv was tested along with test specimens each week and for each new lot number of reagents that was used.

Drug Susceptibility Testing using BACTEC 460 TB System: Drug susceptibility tests (DSTs) using the BACTEC 460 TB system was performed on all isolates that belonged to the MTBC group. Only DST to 4 first line drugs and their concentrations - Streptomycin (2.0mg/L), Isoniazid (0.1mg/L), Rifampicin (2.0mg/L) and Ethambutol (2.5mg/L) were used for the study. For DSTs, 0.1 ml of broth from each positive specimen was inoculated to 12B vials containing fixed concentrations of the antibiotics listed above. A control vial without antibiotics was also inoculated with a 1:100 dilution of the respective growth media. All vials were incubated at 37ºC and read daily in the BACTEC 460 machine until the control tube read 30 growth units.

The result of each test was determined as resistant if they were above or susceptible if below of the control GI reading. For quality control, once a month and when new antibiotics were prepared, cultures with known resistance patterns were tested along with the test specimens.

Identification of Mycobacteria using Hain Genotyping Assay: This procedure consisted of the following summarized steps: (a) DNA extraction from mycobacterial culture;   (b) Preparation of Master Mix for PCR procedure; (c) Amplification Procedure; (d) Hybridization and Detection and; (e) Interpretation of results

DNA extraction: DNA extraction was performed using mycobacteria from liquid cultures (i.e. from positive 12B BACTEC culture vials). DNA extraction was performed when there was heavy growth of mycobacteria (when the liquid culture read at least 900 growth units). In a BSC 1.0ml of the culture was removed from the vial with a tuberculin needle and syringe and placed in a 2.5ml micro-centrifuge tube. The tube was then closed and centrifuged in a micro-centrifuge for 15 minutes at 13,000 r.p.ms. After centrifugation the supernatant was removed and the sediment re-suspended in 300µl molecular grade water. This suspension was then boiled at 96ºC in a water bath for 15 minutes to lyse and inactivate the bacilli. After boiling the suspension was then placed in a sonicating water bath for a further 15 minutes. 5µl of this supernatant was used for the amplification reaction.

Preparation of Master Mix: In a sterile room specifically used for preparing master mixes, the master mix was prepared by combining the following reagents in a micro tube: 35µl of PNM (containing a mixture of triphosphate deoxynucleoside and primers marked with biotin). PNM is included in kit; 5μl of 10X buffer for polymerase incubation; 2.0μl of 2.5mM MgCl$_2$; 0.2μl of HotStart Taq polymerase (Qiagen, Germany); 2.0μl of distilled water. The final volume was 45μl and this is the amount used for 1 sample. This amount was multiplied by the number of samples and controls. After preparation, 45μl amounts of the master mix were aliquoted in 0.5ml centrifuge tubes and labeled with the specimen number before the addition of DNA.

Amplification Procedure: In another room and under a BSC, 5μl of each DNA solution was added to the respective labeled tube containing the master mix prepared above to reach a final volume of 50μl. After addition of the DNA, the tubes were mixed properly by vortexing for 10 seconds. Amplification was performed in a thermal cycler (Perkin Elmer 9600 thermal cycler; Applied Biosystem, CA, USA) using the following amplification protocol: one denaturation cycle of 15 min at 95°C, followed by 10 denaturation cycles of 30s at 95°C and ten elongation cycles of 2 min at 58°C, followed by 20 additional denaturations of 25s at 95°C and annealing of 40s at 53°C, continuing with an elongation step of 40s at 70°C and finishing with an extension cycle of 8 minutes at 70°C. After amplification the amplified DNA was kept at 4°C until hybridization was done.

Hybridization and Detection: Hybridization and detection were performed as described by the manufacturers using a semi-automated method in a TwinCubator (Hain Lifesciences, Nehren, Germany).

Reverse Hybridization Process: In the Reverse Hybridization process, each strip has a total of 17 reaction zones. The first band contains the conjugate control designed to indicate that the conjugate has been effectively united with the substrate, thereby facilitating correct visualization. The second band includes a universal control designed to detect all known mycobacteria and members of the group of gram-positive bacteria with a high G+C content. This band is used for checking the presence of the amplified product after hybridization. The third band contains a sequence that amplifies a fragment of the 23S rRNA region, which is common to all known members of the tuberculosis complex. Amplification bands 4-17 include probes specific for each of the mycobacteria species. A combination of these bands enables identification of the different species of mycobacteria, including *M. tuberculosis* complex.

Drug susceptibility using MTBDRplus (Line probe assay): This procedure was performed exactly as that for identification of mycobacteria except for the difference in the primers used and the type of specimen. While cultured material was used for the Common Mycobacterium CM assay, clinical specimens were used for the MTBDR*plus* assay. The primers used were specific to detect presence of wild types and mutations. Each strip contained bands that detected *M. tuberculosis* Complex, locus controls (*rpo*B, *kat*G and *inh*A) as well as Wild Types (WT) and mutations for *rpo*B, *kat*G and *inh*A. There were eight WT for *rpo*B gene (WT 1-8) and four mutations (MUT 1, 2A, 2B and 3). For *kat*G gene there was one WT and 2 mutations (MUT 1and 2) and for *inh*A gene 2 WT (1 and 2) and 4 mutations (MUT 1, 2, 3A and 3B). The isolate was identified as *M. tuberculosis* complex when the TUB band was present. Resistance was determined when a wild type was missing and or a mutation present for each of the gene on the strip.

ELISA test for detection of gamma interferon (IFN-γ): For each ELISA test run, two strips or 16 wells were required for standards and 4 wells were required for each patient sample.

All reagents except the conjugate were brought to room temperature before the test. For each run the required number of strips were removed from the kit and placed on a strip holder. The standard dilutions were prepared (8.0IU/ml – 0.125IU/ml) as well as the conjugate dilution (5µl conjugate concentrate to 1.0ml of diluent). To each well 50µl conjugate dilution was added followed by 50µl standard dilution and 50µl respective patient samples. The contents of the wells were mixed for 1-2 minutes using a plate shaker and then incubated for 2 hours at room temperature to enable the antigen-conjugate complex to adhere to the surface of the microwells. After incubation, the wells were washed with wash buffer 5 times using an automated plate washer to remove excess conjugate complex. This was followed by the addition of 100µl enzyme substrate (kit component). The wells were mixed as before and incubated for a further 30 minutes at room temperature. The reaction was stopped after this time with 50µl enzyme stop solution and the optical densities of each well measured using wavelengths of 450 and 620. Results were calculated by plotting the results on a graph using Microsoft Office Excel. Results greater than 0.35 in the ESAT-6 and CFP-10 wells were recorded as positive while results less than 0.35 were recorded as negative.

Data Analysis: Statistical analysis of results of culture, identification, DST as well as questionnaire information were performed using Epi Info 3.5.1 version, Centers for Disease Control & Prevention software [10] and Open Epi version 2.3 [11]. Associations between variables were assessed using Chi-square analysis and Fisher's exact test. P-values of ≤0.05 were considered statistically significant.

Ethical approval: The Ethics committee of the Faculty of Medical Sciences, The University of the West Indies, St. Augustine, Trinidad and Tobago, approved the study while written permission for use of the specimens was received from the Chief Medical Officers in the Ministry of Health from each of the countries represented in the study.

3. Results

Specimens and patients: A total of 1,262 specimens comprising 43% culture materials and 57% clinical samples obtained from 15 Caribbean countries were used for this study. The highest number of specimens 28% were obtained from Trinidad & Tobago and the least 0.2% was from Dominica as depicted on Table 1. For latent TB detection, 560 subjects were recruited from Trinidad and Tobago.

Culture and Identification: The BACTEC 460-TB culture method used for culturing the specimens yielded 773 positive cultures and from this, 79.04% (611/773) were identified to belong to the *Mycobacterium tuberculosis* complex group, while 20.96% (162/773) were NTMs using NAP test. The Hain Common Mycobacteria (CM) genotyping assay was used to further identify the NTMs isolates that consisted of *Mycobacterium fortuitium* (34.6%), followed by *Mycobacterium intracellulare* (12.3%), *Mycobacterium gordonae* (6.8%), and *Mycobacterium kansassi* (6.2%). The genotyping assay was unable to identify 16.7% of the NTMs, while 7.4% showed characteristics of mixed infection with *M. tuberculosis* and *M. fortuitium* (referred to Hain Lifesciences for confirmation). The distribution of the NTMs isolates from the various Caribbean countries is highlighted in Table 2.

Laboratory Diagnosis of Latent and Active Tuberculosis Infections in Trinidad & Tobago and Determination of Drug
Susceptibility Profile of Tuberculosis Isolates in the Caribbean

9

| Country | Specimens | | Total (%) |
	Clinical samples	Culture materials	
Antigua	3	-	3 (0.24)
Bahamas	-	28	28 (2.22)
Barbados	-	26	26 (2.06)
Belize	54	-	54 (4.28)
Dominica	2	-	2 (0.16)
Guyana	-	214	214 (16.96)
Jamaica	208	-	208 (16.48)
Montserrat	25	-	25 (1.98)
St. Kitts	3	-	3 (0.24)
Nevis	5	-	5 (0.40)
St. Lucia	77	-	77 (6.10)
St. V &G	7	-	7 (0.55)
Suriname	-	240	240 (19.02)
T&T	328	34	362 (28.68)
TCI	8	-	8 (0.63)
TOTAL	720 (57.05)	542 (42.95)	1,262 (100)

St. V&G = St. Vincent and the Grenadines, T&T = Trinidad & Tobago, TCI = Turks & Caicos Islands

Table 1. Distribution of specimens (clinical samples and cultures) received from fifteen (15) Caribbean countries used for this study (%).

Species	N (%)	Countries
M. fortuitium	56 (34.6)	BDS, BLZ, GUY, SUR, T&T
M. intracellulare	20 (12.3)	ANT, GUY, JAM, STL, SUR, T&T
M. gordonae	11 (6.8)	BRB, GUY, SUR
M. kansassi	10 (6.2)	BRB, JAM, T&T
M. abscessus	8 (4.9)	BRB, JAM, SUR
M. avium	6 (3.7)	JAM, SUR, TCI, NVS
M. intermedium	4 (2.5)	SUR
M. scrofoleceum	3 (1.9)	BLZ, SUR, T&T
M. interjectum	3 (1.9)	SUR, TCI
M. simiae	1 (0.6)	JAM
M. chelonae	1 (0.6)	SUR
Mycobacterium species	27 (16.7)	GUY, JAM, SUR, MNT
Mixed infection (MTB and *M. fortuitium*)	12 (7.4)	JAM, SUR
TOTAL	162(100)	

N = total number, MTB = Mycobacterium tuberculosis, T&T = Trinidad & Tobago, TCI = Turks and Caicos Islands, JAM = Jamaica, SUR = Suriname, GUY = Guyana, MNT = Montserrat, BLZ = Belize, NVS = Nevis, BRB = Barbados, ANT = Antigua

Table 2. Distribution of non tuberculosis mycobacteria (NTM) species identified in specimens from Caribbean countries using the Common Mycobacteria (CM) genotyping assay

3.1 Tuberculin Skin Test and QuantiFERON-TB Gold for the detection of Latent TB infection

A total of 560 subjects were recruited from Trinidad & Tobago for this component of the study. They all had blood samples drawn from them and equally had TST administered on their forearm. Of these 560, only 530 of the subjects met the study criteria and were therefore included in the final analysis of the results. Summary of the result of the detection of latent TB infection using the tuberculin skin test (TST) and the QuantiFERON-TB Gold assay is given on Table 3.

The majority of the subjects were males (73.5%) and between the ages of 40 and 49 years (32.8%), The TST results surprisingly revealed that only 1.8% (3/165) of the TB patient (control group) readings were <5 mm and only 3% (5/165) were 5-9 mm. As expected, 95.2% of the TB patients had a wheal reaction ≥10 mm. None of the HIV subjects had a reaction of ≥ 10 mm but most of them (90.6%) had a reaction < 5 mm; the rest (9.4%) had a reaction measuring 5-9 mm. Among the health care workers, there were no TST readings ≥ 15mm, but most (73.2%) were <5 mm. In Trinidad and Tobago, a TST reading ≥ 10 mm among uncompromised individuals is considered a positive result. For individuals with HIV or any other underlying condition, such as malignancy, the positive cutoff threshold drops to 5-9 mm. Therefore, the 9.4% of HIV-positive subjects in the current study with readings at that level were considered to have positive TST results. Cutoff thresholds for interpretation of actual TST results (which are not considered biologically meaningful) range from 5 mm to 15 mm, depending on the type of high-risk group being surveyed and the level of TB prevalence in the study setting. The positive cutoff values used in the current study are relatively high but did not affect the final study results due to the clustered distribution of the induration values described above.

The comparative results of the two test methods used for the diagnosis or screening for latent TB infection among high risk groups in Trinidad & Tobago (Table 3) revealed that the QFT-G assay detected a significantly higher proportion of latent TB infected individuals than the TST in all high-risk groups except TB patients (the study controls), among whom the TST appeared to be more effective. The differences were statistically significant among all target groups studied for each testing method.

There was no significant age difference between the TST positive subjects and those with positive results for the QFT-G assay, who ranged from 20 to 60 years and 21 to 59 years respectively (with a mean age of 33.1 versus 34.5 years; p > 0.05). Most of the HIV and TB positive subjects (68.8% and 69.7% respectively) were in the 30-59 year age group.

The average number of hours required to complete the TST was 70.1 hours versus 23.4 hours for the QFT-G assay (p <0.0001). The average cost to perform each TST was US $3.70 (for a total cost of US $2,065.00), whereas US $18.60 was required to carry out the QFT-G assay (total cost of US $10,440.00). These differences were significant (US$3.70 versus US$18.60; p =0.0008) and favored use of the TST method for latent TB infection (LTBI) detection.

When the results of both tests were combined, the rate of LTBI detection increased to 88.7%. In the prison inmate group, concomitant results for both tests were available for 62 subjects. Of these, 24.2% (15/62) tested positive based on the TST and 56.5% (35/62) tested positive based on the QFT-G assay. The rate of concordance between the two tests for this target group was 49.7% (32/62) for negative results, and 15.6% (10/62) for positive results, and overall agreement of 76%. For all discordant results, subjects were more likely to be TST-positive and QFT-G – negative (92.1%) versus TST-negative and QFT-G – positive (7.0%). Overall, 39.6% of all subjects had a positive TST result and 51.3% had a positive QFT-G assay result. The significant differences obtained for TAT favored the QFT-G assay, whereas the cost of material required to perform the tests favored the TST.

High risk group	N	No. cases detected (%)		P-value
		TST	QFT-G	
TB patients' contacts[a]	200	35 (17.5)	78 (39.0)	<0.001
Health Care Workers	40	3 (7.5)	15 (37.5)	<0.003
Prison inmates	62	15 (24.2)	35 (56.5)	<0.006
HIV+ patients	60	12 (20.0)	26 (43.3)	<0.0006
TB Patients (controls)	168	157 (93.5)	118 (70.2)	<0.008
Total	530	210 (39.6)	272 (51.3)	0.08
Cost per test[b]		$3.70	$18.60	<0.0008
Turnaround time[c]		70.0	23.0	<0.0001

N = total number of subjects tested. [a] Individuals who came into contact with active TB patients - friends and family members. [b] In 2010 US dollars ($1 = 6.35 TTD). [c] Average number of hours from time of intradermal injection of tuberculin on subjects' forearms to the time wheal reaction at puncture was read within 72 hours.

Table 3. Comparison of QuantiFERON® TB-Gold (QFT-G) assay and tuberculin skin test (TST) in diagnosis/screening for latent tuberculosis (TB) infection among high-risk groups from Trinidad & Tobago

The average number of hours required to complete the TST was 70.0 hours versus 23.0 hours for the QFT-G assay (p <0.0001). The average cost to perform each TST was US $3.70 (for a total cost of US $2,065.00), whereas US $18.60 was required to carry out the QFT-G assay (total cost of US $10,440.00). These differences were significant (US$3.70 versus US$18.60; p =0.0008) and favored use of the TST method for LTBI detection.

Drug Susceptibility Testing (DST): The BACTEC 460 TB System was used to successfully determine the drug susceptibility tests (DST) of 91.3% (558/611) cultures identified as *M. tuberculosis* Complex from 12 of the Caribbean countries as revealed on Table 4. Overall, a total of 42 (7.5%) isolates from 8 countries showed resistance to at least one or more anti-TB drugs.

Analysis of the susceptibility pattern to the anti TB agents revealed that 73.8% (31/42) of the isolates were resistant to isoniazid (INH), 66.7% (28/42) were resistant to rifampicin (RIF), 38.9 (16/42) were resistant to both RIF and INH while 28.6% (12/42) were either resistant to streptomycin or ethambutol. The highest number of isolates subjected to DST analysis were obtained from Trinidad & Tobago and then followed by Guyana. Although no multidrug resistance was seen in isolates from several of the Caribbean countries, the highest frequency of resistance and multidrug resistance were noted among isolates from Guyana.

The Hain Genotyping line probe assay (MTBDR*plus*) was further used to genotypically analyze a total of 33 isolates that had initially been identified to be resistant to INH (26 isolates) and/or RIF (24 isolates) by the phenotypic method. This result is shown on Table 5. Overall, of the 24 isolates showing resistance to RIF using the phenotypic method, 23 (95.8%) showed resistance with the genotypic method. Of the 26 isolates showing resistance to INH with the phenotypic method, 9 (34.6%) showed resistance with the genotypic method. Additionally, 2 isolates sensitive to INH with the phenotypic method showed resistance with the genotypic method and 1 isolate resistant to RIF with the phenotypic method was sensitive with the genotypic method.

Resistance to RIF was identified genotypically by the presence or absence of mutations in the *rpo*B gene, while resistance to INH was identified by the presence or absence of mutations in the *kat*G and *inh*A genes. The codons most frequently involved in RIF mutations were S-531L (57.1%) and codon S-516L (20%). Twenty (20) isolates carried the most common mutation, Ser531 → Leu. As for INH resistance, of the 9 isolates that the Genotype MTBDR*plus* detected, 78% of them carried mutation at S315T1 codon of the *kat*G gene, showing AGC → ACC mutation, and 22% showed AGC → ACA mutation. Equally, 64.7% of these mutation occurred at these bands at the *inh*A gene in the MDR isolates from the region.

Country	N	S	R	MDR
Bahamas	21	15	6 (14.3)	0
Barbados	14	12	2 (4.8)	1 (6.25)
Belize	5	3	2 (4.8)	1 (6.25)
Dominica	1	1	0	0
Guyana	141	117	24 (57.1)	13 (81.25)
Jamaica	95	92	3 (7.14)	0
St. Lucia	10	10	0	0
St. Kitts	2	2	0	0
St. V&G	6	6	0	0
Suriname	115	112	3 (7.1)	1 (6.25)
T&T	145	144	1 (2.4)	0
TCI	3	2	1 (2.4)	0
Total	558	516	42 (100)	16 (100)

N = number of isolates tested, S = isolates fully susceptibile to all first line drugs, R = isolates resistant to any of the first line drugs, MDR = isolates resistant to both isoniazid and rifampcin, T&T – Trinidad and Tobago, TCI – Turks and Caicos Islands, St. V&G – St. Vincent and the Grenadines.

Table 4. BACTEC 460 TB System susceptibility results of 558 TB isolates (patients) from the Caribbean (%)

BACTEC 460 MTBDRplus	rpoB		katG		InhA		RIF	INH
	MWT	Mut	MWT	Mut	MWT	Mut	RIF	INH
RIF	WT7	2A	-	-	-	-	R	-
R	WT8	3	-	-	-	-	R	-
R	N	2A, 3	-	-	-	-	R	-
R	WT8	3	-	-	-	-	R	-
R	WT8	3	-	-	-	-	R	-
RE	WT8	3	-	-	-	-	R	-
I	WT8	3	N	N	N	N	R	S
I	-	-	N	N	N	N	-	S
I	-	-	N	N	N	N	-	S
I	-	-	WT1	1	N	N	-	R
I	-	-	N	N	N	N	-	S
I	W3,4	-	N	N	N	N	R	S
I	-	-	N	N	WT1	1	-	R
IE	_	-	N	N	N	N	-	S
IR	WT8	3	N	N	N	N	R	S
IR	WT8	3	N	N	W	1	R	R
IR	WT4,5,7,8	N	N	N	N	N	R	S
IR	WT7	2B	N	N	N	N	R	S
IR	N	N	N	N	WT1	1	S	R
IR	WT8	3	N	N	N	N	R	S
IR	WT2.3N		WT1	N	N	N	R	R
IRE	WT8	3	N	N	N	N	R	S
IRE	WT3.41		N	N	WT1	1	R	R
IRE	WT8	3	N	N	N	N	R	S
IRE	WT8	N	WT1	1	N	N	R	R
SIR	WT3, 4		N	N	N	N	R	S
SIRE	WT3, 4		1	N	N	N	R	S
SIRE	WT8	3	N	N	N	N	R	S
SIRE	WT8	N	WT1	1	N	N	R	R
IRE	WT8	N	WT1	1	N	N	R	S
SIR	WT3, 4		N	N	N	N	R	S
SIRE	WT3, 4		1	N	N	N	R	S
SIRE	WT8	3	N	N	N	N	R	S
SIRE	WT8	N	WT1	1	N	N	R	R

MWT = Missing wild type, MUT = mutation, N = none, R = resistant, S = susceptible, R-IRE = resistant to isoniazid, rifampicin and Ethambutol, R-SIRE = resistant to Streptomycin, isoniazid, rifampicin and ethambutol

Table 5. Results of MTBDR*plus* for isolates that showed resistance to INH and RIF using BACTEC 460 assay

4. Discussions

One of the major objectives of this study was to evaluate the tuberculin skin test (TST), the method currently being used in Trinidad & Tobago, with that of the Quantiferon TB-Gold Test (a new IFN-γ based test that has now been introduced in the market for LTBI detection) to determine the cost and efficiency of these methods in detecting latent TB infection (LTBI). Unlike the TST and IFN-γ analysis, most diagnostic assays for detecting *M. tuberculosis* infection are based on either isolation or identification of the bacteria, which makes them inapplicable for diagnosis of latent infection. The development of IFN-γ tests to detect T-cells specific for *M. tuberculosis* antigens addressed this important issue. The current study was carried out among individuals from various groups with a high risk of developing TB due to either exposure to or contact with TB patients, lack of isolation facilities, or weak infection control. In the current study, the two selected testing methods (QFT-G and TST) detected LTBI among the various target groups at different rates.

Among the TB patient [control] group, the rate of TB detection by the QFT-G assay (70.2%) was significantly different from that of the TST. This rate of detection was similar to that observed by Lee *et al.*, who reported a sensitivity of 70% among 87 patients diagnosed with TB [12], and higher than both the 64.4% rate of detection observed by Kobashi *et al.* in Japan [13] and the rate observed by Dewan *et al.*, who reported a sensitivity of 60% in culture-confirmed cases [14]. However, the 70.2% rate was lower than that reported by both Kang *et al.* (81% sensitivity in 54 patients) and Mori *et al.* (89% sensitivity among 118 patients) [15, 16]. More recently, Kobashi *et al.* demonstrated significant differences in the quantitative responses of IFN-γ to *M. tuberculosis* between patients with active TB disease and those with LTBI [13].

Combining the results for the QFT-G assay and the TST in the current study increased the overall sensitivity for detection of LBTI among the culture-confirmed TB-infected control group. This confirms and reinforces recommendations that negative results should not be used alone to exclude active TB but should be interpreted in conjunction with other clinical and diagnostic findings [17]. It also underscores the fact that the QFT-G assay has a limited role in the evaluation of patients with culture-confirmed TB. The authors of the current study agree with Kobashi *et al.*'s conclusion that it would be difficult to use the QFT-G assay to completely discriminate active TB disease from LTBI [13].

In the current study, 43.3% of all HIV patients included in the analysis had a positive result for the QFT-G assay. This was in huge contrast to the earlier study by Kobashi *et al.* [13], in which all HIV patients produced QFT-G–positive results. The indeterminate or nonreactive results observed in some of the HIV-positive subjects in the current study also contrast with those found by Ferrara *et al.* [17]. In the current study, the QFT-G assays were run several times to minimize the effect of laboratory and procedural errors. However, the indeterminate and nonreactive results persisted, with test results continuing to produce low mitogen levels. Although all indeterminate or nonreactive results were excluded from the final analysis, the QFT-G assay results should be interpreted with caution, bearing in mind the high prevalence of HIV in Trinidad & Tobago and the Caribbean region. Several possible explanations for a high rate of indeterminate and nonreactive results have been adduced and these include the presence of lymphocytopenia and/or inflammatory and immunosuppressive conditions, as well as hypoalbuminemia, which suggests poor nutritional status [13], and there is a high probability that some of these conditions could have existed among the subjects of the current study. Lymphocytopenia (especially the CD4 strain) has been shown to depend on the elaboration of inflammatory cytokines by T-cells previously sensitized to *M. tuberculosis*–specific antigens in QFT-G assays. In the blood, mononuclear cells from peripheral blood are stimulated in vitro, and the production of IFN-γ from sensitized T-lymphocytes by *M. tuberculosis*–specific antigen is measured by ELISA in the QFT-G [18,19].

In the current study, however, only 58% of TST-positive subjects had a positive QFT-G result. More than half of this group consisted of prison inmates with a documented TST > 10 mm. In Trinidad & Tobago, TST is likely to be a very good indicator of latent infection in recently exposed individuals because of the following reasons (a) most individuals under the age of 20 years did not receive the BCG vaccination, which was discontinued during the early 1990s, and (b) BCG vaccination has been observed to significantly increase the likelihood of a positive TST in subjects without LTBI.

Multiple outbreaks of TB, including those involving the multi-drug-resistant strain (MDR-TB), have been reported in prisons and jails, especially among HIV-infected inmates, a population regarded as having moderate risk of acquiring TB [20]. The results of the current study from this moderate-risk population show that prevalence of LTBI was 24.2% and 56.5% based on the TST and the QFT-G assay respectively. These values were quite high compared to those observed in correctional facilities in the United States, where prevalence was less than 10%. However, the QFT-G values obtained in the current study were in line with the current rate of TB in Trinidad & Tobago, which is estimated to be about 17 per 100 000 population [21]. It has been suggested that annual TB screening of prison inmates using the TST may account for the increase in the number of TST-positive results, due to the "boosting" effect caused by repeat use of the test. However, this type of screening is not carried out among prison inmates in Trinidad & Tobago. Therefore, the high rate of TST-positive results in the current study could be attributed mainly to exposure to the disease.

The prevalence of LTBI among health care workers using the TST in the current study was a mere 7.5%. This value was very low compared to those reported by studies in Portugal (33%) and Germany (10%)[22, 23]. The low value found in the current study may have been due to a smaller sample size and the use of a higher positive cutoff. Like the studies in Portugal and Germany, the current study showed that the QFT-G assay was more useful than the TST in identifying LTBI among health care workers. As this target group may be exposed to TB more frequently than the local population, screening of staff exposed to the disease is frequently recommended to identify infected individuals and treat them adequately and promptly. Because the QFT-G assay was more sensitive than the TST in detecting LTBI, the authors of the current study strongly support its use in screening health care workers in Trinidad & Tobago.

The TST may also be less desirable due to complications in interpreting its results caused by the above-mentioned boosting effect (from repeat testing) as well as conversions and reversions (changes in results from negative at baseline to positive and vice versa, respectively). In a study on health care workers in India, Pai *et al.* suggested that individuals with recent exposure to TB usually presented with large increases (≥ 10 mm) in TST indurations that were always accompanied by substantial increases in IFN-γ [24]. This finding was in line with the results of the current study.

The QFT-G assay also fared better than the TST in terms of TAT. In terms of cost, however, the TST appears best suited for the resource-strapped environment of Trinidad & Tobago (if the calculation of this variable is based mainly on the cost of the materials required to perform the test versus the cost of labor and other inputs). This argument is partly supported by Pooran *et al.*, who concluded in a recent report that screening for LTBI using TST alone was the most cost-effective testing strategy but ultimately incurred the highest cost due to test inaccuracies [25]. Another factor that may make the TST less cost-effective over time is high replacement costs, since the Mantoux test solution is often not accessible in developing countries and would have to be replaced with the relatively labor-intensive IFN-γ release assay. Minimizing cost for TB testing has become increasingly important because prevalence of the disease has fallen dramatically in developed countries and more than 90% of all cases worldwide occur in resource-strapped developing countries [26]. However, as pointed out by both Diel *et al.* and Marra *et al.*, use of the IFN-γ release assay alone or in combination with the TST for screening close TB contacts prior to LTBI treatment is highly cost-effective in reducing the TB disease burden [27, 28, 29].

4.1 Profiles of drug susceptibility patterns of *Mycobacterium tuberculosis* isolates encountered in the Caribbean

Drug resistance using the Hain Lifescience MTBDR*plus* line probe assay revealed that this method performed very well for the detection of RIF resistance isolates in the region. This is in agreement with the high sensitivity reported elsewhere [30, 31, 32]. However, the results for detection of resistance to INH were much lower using this assay. This observation is not unique since the molecular mechanisms for INH resistance are not fully understood and about 25-30% of phenotypic INH-resistance associated mutations are still unaccounted for [32].

This study revealed that the codon most frequently involved in the mutation was the S-531L of the *rpo*B gene among the RIF resistant isolates. Similar result has been reported by Cavusoglu *et al.*, 2007 [34], but Barnard *et al.*, 2008 [35], reported that most mutations in the isolates tested in their study occurred at several other codons. Also, a high proportion of the mutational changes were detected in the S-315T1 codon of the *kat*G gene for the INH and RIF monoresistant isolates in this study in contrast to regions reported elsewhere [35]. This was a trend reported in a high burden setting that seem to be a different trend among the *M. tuberculosis* isolates seen here in the Caribbean region.

The MTBDR*plus* genotype assay allowed for the rapid and specific detection of most mutations conferring resistance to RIF and to a lesser extent INH. Collective observations have indicated that mutations to the *rpo*B gene may account for the greater than 96% of the resistance to RIF [30,35]. This present study indicated that this is also true for Caribbean TB isolates that showed an overall resistance detection of 95.8% with the MTBDR*plus* assay.

Detection of INH resistance using the MTBDR*plus* assay for the *kat*G and *inh*A gene was disappointing. In this study, only 34.6% resistance to INH was detected using the MTBDR*plus* assay which is less than that reported by Johnson *et al.*, 2008 [36]. Other studies showed detection of 60-90% within the *kat*G gene and 15-43% within the *inh*A gene [32, 31]. Nonetheless, it must be kept in mind that the isolates used in this study were screened using the single drug concentration of 0.1µg/ml of INH in the BACTEC 460 TB system (which detects low levels of resistance to INH at this concentration, mainly useful for therapeutic purposes). The study did not discriminate between strains with low levels of INH resistance with those harboring a high level of resistance, a fact that may indirectly explain the poor agreement between the number of INH-resistant isolates detected using the gold-standard BACTEC 460 TB as compared to the MTBDR*plus* (26 instead of 9). In fact, it has been shown that the MTBDR*plus* assay was unable to detect low levels of INH resistance that was commonly detected using the BACTEC 460 TB system [32].

Previous reports have confirmed that high INH concentration levels of more than 0.4µg/ml can be detected in the *kat*G genes among *M. tuberculosis* isolates that are resistant to the drug [32]. This detection of low INH resistance among the *M. tuberculosis* isolates seen in this study could perhaps be because of the low concentration of the INH drug used. In addition, the MTBDR*plus* assay only detects those resistances of *M. tuberculosis* that have their origins in the *rpo*B, *kat*G and *inh*A regions (MTBDR*plus* kit insert). Since resistance originating from mutations of other genes or gene regions as well as other RIF and INH mechanisms are not detected by the MTBDR*plus*, it could be that other mechanisms of resistance possessed by the isolates from the Caribbean were not detected. This will definitely require further studies since such was outside the scope of this study.

With the MTBDR*plus* assay, clinical specimens that are AFB positive with moderate to many AFBs, can be reliably tested for drug resistance. Furthermore, the genotypic DST method was able to detect drug resistance in samples that were contaminated as well as in those that had lost viability, circumventing the need to request follow-up sputum thus decreasing the time between specimen collection, results and treatment of the patient. This study also showed that less time was spent using the MTBDR*plus* in detecting INH and RIF resistance in TB isolates in the Caribbean. Using the BACTEC 460 TB system, the mean time for reporting results showing any drug-resistance was 32 days for cultures and 40 days for clinical specimens. This time represented repeating all drug-sensitivities for specimens showing any resistance. For specimens that were sensitive to anti-TB drugs, the mean time was 21 days for clinical specimens and 14 days for isolates.

Determination of drug resistance is difficult due to technical reasons and in several cases; these results are not always accurate [37]. In addition, it can take up to 6 weeks to get a phenotypic DST result and during this time many transmission events may take place. Therefore, alternative methods need to be evaluated to improve the speed of diagnosis especially drug resistant TB and this is what was achieved using the MTBDR*plus* assay in this study. With the BACTEC 460 system, culture material was not able to give results for non viable or contaminated materials; however in this study the MTBDR*plus* system gave identifiable results. This is in agreement with what has been reported as these tests are able to perform on specimens that contain non viable bacilli or from specimen that were contaminated by other bacteria and fungi [32, 35, 36].

Although MTBDR*plus* assay has limitations as with any DNA-based screening nucleic acid sequence, it is possible that mutations that do not cause an amino acid exchange (silent mutations) will still produce the absence of one of the wild type probes. In addition, this assay only detects those resistance of the M. *tuberculosis* that have origins in the *rpoB*, *katG* and *inh*A regions, yet the high sensitivity of RIF resistance detection is a plus point since this test can be used for detecting RIF resistance, a surrogate marker for multiple drug resistance in M. *tuberculosis* isolates. This assay is an excellent test to use on selected clinical samples because the amount of time required in generating a result was within 24 hours after receipt of specimen, culturing of the specimen is not required and contaminated as well as non-viable cultures can be used. Finally, the test method was also cheaper to use in resource-poor countries like in the Caribbean region.

Despite the global expansion in coverage of drug-resistance surveillance, data on drug resistance are still unavailable for more than 100 countries throughout the world [38]. Even in the Caribbean there is a paucity of information or data on the anti TB susceptibility pattern. This study was very important as it provided data on drug resistance that was lacking for most of the countries in the Caribbean. The level of drug resistance observed in most of the countries in this study was quite low with the exception of Guyana. Although drug resistance has been reported from several countries in the Caribbean, data reported to WHO on drug resistance is lacking as only Trinidad and Tobago reported 1 case of MDR-TB to the WHO in 2006 [39].

In this study, resistance to anti-TB medications was seen in seven countries, five of which had >5 cases of TB/100,000 population and with one country (Guyana) accounting for 85% of the MDR-TB strains seen. This data confirms the continued existence of drug resistance in Guyana, as an earlier report by Menner *et al.*, 2005 [40] also reported a high frequency of drug resistance in this country with 22.2% of the isolates tested showing resistance to at least one anti-tuberculosis drug and 11.1% showing resistance to INH and RIF [40]. The reason for the continued persistence of MDR-TB in Guyana according to Menner *et al* is the lack of human resources to adequately follow up and monitor patient treatment as well as poor management of the tuberculosis control programme [40]. In this present study similar results were seen as 20.5% of isolates tested showed resistance to at least one anti-TB drug and 14.5% showed resistance to INH and RIF (MDR-TB).

Unlike previous studies from Africa, Haiti and Guyana that showed high levels of drug-resistance with high TB/HIV co-infection rates [40, 41, 42, 43, 44], the moderate TB incidence seen in the rest of the Caribbean was not accompanied by any substantial level of drug-resistance. For example, there was no case of drug resistance among TB isolates from Trinidad and Tobago. This was very surprising especially with the high levels of TB/HIV co-infection (30.6% of the TB positive cases) and the high defaulter rate (22.7% of the TB positive cases). As reported in the literature, drug resistance was commonly seen in other countries where there was inadequate chemotherapy and also where HIV co-infections was present [45, 46]; but this is in contrast to Trinidad & Tobago where despite the high prevalence of HIV co-infection with TB, drug resistant cases were almost non- existent.

The absence of drug resistance in Trinidad and Tobago may be attributed to the excellent care and treatment TB programme such as direct observed treatment (DOT), adequate provision and supply of TB drugs that exists in the country. Additionally, all patients with tuberculosis are admitted and managed at the Caura Chest hospital until they become non-infectious, after which they are monitored on a regular basis by public health officials from the TB programme.

In Suriname drug resistance was rarely seen and when it occurred, only mono-resistance was seen. Mono-resistance was also recorded for isolates from Jamaica and The Bahamas, two countries where HIV infection is also relatively high and where low levels of resistance are seen. As in Trinidad and Tobago, the TB programmes in these countries are well managed and there is a very good collaboration between the TB and the HIV programmes.

A review of the literature for drug resistance in other parts of the Caribbean showed that similar low levels of drug resistance have been seen in the French Caribbean Islands of Guadeloupe and Martinique where there is significant migrant population from Haiti, an area of high drug resistance. The incidence of monoresistance in the French Caribbean Islands was 12.9%, however the incidence of MDR-TB was much lower with a rate of 0.9% [47].

Limitations of the study: An inherent limitation designed to compare cost and turnround time against an imperfect conventional test such as TST is that no gold standard has been established for resolution of discordant results. The MTBDR*plus* assay has the limitation that as a DNA assay based procedure that screens for nucleic acid sequence and not amino acid sequence, it is possible that mutations that do not cause amino acid exchange (silent mutations) will result in the absence of one of the wild types probes. Besides the assay detects only resistance that originate in the *rpo*B, *kat*G and *inh*A regions of the *Mycobacterium tuberculosis*. Hence other regions where resistance occurs will completely be missed.

The lack of adequate facilities for manipulation of solid and liquid cultures of *M. tuberculosis* is a major challenge in the Caribbean. Because of this drug susceptibility testing information for proper management of patients infected with TB as well as identification of species is limited.

5. Conclusions

Despite the several constraints and limitations, this study demonstrated that the QFT-G test was more effective and a quicker turnaround time was achieved over the TST in detecting LTBI among several target groups in the population studied. However, because the QFT-G appears more costly as well as showing indeterminate and non reactive response for immuno-compromised subjects such as HIV positive patients, care must be taken when screening or making a diagnosis of LTBI based on QFT-G results in a poor resource and high HIV prevalence setting like Trinidad & Tobago or any other Caribbean country.

The turnaround time for results for line probe assays is also a major asset. Additionally, the identification of organisms and DST can be performed on contaminated as well as non-viable specimens. Finally, the cost of this assay makes it ideal for use as it is less than 2 times that of traditional culture methods.

Although the Quantiferon Gold TB test results were comparable in many aspects with other published international studies the use of this test for the Caribbean may still be limited due to the cost involved when compared to the Tuberculin Skin Test. This is so because of the cost of the kit, transportation issues and the laboratory component of the test.

6. Recommendations

The authors therefore support the recommendation that Quantiferon Gold TB test be used in conjunction with the well established TST for the screening of patients suspected of infection. Confirmation of positive TST can then be performed using the QFT-G test if warranted. In cases where the patient is co-infected with HIV, the interpretation of the test should be made in collaboration with the CD4+ count of the patient as this test is dependent on the reaction of T-cells and if the CD4 count is low then the result can be falsely negative.

7. Acknowledgement

The authors would like to express their gratitude to all the subjects who volunteered for this study, the staff at Caura Chest hospital, Eric Williams Medical Sciences, Complex, CAREC, Trinidad & Tobago Public health laboratory for all their technical assistance and support in several ways. Fund for the study was partly provided by the University of the West Indies, St. Augustine.

8. References

[1] New Jersey Medical School (NJMS), National Tuberculosis Centre [Online]. Brief History of Tuberculosis, July 23, 1996 [Assessed online March 27, 2009 from: http://www.umdnj.edu-ntbcweb/history.html].

[2] World Health Organization. TB/HIV Research priorities in resource-limited setting: Report of an expert consultation, 2005. WHO/HTM/TB/2005.355.

[3] Health Agenda for the Americas 2008-2017. Text document distributed at the launching ceremony in Panama City, 3 June, 2007.

[4] Getahun, H., Harrington, M., O'Brien, R., Nunn, P. (2007). Diagnosis of smear-negative pulmonary tuberculosis in people with HIV infection or AIDS in resource-constrained settings: informing urgent policy changes. Available at www.thelancet.com. Published online on February 28, 2007. DOI:10.1016/S0140-6736(07)60284-0.

[5] Hale YM, Pfyffer GE and Salfinger M, 2001. Laboratory diagnosis of mycobacterial infections: new tools and lessons learned. Clin. Infect. Dis. 33:834-846.

[6] Akpaka PE; Baboolal S, Clarke D, Francis L, Rastogi N. (2008) Evaluation of methods for rapid detection of resistance to isoniazid and rifampicin in Mycobacterium tuberculosis isolates collected in the Caribbean. Journal of Clinical Microbiology; 46 (10):3426-3428

[7] Baboolal S, Ramoutar D, Akpaka PE. (2010). Comparison of QuantiFERON®-TB Gold assay and Tuberculin skin test to detect latent tuberculosis infection among among target groups in Trinidad & Tobago. *Pan American Journal of Public Health/ Rev Panam Salud Publica; 28(1):36-42*

[8] Mathew, P., Kuo, Y.H., Vazirani, B., Eng, R.H.K and Weinstein, M.P. (2000). Are Three Sputum Acid Fast Bacillus Smears Necessary for Discontinuing Tuberculosis Isolation? J Clin Microbiol 40(9) 3482-3484.

[9] Herman, P., Fauville-Dufaux, M., Breyer, D., van Vaerebergh, B., Pauwels, K., Dai Do Thi, Chuong., Sneyers, M., Wanlin, M., Snacken, R and Moens, W. (2006). Biosafety recommendations for the contained use of *Mycobacterium tuberculosis* complex isolates in industrialized countries. Royal Library of Belgium Deposit Number: D/2006/2505/22.175. Supply, P., Lesjean, S., Savine, E., Kremer, K., van Soolingen, D., Locht, C. (2001). Automated high-throughput genotyping genotyping for study of global epidemiology of *Mycobacterium tuberculosis* based on mycobacterial interspersed repetitive units. J. Clin. Microbiol. 39. 3563-3571.

[10] Centers for Diseases Control and Prevention. Epi Info 3.5.1 version software. Atlanta Georgia, USA

[11] Dean, A.G., Sullivan, K.M., Soe, M.M. OpenEpi. Open Source Epidemiologic Statistics for Public Health version 2.3. www.OpenEpi.com. Updated 2009/20/05

[12] Lee, J. Y., Choi, H. J., Park, I-N., Hong, S-B., Oh, Y-M., Lim, C-M., Lee, S. D., Koh, Y., Kim, W. S., Kim, D. S., Kim, W. D., Shim, T. S. (2006). Comparison of two commercial interferon-γ assays for diagnosing *Mycobacterium tuberculosis* infection. Eur Respir J; 28:24-30.

[13] Kobashi, Y., Mouri, K., Obase, Y., Fukuda, M., Miyashita, N., Oka, M. (2007). Clinical evaluation of QuantiFERON TB-2G test for immunocompromised patients. Eur Respir J; 30:945-950.

[14] Dewan, P. K., Grinsdale, J., Kawamura, L. M. (2007). Low Sensitivity of a Whole-Blood Interferon-γ Release Assay for Detection of Active Tuberculosis. Clin Infect Dis; 44:69-73.

[15] Kang, Y. A., Lee., H. W., Yoon, H. I., Cho, B. L., Han, S. K., Shim, Y-S., Yim, J-J. (2005). Discrepancy Between the Tuberculin Skin Test and the Whole-Blood Interferon γ Assay for the Diagnosis of Latent Tuberculosis Infection in an Intermediate Tuberculosis-Burden Country. JAMA; 293:2756-2760.

[16] Mori, T., Sakatani, M., Yamagishi, F. et al. (2004). Specific detection of tuberculosis infection: an interferon-gamma-based assay using new antigens. Am J Resp Crit Care Med; 170:59-64.

[17] Ferrara, G., Losi, M., Meacci, M., Meccugni, B., Piro, R., Roversi, P., Bergamini, B. M., D'Amico, R., Marchegiano, P., Rumpianesi, F., Fabbri, L. M., Richeldi, L. (2005). Routine Hospital Use of a New Commercial Whole Blood Interferon-γ Assay for the Diagnosis of Tuberculosis Infection. Am J Respir Crit Care Med. 172:631-635.

[18] Stuck, A. E., Minder, C. E., Frey, F. J. (1989). Risk of infection complication in patients taking glucocorticosteroids. Rev Infect Dis; 11: 954–963.

[19] Andersen, P., Munk, M. E., Pollock, J. M., Doherty, T. M. (2000). Specific immune based diagnosis of tuberculosis. Lancet; 256:1099–1104.

[20] Porsa, E., Cheng, L., Seale, M. M., Delclos, G. L,. Ma, X., Reich, R., Musser, J. M., Graviss, E. A. (2006). Comparison of a New ESAT-6/CFP-10 Peptide-Based Gamma Interferon Assay and a Tuberculin Skin Test for Tuberculosis Screening in a Moderate-Risk Population. Clin Vaccine Immunol; 13:53-58.

[21] Francis, M. and Rattan, A. (2006). Tuberculosis in CAREC Member Countries. CAREC Surveillance Report, Vol 26; No. 3

[22] Torres Costa J, Sá R, Cardoso MJ, Silva R, Ferreira J, Ribeiro C, et al. Tuberculosis screening in Portuguese healthcare workers using the tuberculin skin test and the interferon-gamma release assay. Eur Respir J. 2009;34(6):1423–8.

[23] Schablon A, Harling M, Diel R, Nienhaus A. Risk of latent TB infection in individuals employed in the healthcare sector in Germany: a multicentre prevalence study. BMC Infect Dis. 2010;10(1):107.

[24] Pai, M., Kaustubh, G., Joshi, R., Dogra, S., Kalantri, S., Mendiratta, D.K., Narang, P., Daley, C.L., Granich, R.M., Mazurek, G.H., Reingold, A.L., Colford, J.M. (2005). Mycobacterium tuberculosis Infection in Health Care Workers in Rural India. Comparison of a Whole-Blood Interferon γ Assay with Tuberculin Skin Testing. JAMA; 293 (22):2746-2754.

[25] Pooran A, Booth H, Miller RF, Scott G, Badri M, Huggett JF, et al. Different screening strategies (single or dual) for the diagnosis of suspected latent tuberculosis: a cost effectiveness analysis. BMC Pulmo Med. 2010;10(1):7.

[26] Mathema, B., Kurepina, N.E., Bifani, J. and Kreiswirth, B.N. (2006). Molecular Epidemiology of Tuberculosis: Current Insights. Clin Microbiol Rev; 19(4):658-685.

[27] Diel, R., Wrighton-Smith, P. and Zellweger, J-P. (2007). Cost-effectiveness of interferon-c release assay testing for the treatment of latent tuberculosis. Eur Respir J; 30: 321-332.

[28] Marra F, Marra CA, Sadatsafavi M, Morán-Mendoza O, Cook V, Elwood RK, et al. Cost-effectiveness of a new interferon-based blood assay, QuantiFERON-TB Gold, in screening tuberculosis contacts. Int J Tuberc Lung Dis. 2008;12(12):1414–24.

[29] Pai, M., Riley, L.W., Colford, J.M. Jr. (2004). Interferon-gamma assays in the immune diagnosis of tuberculosis: a systematic review. Lancet Infect Dis; 4: 761–776.

[30] Hilleman, D., Rush-Gerdes, S., Richter, E. (2007). Evaluation of the GenoType MTBDRplus Assay for Rifampin and Isoniazid Susceptibility Testing for Mycobacterium tuberculosis strains and Clinical Specimens. J Clin Microbiol 45(8): 2635-2640.

[31] Somoskovi, A., Dormandy, J., Mitsani, D., Rivenburg, J., Salfinger, M. (2006). Use of smear-positive samples to assess the PCR-based Genotype MTBDR assay for rapid, direct detection of the Mycobacterium tuberculosis Complex as well as its resistance to Isoniazid and Rifampicin. J Clin Microbiol 44(12):4459-4463.

[32] Bang, D., Anderson, A.B., Thomsen, V.Q. (2006). Rapid Genotypic detection of Rifampin- and Isoniazid- resistant Mycobacterium tuberculosis directly in clinical specimens. J Clin Microbiol 44(7):2605-2608.

[33] Wade., M.M., Zhang, Y., (2004). Mechanisms of drug resistance in Mycobacterium tuberculosis. Front Biosci 9975-994.

[34] Cavusoglu, C., Turhan, K., Akinci, P., Soyler, I. (2007). Evaluation of the Genotype MTBDR assay for rapid detection of rifampin and isoniazid resistance in Mycobacterium tuberculosis isolates. J Clin Microbiol 44; 2338-2342.

[35] Barnard, M., Albert, H., Coetzee, G., O Brien, R., Bosman, M.E. (2008). Rapid Molecular screening for multidrug-resistant tuberculosis in a high-volume health laboratory in South Africa. Am J Respir Crit Care Med 177:787-792.

[36] Johnson, R., Jordaan, A.M., Warren, R., Bosman, M., Young, D., Nagy, J.N., Wain, J.R., van Helden, P.D., Victor, T.C. (2008). Drug susceptibility testing using molecular techniques can enhance tuberculosis diagnosis. J Inf dev Countries 240-45.

[37] Parsons, L.M., Salfinger, M., Clobridge, A., Dormandy, J., Mirabello, L., Polletta, V.L., Sanic, A., Sinyavskiy, O., Larsen, S.C., Driscole, J., Zickas, G., Taber, H.W. (2005). Phenotypic and molecular characterization of Mycobacterium tuberculosis isolates resistant to both Isoniazid and Ethambutol. JCM 49(6) 2218-2225.

[38] Zignol, M., Hosseini, M.S., Wright, A., Weezenbeek, C.L., Nunn, P., Watt, C.J., Williams, B.G. and Dye, C. (2006). Global Incidence of Multidrug-resistant tuberculosis. J. Infect Dis. 194:479-85.

[39] World Health Organization. Global Tuberculosis Control, Surveillance, Planning and Financing. WHO Report, 2008. WHO/HTM/TB/2008.393

[40] Menner, N., Gunther, I., Orawa, H., Roth, A., Rambajan, I., Wagner, J., Hahn, H., Persaud, S., Ignatius, R. (2005). High frequency of multidrug-resistance Mycobactium tuberculosis isolates in Georgetown, Guyana. Tropical Medicine and International Health 10 (12) 1215-1218.

[41] Diguimbaye, C., Hilty, M., Ngandolo, R., Mahamat, H.H., Pfyffer, G.E., Baggi, F., Tanner, m., Schelling, E, Zinsstag. J. (2006). Molecular characterization and drug resistance testing of *Mycobacterium tuberculosis* isolates from Chad. J Clin Microbiol 44:1575-1577.186. Ferdinand, S., Sola, C., Verdol, B., Legrand, E.Goh, K.S., Berchel, M., Aubery, A., Timothee, M., Joseph, P., Pape, J.W., Rastogi, N. (2003). Molecular characterization and drug resistance patterns of strains of *Mycobacterium tuberculosis* isolated from patients in an AIDS counselling center in Port-au-Prince, Haiti: a 1-year study. J Clin Microbiol 41(2):694-702.

[42] UNAIDS/WHO/ AIDS Epidemic Update (2009). www.unaids.org/en/knowledgeCentre/HIVData/EpiUpdate/EpiUpdArchive/20 09. [downloaded 18/02/11]

[43] Pratt, R., Robinson, V., Navin, T. (2009). Trends in Tuberculosis – United States, 2008. JAMA 301 (18): 1869-1871.

[44] Streicher, E.M., Warren, R.M., Kewlwy, C., Simpson, J., Rastogi, N., Sola, C., van der Spuy, G.D., van Helden, P.D., Victor, T.C., 2004. Genotypic and phenotypic characterization of drug resistant *Mycobacterium tuberculosis* isolates from rural districts of Western Cape Province of South Africa. J Clin Microbiol. 42, 891-894.

[45] Zagar, E. M., Mc Nerney, R., 2008. Multidrug-resistant tuberculosis. BMC Infectious Diseases 8:10 doi:10.1186/47 1-2334-8-10.

[46] Khue, P.M., Phue, T.Q., Hung, N.V., Jarlier, V., Robert, J. (2008). Drug resistance and HIV co-infection among pulmonary tuberculosis patients in Haiphong City, Vietnam. Int J Tuberc Lung Dis 12(7): 763-768.

[47] Brudey, K., Driscoll, J.R., Rigouts, L., Prodinger, W.M., Gori, A., Al-Hajoj, S.A., Allix, C., Aristimuno, L., Arora, J., Baumanis, V.,et al (2006). *Mycobacterium tuberculosis* complex genetic diversity: mining the fourth international spoligotyping database (SpolDB4) for classification, population genetics and epidemiology. BMC Microbiol. 6:6-23.

Clinical Laboratory Diagnostics for *Mycobacterium tuberculosis*

N. Esther Babady[1] and Nancy L. Wengenack[2]
[1]Memorial Sloan-Kettering Cancer Center, New York, New York,
[2]Mayo Clinic, Rochester, Minnesota,
USA

1. Introduction

This chapter highlights current state-of-the-art methods for the detection and identification of *Mycobacterium tuberculosis* (*Mtb*) complex in the clinical diagnostic laboratory. Methods discussed include stain and culture which traditionally would have been followed by phenotypic-based identification methods. At this point in time however, molecular methods are considered the gold standard for both the rapid detection of *Mtb* directly from patient specimens as well as for the identification of *Mtb* following growth in culture. There are also instances where speciation of *Mtb* in order to distinguish it from other members of the *Mtb* complex is clinically important and these will be discussed. In addition, this chapter provides an overview of methods used in the clinical laboratory for *Mtb* drug resistance testing and suggests what the future might hold for *Mtb* diagnostics.

2. *M. tuberculosis* and biosafety in the clinical laboratory

M. tuberculosis presents a risk of laboratory-acquired infection due to its transmission via aerosol routes, ability to withstand common laboratory processing techniques such as heat-fixation or frozen section preparation and a extremely low ID_{50} of <10 bacilli. The United States Centers for Disease Control and Prevention (CDC) estimates that laboratory workers are three times more likely than non-laboratory workers to become infected with *Mtb*. Therefore, biological safety organizations have defined a number of safety practices and procedures that must be strictly followed when working with *Mtb* which is classified as a risk group 3 organism. Specimens and cultures of unknown isolates shall be handled as if they contain *Mtb* until proven otherwise. Only non-aerosol generating processes such as accessioning of specimen or reading of acid-fast smears can be done under BSL-2 conditions outside of a BSC. All other specimen-handling including opening/closing of tubes, pipeting and transfer must be done in a BSC. Personnel must exercise caution to avoid aerosol generation. More specifically, smear preparation, culture decontamination and concentration, and culture plating must be done inside a BSC with the possible exception of the centrifugation step. However, centrifugation must be done using aerosol-proof containers which are opened, loaded and closed inside the BSC to reduce the risk of personnel exposure. All laboratory surfaces must be decontaminated with a tuberculocidal reagent before and after working with specimens and cultures. Propagation and manipulation of *Mtb* complex cultures (e.g., identification and susceptibility testing) requires BSL-3 practices, equipment and facilities. Clinical laboratories without BSL-3 facilities must refer all positive mycobacterial cultures to another laboratory with BSL-3 capabilities for identification and, if necessary, susceptibility testing. Acid-fast smears must not be prepared from positive mycobacterial cultures of unknown identity without BSL-3 facilities. Identification methods (e.g., biochemical analysis, nucleic acid hybridization probes, sequencing, PCR) required initial specimen processing under BSL-3 conditions until any viable mycobacteria have been rendered non-viable by heating and/or lysis via chemical or physical means. Laboratories must verify that their processing methods are effective in rendering *Mtb* nonviable prior to conducting any activities outside of a BSL-3 laboratory.

BSL-3 facilities have highly specialized requirements some of which include restricted laboratory access, self-closing double door entry, directional airflow with a specified number of air exchanges over time, BSCs exhausted to the outside, and posted signage regarding the hazard (in this case *Mtb*). Class II BSCs are one of the most important pieces of equipment in the mycobacteriology laboratory and they must be maintained in good working order at all times. Frequent (at least daily) checks of function by means such as magnehelic gauge monitoring is needed. Regular maintenance and certification programs must be undertaken and documentation of cabinet performance must be maintained by the laboratory. Specimens should be covered before transport and should be transported in well-sealed, leak-proof containers. All biohazard waste should be autoclaved prior to leaving the facility.

BSL-3 personnel safety practices include the use of fluid-resistant, cuffed, solid-front gowns, gloves, eye protection, respiratory protection (N-95 or better fitted respirator or powered air purifying respirator (PAPR)). Each laboratory must perform a risk assessment to define the personal protective equipment, facilities and engineering practices that are appropriate for their institution and that comply with applicable regulations. The risk assessment is the responsibility of the laboratory director but it should be done in collaboration with institutional biosafety officials as this is helpful in making certain that no safety practice has been overlooked. A sample risk assessment is provided in Table 1 but each laboratory must perform their own assessment as situations may differ between laboratories. The laboratory must have a written spill procedure and must review the procedure with lab staff regularly to assure competency. Spill "drills" in which staff physically respond to a simulated spill are highly recommended as they routinely point out any potential gaps in procedures or staff knowledge.

Strict regulations exist in many countries concerning the shipping and transportation of diagnostic specimens that are known to contain or that potentially contain *Mtb* complex and for shipment of known *Mtb* complex isolates. Personnel who package these specimens and isolates must have specialized training that is updated at prescribed intervals. Packaging materials must be leak-proof, able to withstand unpredictable handling throughout the transportation chain and must be properly labeled in order to alert transportation workers of hazards contained within the package. Individuals involved in the shipping of specimens and isolates should be knowledgeable about the regulations within their country and if, sending specimens or isolates internationally, within the destination country.

Procedure	Aerosol Potential	Biosafety Level Required	Personal Protective Equipment Required	Engineering Controls Required	Special Practices or Equipment Required
Reading of smears (AR, Kinyoun, Modified Acid Fast)	Slight	BSL 2	Gown, gloves	May be done on bench top	
Manipulation of mycobacterial cultures for identification (e.g. subculturing)	Significant	BSL 3	Gown, shoe covers, eye protection, gloves and respirator/head cover or PAPR	Work in biological safety cabinet	Use disposable loops; Use racks to prevent tipping/spilling; Work over disinfectant-soaked towel
Susceptibility testing of mycobacteria	Significant	BSL 3 for setup BSL 2 for incubation and reading of closed bottles/ plates/ tubes	Setup - Gown, shoe covers, eye protection, gloves and respirator/head cover or PAPR	Work in biological safety cabinet to inoculate bottles, tubes or plates with organism	Use extreme care to avoid aerosol generation when inoculating bottles/plates/tubes

Table 1. Sample partial risk assessment – this table is intended as an example of one style of risk assessment that can be developed. Each laboratory must develop a laboratory-specific risk assessment in conjunction with their institutional safety officer(s).

3. Stains for mycobacteria

Mycobacteria, including Mtb complex, can be rapidly and inexpensively detected directly from pretreated and concentrated respiratory specimens, body fluids, and tissue using acid-fast stains. A Gram stain is not able to reliably detect mycobacteria which can appear as non-stained "ghosts" or as beaded Gram-positive bacilli. Therefore, acid-fast stains, such as the Ziehl-Neelsen stain or the fluorescent auramine-rhodamine stain are recommended for mycobacteria. The acid-fast stain forms a complex between the unique mycolic acids of the mycobacterial cell wall and the dye (e.g., fuchsin). Complex formation makes the mycobacteria resistant to destaining by acid-alcohols providing the basis for the "acid-fast" terminology. Non-acid fast bacteria do not retain the acid-fast dye in the presence of the acid-alcohol decolorizer and are often stained in a subsequent step using a counterstain such as methylene blue. Commonly utilized acid-fast stains contain carbol-fuchsin dye and are the Ziehl-Neelsen stain which utilizes phenol plus heat to aid in dye penetration, and the Kinyoun stain which uses phenol in the absence of heat. The Ziehl-Neelsen stain is considered the more sensitive of the two (Somoskovi et al., 2001). Fluorescent stains such as auramine O are also used alone or in combination with rhodamine B. The fluorescent stains exhibit increased fluorescence upon binding DNA and RNA providing enhanced sensitivity for examining concentrated direct specimens by staining the bacilli while avoiding non-specific staining of artifacts and background more typical of the non-fluorescent stains.

Mycobacteria appear as long slender rods (1-10μm long x 0.2-0.6μm wide) and are often slightly curved or bent. At least 300 fields should be examined under high power (1000X) when using a carbol-fuchsin stain and light microcopy. The fluorochrome stain can be examined using a lower power (250X) and a minimum of 30 fields should be examined under the lower power (Pfyffer & Palicova, 2011). When positive, an indication of the quantity of acid-fast bacilli present should be provided. Factors which influence the sensitivity of acid-fast smears include the amount of acid-fast bacilli present in the specimen, the experience of the reader, the stain used, the number of fields examined, the type of specimen (e.g., generally respiratory specimens have higher yield than non-respiratory), the patient population being examined, volume of the specimen and smear pre-treatment (direct vs. pre-treated, concentrated). Rigid quality control processes must be followed to prevent cross-contamination and false results. Laboratories should use a positive and negative control slide for each batch of acid-fast smears prepared and should have a second reader confirm positive results and at least 10% of negative slides to reduce the potential for incorrect results. Staining jars or dishes should not be used to prevent potential cross-contamination and care should be taken to avoid the transfer of bacilli via the microscopy oil used for examining the slide. Laboratories must also participate in a proficiency testing programs (e.g., College of American Pathologists) to ensure continued competency.

Acid-fast stains lack sensitivity and a large number of bacilli (10^4-10^6/mL) are required for a positive stain. Therefore, a positive stain from a respiratory specimen is typically thought to correlate with a higher infectivity potential and patients are routinely placed in airborne isolation rooms until their acid-fast smears convert to negative. Immunocompromised individuals often present with lower bacterial loads making detection by smear difficult (Chegou et al., 2011). Up to 30% of persons (commonly children) are unable to produce sputum for a smear requiring the use of more invasive methods (gastric washing, bronchoalveolar lavage, etc). Smears can be used to follow the response to treatment in smear-positive individuals. A concentration step provides increase sensitivity over direct smear microscopy (Steingart et al., 2006).

Acid-fast stains are also non-specific and the reader cannot determine the species of mycobacteria present in a positive smear. Mycobacteria tend to clump and produce cord-like strands of bacilli and there may be some indication of which species is present based on characteristic cording but this is highly subjective and not recommended as a routine method of determining species (Attorri et al., 2000; Julian et al., 2010).

4. Culturing of *M. tuberculosis*

The growth of *Mtb* in culture is considered the gold standard for identification of a case of tuberculosis. The sensitivity of culture is much better than an acid-fast smear with only 10-100 viable organisms/mL of specimen required for a positive culture. Media for the growth of *Mtb* is the same as that used for other mycobacteria species and generally includes both a solid and a liquid-based medium. Solid media utilized is typically either egg-based such as the Lowenstein-Jensen (L-J) medium or agar-based such as Middlebrook 7H10 medium.

Antimicrobial agents can be added to help with elimination of contaminating organisms which may have a more rapid growth rate than *Mtb* and which may therefore obscure any *Mtb* present on the plate. In general, *Mtb* colonies are seen more rapidly on agar-based medium (10-12 days) as opposed to egg-based medium (18-24 days) (Liu et al., 1973). Care must be taken to protect Middlebrook medium from excessive light and heat which results in breakdown of the medium and release of a formaldehyde byproduct which is toxic to *Mtb* (Miliner et al., 1969). Use of Middlebrook 7H11 medium containing casein is reported to improve the recovery of isoniazid-resistant isolates of *Mtb* (Pfyffer & Palicova, 2011). Broth medium such as Middlebrook 7H9 medium is reported to provide a more rapid recovery of *Mtb* compared with solid medium. There are several commercially-available semi-automated broth culture systems for mycobacteria including *Mtb* complex. The BACTEC 460 radiometric and BACTEC 960 Mycobacterial Growth Indicator Tube (MGIT) fluorimetric systems (Becton, Dickinson, Sparks, MD) and the VersaTREK culture system (TREK Diagnostics Systems, Cleveland, OH) are FDA-cleared in the United States. The BACTEC 460 system is currently being phased out by the manufacturer in favor of the non-radiometric MGIT system. Other culture systems include Septi-Chek biphasic System (Becton, Dickinson,) and the MB/BacT Alert 3D system (bioMérieux, Marcy l'Etoile, France) which has a colorimetric CO_2-based sensor to detect mycobacterial growth. There are numerous publications in the literature which compare the performance of the commercially-available broth systems but in general, these systems have a sensitivity of 88-93% for the detection of *Mtb* complex (Cruciani et al., 2004).

Cultures for *Mtb* complex should be incubated at 35-37°C in an atmosphere of 5-10% CO_2 for primary cultures on solid medium. Since *Mtb* complex grows slowly in culture, many laboratories choose to examine culture plates for growth twice per week during early stages of growth and then weekly for older cultures. The advantage of semi-automated broth systems such as the MGIT and VersaTREK are that CO_2-supplementation is not generally required and the cultures are continuously monitored without the need for laboratory technologist intervention unless a culture is flagged by the instrument as positive. After either a solid or broth culture shows growth, the presence of acid-fast bacilli must be confirmed as described below in order to rule out non-mycobacterial contaminants.

5. Identification of *M. tuberculosis* from culture isolates

5.1 Microscopy

The first step in the examination of organisms growing on either solid media or liquid media is to confirm their identity using various staining methods as discussed in section 3. Depending on the stain used, the identification of *Mycobacterium* bacilli is done using either a light microscope under 100 x oil immersion objective or a fluorescent microscope under 25x or 40x objective. Microscopy however is not specific and cannot differentiate *Mtb* from other *Mycobacterium* and further analysis is required for final identification which can take up to 4-6 weeks.

Recently, the Microscopic Observation Drug Susceptibility (MODS) assay has been reported for the detection of *Mtb* complex in liquid culture through microscopic observation of characteristic cording and this method is characterized as in "late stage development/evaluation" for use in high TB burden settings by the World Health

Organization (WHO) (Caviedes & Moore, 2007; Moore, 2007; WHO, 2008; Ha et al., 2009; Limaye et al., 2010).

5.2 Biochemical analysis

Following microscopic and microscopic examination of culture isolates, final identification to the species level of *Mtb* complex is performed using a set of conventional biochemical reactions in combination with growth temperature. Although conventional biochemical assays are relatively inexpensive and simple to perform, they are time-consuming due to required incubation periods of up to 4 weeks, resulting in major delays in identification. Furthermore, with greater than 130 mycobacterial species identified to date, the use of phenotypic methods is limited and biased to identify only the most common species of mycobacteria, underestimating the complexity of the genus and resulting in misidentification of unfamiliar species (Kirschner et al., 1993; Springer et al., 1996). *M. tuberculosis*, as with other members of the *Mtb* complex, is a slow growing mycobacterium, requiring in general 15 days to 40 days to grow in culture. The optimal isolation temperature for the organism is 35-37°C and the organism does not produce pigmentation even following exposure to light (non-chromogen). The most useful biochemical tests used for identification of a nonchromogenic, slow-growing mycobacterium such as *Mtb* complex includes: niacin accumulation, nitrate reduction, pyrazinamidase activity, inhibition of thiophene-2-caroxylic acid hydrazide, urease activity and catalase activity. Other tests that can provide additional information include tellurite reduction, Tween 80 hydrolysis, the arylsulfatase test, iron uptake and NaCl tolerance. In general, a mature growth (2-3 weeks) is required for biochemical tests, they are often performed on a LJ slants and require up to 3 weeks for final read of results.

5.2.1 Niacin accumulation

Niacin (nicotinic acid) is produced by all species of mycobacteria and further metabolized to nicotinamide adenine dinucleotide (NAD). However, *Mtb* complex, *M. simiae* and some strains of *M. chelonae*, *M. bovis*, and *M. marinum* do not have the enzyme responsible for metabolizing niacin, resulting in its accumulation in the culture media. A water extract is prepared by adding 1 mL of sterile water to the surface of an LJ slant with a growth of mycobacteria species at least three weeks-old. An aliquot of this extract is then added to a tube containing a niacin strip, incubated for up to 30 minutes with gentle shaking. A positive reaction (presence of niacin) is read as the development of a yellow color. Since species other than *Mtb* complex can accumulate niacin, additional biochemical testing is required for the final identification of *Mtb* complex.

5.2.2 Nitrate reduction

M. tuberculosis complex contains the enzyme nitroreductase which is able to reduce nitrate (NO_3) into nitrite (NO_2). This reaction is detected in the laboratory by inoculating a nitrate broth with a loopful of a 3-4 weeks old mycobacterial culture and α-napthalamine, and sulfanilic acid that will react with the released NO_2 to produce a red or pink color. A negative result (lack of color) is further confirmed by the addition of zinc dust. If a red color (nitrate reduced) develops following addition of zinc dust, then the original result is confirmed as negative.

5.2.3 Pyrazinamidase

The deamination of pyrazinamide into pyrazinoic acid and ammonia by the enzyme pyrazinamidase (PZA) is an essential test to distinguish *Mtb* complex (PZA positive) from *M. bovis* (PZA negative). Other non-tuberculous mycobacteria species including *M. marinum* and *M. avium* complex can also be positive for PZA. The test is performed by inoculating two LJ slants with the mycobacterium species and incubating them for 4 days at 35-37°C in a non-CO_2 incubator. After 4 days, 1% ferric ammonium sulphate is added to one of the tube and incubated at room temperature for 30 minutes. The PZA reaction is positive if a pink band forms on the surface of the LJ slant. If the reaction is negative, the LJ slant is incubated for an additional 4 hours at 2-8 °C and observed for the appearance of the pink band. If the test is still negative after 4 hours, the second tube will be tested on day 7 to finalize the test.

5.2.4 Urease

The presence of urease, the enzyme that hydrolyzes urea into ammonia and carbon dioxide, can be detected in mycobacterial species by incubating an actively growing culture to a urea broth for up to 7 days at 35-37°C in a non-CO_2 incubator, with readings done at days 1, 3 and 7. *M. tuberculosis* complex is positive for urease and will produce a dark pink to red color following incubation in urea broth.

5.2.5 Inhibition of thiophene-2-caroxylic acid hydrazide (TCH)

M. tuberculosis complex can be differentiated from *M. bovis* by its ability to grow in the presence of TCH, a property shared by most mycobacteria species except for *M. bovis*. This test uses quadrant Petri dishes with one of the quadrant containing TCH. A dilute suspension of the mycobacterial growth (10^{-3} to 10^{-4} in sterile water) is added to each quadrant and the plate incubated for 3 weeks at 35-37°C in a 10 % CO_2 incubator. A resistant organism shows greater than 1% growth in the TCH quadrant when compared to growth in the control quadrant.

5.2.6 Arylsulfatase test

Arylsulfatase is an enzyme that hydrolyzes free phenolphthalein from the tri-potassium salt of phenolphthalein disulfite. A suspension of a pure mycobacterium culture in sterile water is incubated with phenolphthalein in oleic acid agar for either 3 days (rapid growers) or 14 days (slow growers) at 35-37°C in a non-CO_2 incubator. The appearance of a pink or red color after addition of sodium bicarbonate (Na_2CO_3) indicates a positive reaction. All members of the *Mtb* complex lack the arylsulfatase enzyme and are therefore negative for that reaction (Koneman, 2006; Lee, 2010).

5.2.7 Catalase test

Catalase is an enzyme that splits hydrogen peroxide (H_2O_2) into water (H_2O) and oxygen (O_2). Unlike the catalase assay used to identify for other types of bacteria (i.e. *Streptococcus* spp.), the catalase assay for mycobacteria is performed using 30% H_2O_2 (Superoxol) in 10% Tween-80 and the test performed both at 22-25°C and 68°C. *M. tuberculosis* complex has catalase activity at 22-25°C but not at 68°C (ie., heat-labile catalase). In addition to determining catalase activity at 68°C, the strength of the catalase reaction is also evaluated to differentiate *Mtb* complex from other mycobacteria. This semiquantitative test is performed by adding Superoxol to a 2-weeks-old culture of mycobacteria growing on a Lowenstein-Jensen slant at 37°C. Five minutes after addition of the Superoxol, the strength of the catalase reaction is determined by measuring the height of the bubbles, characteristic of the catalase reaction, in the tube. If the height of the bubbles is > 45 mm, the reaction is considered high and if the height of the bubbles is < 45 mm, the reaction is considered low. *M. tuberculosis* complex has low catalase activity.

5.2.8 Iron uptake

Only a few mycobacteria species are able to take up iron from ferric ammonium citrate and convert it to iron oxide (rust). This biochemical reaction is mainly used to identify *M. fortuitum* which when incubated with 20% ferric ammonium citrate for up to 3 weeks on a Lowenstein-Jensen slant at 28-30°C will turn a dark, rusty brown color. *M. tuberculosis* complex does not take up iron.

5.2.9 NaCl tolerance

The ability to grow on media containing 5% NaCl differentiates the slow growing mycobacteria from the rapid growers as only *M. triviale* (a slow grower) can grow on this media and only *M. chelonae* and *M. mucogenicum* (rapid growers) fails to grow in the presence of this salt concentration. The test is performed by inoculating an LJ slant containing 5% NaCl with a 1 MacFarland concentration of a mycobacterial culture and incubating it at 28°C in a 5-10% CO_2 incubator for up to 4 weeks (Witebsky & Kruczak-Filipov, 1996; Lee, 2010). *M. tuberculosis* complex does not grow on LJ slant containing 5% NaCl.

5.2.10 Tellurite reduction

Most mycobacterium can reduce potassium tellurite to metallic tellurium in liquid broth within 3 days. The test is performed by inoculating a Middlebrook 7H9 liquid medium containing Tween 80 with a heavy concentration of organisms and incubating at 37°C in a 5-10% CO_2 incubator for up to 7 days. After 7 days, a solution of potassium tellurite is added to the liquid culture and further incubated for 3 days. A positive reaction shows a black precipitate (metallic tellurium) at the bottom of the tube. This test is often used to identify MAC. *M. tuberculosis* complex is negative for tellurite reduction (Witebsky & Kruczak-Filipov, 1996; Lee, 2010).

5.2.11 Tween 80 hydrolysis

This assay tests for the presence of the enzyme lipase which can cleave the oleic acid from the detergent Tween 80 (polyoxyethylene sorbitan monooleate). The release of the oleic acid from Tween 80 results in a change of color of the neutral indicator from yellow to red within 5-10 days after incubation of Tween-80 with a mycobacterium at 37°C in a 5-10% CO_2 incubator. *M. tuberculosis* complex is negative for Tween 80 hydrolysis.

The use of conventional methods for the initial identification of *Mtb* complex is not ideal. This section provided a review of the most common tests used traditionally but the combined use of these various assays results in a significant delay in identification of up to one month after growth of the culture in the laboratory. The following sections will cover the more rapid methods currently in use in most mycobacteriology laboratory for identification of *Mtb* complex.

Biochemical Test	Reaction
niacin accumulation	Positive
nitrate reduction	Positive
pyrazinamidase activity	Positive
urease activity	Positive
inhibition of thiophene-2-caroxylic acid hydrazide (TCH)	Positive
arylsulfatase test	Negative
catalase test	Negative (heat-labile)
iron uptake	Negative
NaCl tolerance	Negative
tellurite reduction	Negative
Tween 80 hydrolysis	Negative

Table 2. Biochemical tests for identification of *Mycobacterium tuberculosis* complex from a culture isolate

5.3 High-Performance Liquid Chromatography

High-performance liquid chromatography (HPLC) of mycolic acids was first proposed for use as a standard test in mycobacteria species identification by the CDC in 1985. This technique had been widely used by clinical chemistry laboratories for the separation and identification of drug compounds (Butler & Guthertz, 2001). HPLC can be used to differentiate mycobacteria based on differences in their mycolic acid profiles. Mycolic acids are high-molecular weight fatty acids with long carbon side chains present in abundance in the cell wall of mycobacteria and other organisms including *Corynebacterium, Dietzia, Rhodococcus, Nocardia, Gordonia, Williamsia, Skermania,* and *Tsukamurella* species with *Mycobacterium* species containing the longest carbon chain (60-90) (Butler & Guthertz, 2001). Mycolic acids samples are prepared through a series of steps involving saponification of the mycobacteria, organic solvent extraction and derivatization of the mycolic acids to UV-adsorbing *p*-bromophenacyl (PBPA) esters (Durst et al., 1975; Butler et al., 1991). The derivatized mycolic acids solution is then separated on a HPLC instrument and the resulting chromatogram interpreted based on the peak pattern which is specific for each species of mycobacterium (Butler et al., 1991; Butler & Guthertz, 2001).

Although sensitive and specific when compared to biochemical tests and other molecular assays, with agreement ranging from 90-99% depending on the mycobacterial species (Guthertz et al., 1993; Thibert & Lapierre, 1993), HPLC is a technically demanding method which is not easily implemented in routine diagnostic laboratories. This method requires a high level of expertise for recognition of species based on the HPLC chromatogram and therefore only limited to a few reference laboratories including the CDC in Atlanta, GA. A commercial HPLC assay, the Sherlock Mycobacteria Identification HPLC system (SMIS; MIDI Inc., Newark, DE), was developed to simplify use of HPLC in the clinical laboratories through automated recognition of mycobacterial species based on software that analyzes HPLC peak patterns comparing them to a library containing several *Mycobacterium* species chromatograms (Kellogg et al., 2001; LaBombardi et al., 2006). Of the 370 isolates tested in a multicenter study by SMIS, 327 (88%) were identified to the species level by the SMIS software with 279 (75%) correctly identified (Kellogg et al., 2001). The sensitivity of the SMIS identification could be increased to 98.9% (366/370) by manual calculation of relative peak height ratios and relative retention times and additional biochemical properties. In another study by LaBombardi et al. (LaBombardi et al., 2006), the SIMS correctly identified 61/90 isolates (67.8%) growing on Middlebrook 7H11 plates (BBL, Sparks, MD) and 73/161 (45.3%) isolates growing in VersaTREK Myco bottles (TREK Diagnostic Systems, Cleveland, OH). This performance was increased by used of a modified library to 91% for isolates growing on solid media and 83.2% for isolates recovered from liquid culture. In both studies, no *Mtb* complex isolates were misidentified and the sensitivity ranged from 83-100% (Kellogg et al., 2001; LaBombardi et al., 2006). Of note, although HPLC is a faster and more sensitive technology than conventional biochemical testing, this method cannot be used directly on clinical specimen and is not able to differentiate between members of the *Mtb* complex, except for the *M. bovis* BCG strain (Butler et al., 1991; Floyd et al., 1992).

5.4 Nucleic acid hybridization probes

The introduction of nucleic acid hybridization probes in the clinical laboratory significantly impacted the turn-around time and workload for identification of mycobacteria species. Nucleic acid hybridization probes are single-stranded or double-stranded DNA/RNA fragments, labeled with a radioactive, chemiluminescent or a fluorescent marker, that are complementary to a target DNA or RNA sequence (Wetmur, 1991). In clinical microbiology, nucleic acid hybridization probes often target ribosomal RNA (rRNA) because of their high copy number present in organisms growing in culture. The first nucleic acid hybridization probes from Gen-Probe (San Diego, CA) for rapid identification of *M. avium* complex and *Mtb* complex were labeled with I^{125} radioactive isotope. Labeled DNA-RNA complexes were separated from non-hybridized DNA using an adsorption suspension containing hydroxyapatite and the I^{125} in the adsorbed labeled complex was counted using a gamma counter. Results were calculated as percentage of input probe hybridized (Drake et al., 1987; Kiehn & Edwards, 1987; Ellner et al., 1988; Musial et al., 1988; Peterson et al., 1989). The introduction of these radioactive probes resulted in a significant decrease in the turn-around time for identification of both *M. avium* complex and *Mtb* complex from weeks to approximately 2 hours with sensitivity and specificity ranging from 83-100% and 99.2-100% respectively (Drake et al., 1987; Kiehn & Edwards, 1987; Ellner et al., 1988; Musial et al., 1988; Peterson et al., 1989).

The I^{125} probes were eventually replaced with non-radioactive probes to reduce staff potential for exposure to radioactive materials. Two types of non-isotopic probes were introduced, the synthetic nucleic acid probes (SNAP) (Syngene, Inc., San Diego, CA) and the AccuProbes (Gen-Probe, San Diego, CA). The SNAP probes utilized DNA probes labeled with alkaline-phosphatase and was performed by spotting the isolate to be tested on a nylon membrane and incubating the membrane with the labeled probes, followed by incubation in a solution of nitroblue tetrazolium chloride, 5-brom-4-chloro-3- indolyphosphate substrates and alkaline phosphatase buffer. A positive reaction was read as the presence of a blue or purple color on the nylon membrane within a few hours (Lim et al., 1991; Woodley et al., 1992). Although 100% sensitive, cross-reactivity was detected with SNAP probes between *Mtb* complex and *M. terrae*, requiring the 68°C catalase test to be performed to differentiate between the two species (Lim et al., 1991; Ford et al., 1993).

AccuProbes are labeled with acridinium ester and hybridization is measured by chemiluminescence following hydrolysis of the label upon addition of H_2O_2 and NaOH. The chemiluminescence is measured using a luminometer and expressed as RLU (relative light units). Unlike the previous version with the I^{125} isotope, no wash steps are necessary as non-hybridized probes are chemically degraded and only acridinium ester-labeled, hybridized probes can produce measurable chemiluminescence (Goto et al., 1991). The AccuProbe for *Mtb* complex can be performed on culture growing from both liquid and solid media and will detect all members of the *Mtb* complex (Gen-Probe, 2011). The sensitivity and specificity of the acridinium ester labeled probes was comparable to that of the radioisotope labeled probes (Goto et al., 1991; Lebrun et al., 1992). Similar to the SNAP probes, detection of some strain of *M. terrae* by *Mtb* complex probes was also observed (Lim et al., 1991; Ford et al., 1993), although increased stringency in the detection method resolved the false-positive detection of *M. terrae* by AccuProbes *Mtb* complex probes.

Although the use of nucleic acid probes has allowed same day identification of *Mtb* complex from culture, the sensitivity of these probes is not high enough for detection of the organisms directly from clinical specimens, which still limits the rapid identification to the time it takes for the organisms to grow in either liquid or solid media. Furthermore, the *Mtb* complex AccuProbes do not distinguish amongst members of the *Mtb* complex.

5.5 Line Probe assays

Line Probe assays were developed to expand the range of mycobacterium species identified using nucleic acid probes since those were only available for *Mtb* complex, *M. avium*, *M. intracellulare*, *M. kansasii* and *M. gordonae* (Gen-Probe, San Diego, CA). The first commercially available LineProbe assay, the INNO LiPa Mycobacteria (Innogenetics, Ghent, Belgium), uses reverse hybridization technology in which probes are immobilized as parallel lines on a membrane strips as opposed to being in solution as is the case with AccuProbes. Amplified, biotinylated DNA fragments of the 16-23S rRNA spacer region of mycobacterial organisms are incubated with the labeled strips; addition of streptavidin-alkaline phosphatase and a chromogenic substrates results in the formation of a precipitate on the membrane where hybridization as occurred (Scarparo et al., 2001; Tortoli et al., 2001). The LiPa assay is able to detect up to 14 different species of mycobacteria (Table 3) and results are interpreted according to a flowchart decision scheme (Tortoli et al., 2001). A multicenter evaluation of LiPa assay conducted in Italy tested 238 mycobacterial organisms from both solid and liquid media as well as two Nocardia strains (Tortoli et al., 2001). All 238 mycobacterial strains reacted with the genus specific probes for a sensitivity of 100% and 61 of the 238 strains were identified to the species level. The other 177 strains were outside of the detection range of the LiPa assay. Additional studies using only liquid culture media, MB/BacT Alert 3D (Organon Teknika, Boxtel, The Netherlands), and BACTEC 12B Bottles (BACTEC; Becton Dickinson, Sparks, MD), showed similar sensitivity of 100% for detection of mycobacterial strains by the genus specific probes as well as correct identification at the species levels and specificity of 100% (Miller et al., 2000; Scarparo et al., 2001).

The LiPa test is a more complex assay than the AccuProbe, requiring highly skilled technologists and has a turn-around time of at least 6 hours, including a PCR amplification step. Furthermore, control of the hybridization temperature is key to preventing formation of non-specific bands. However, in addition to its ability to detect several mycobacterial species compared to AccuProbes, the Inno-LiPa assay has the advantage of being able to detect mixed mycobacterial infections which often results in decreased sensitivity of the AccuProbes (Scarparo et al., 2001). Both assays still have to be performed from organisms growing in culture and are not able to differentiate among the members of the *Mtb* complex.

Another line probe assay, the GenoType Mycobacterium (Hain, Nehren, Germany) was developed and made available in two different kit formats. One kit, the Genotype Mycobacterium CM (Common Mycobacteria) was designed to detect the most frequently isolated mycobacteria species in clinical laboratories while the other kit, the Genotype Mycobacterium AS (Additional Species), was designed for the detection of less frequently encountered mycobacteria species (Makinen et al., 2006; Richter et al., 2006; Russo et al., 2006). Russo and colleagues tested 197 isolates including genera other than mycobacteria previously identified by conventional biochemical tests, HPLC, Inno-Lipa and 16S rRNA sequencing (Russo et al., 2006). The sensitivity of the assay for the mycobacterium genus was 98.9 and 99.4% for the CM and AS kits respectively with a specificity of 100% for the AS kit and 88.9% for the CM kit due to weak cross-reaction of several strains of the genus *Tsukamurella*. The overall sensitivity and specificity for species identification was 97.9% and 92.4% for the CM kit and 99.3% and 99.4% for the AS kit with all members of the *Mtb* complex correctly identified as *Mtb* complex by the CM kit and *Mtb* species by the AS kit. Similar performance were established in other independent studies evaluating the GenoType CM and AS kits, with the sensitivity and specificity for *Mtb* complex members approaching 100% when compared to 16S rRNA sequencing and biochemical testing (Makinen et al., 2006; Richter et al., 2006).

A third kit from Hain LifeScience, the Genotype MTBC DNA strip assay was designed specifically for the differentiation of members of the *Mtb* complex and identification of *M. bovis* BCG. Similar to the LiPa assay, the MTBC DNA strip assay uses reverse hybridization technology on a solid membrane matrix. The DNA probes immobilized on the membranes target polymorphisms in the *gyrB* DNA sequence of the *Mtb* complex and the RD1 deletion of *M. bovis* BCG (Richter et al., 2003). Ritcher and colleagues (Richter et al., 2003) evaluated the performance of the MTBC assay using well-characterized strains of *Mtb* complex including *Mtb*, *M. bovis* subsp. *bovis*, *M. bovis* subsp. *caprae*, *M. bovis* BCG, *M. africanum* subtype I , *M. africanum* subtype II , *M. canetti*, and *M. microti* as well as clinical isolates of *Mtb* complex identified by conventional methods and other molecular tests (PCR-Restriction fragment length polymorphism). The MTBC assay was able to differentiate all species of the *Mtb* complex except for separating *Mtb* from some strains of *M. africanum* subtype II and *M. canetti* (sensitivity of 94%). A similar study conducted by Neonakis and colleagues showed 100% agreement between conventional methods/AccuProbes and MTBC assay for the identification and differentiation of 120 clinical isolates of the *Mtb* complex (Neonakis et al., 2007).

Species	AccuProbes	Inno-LiPa	GenoType CM	GenoType AS	GenoType MTBC
Mycobacterium spp.		X	X		
M. tuberculosis complex	X	X	X		
M. tuberculosis					X
M. bovis subsp. *bovis*					X
M. bovis BCG					X
M. bovis subsp. *caprae*					X
M. africanum					X
M. microti					X
M. kansasii	X	X	X	X	
M. avium	X	X	X		
M. intracellulare	X	X	X		
MAI-X		X			
M. malmonense		X	X		
M. haemophilum		X		X	
M. scrofulaceum		X	X		
M. paratuberculosis		X			
M. silvaticum		X			
M. chelonae		X	X		
M. gastri		X		X	
M. xenopi		X	X		
M. gordonae	X	X	X		
M. abscessus			X		
M. fortuitum			X		
M. marinum			X		
M. ulcerans			X	X	
M. peregrinum			X		
M. simiae				X	
M. mucogenicum				X	
M. goodii				X	
M. celatum				X	
M. smegmatis				X	
M. genavense				X	
M. lentiflavum				X	
M. heckeshornense				X	
M. szulgai				X	
M. phlei				X	
M. asiaticum				X	
M. shimoidei				X	

Table 3. Mycobacterium species detected by commercially available probe assays

5.6 DNA sequencing

The first report of nucleic acid sequencing for the identification of mycobacteria appeared in the literature in the early 1990s. Rogall et al. (Rogall et al., 1990) described the use of a 1 kb gene fragment targeting the 5′ region of the 16S rRNA to detect and differentiate among the various species of mycobacteria, including the *Mtb* complex. In this study, amplified sequences were electrophoresed on a 6% sequencing gel, dried and the gel was exposed to X-rays film for 12 hours. Sequences obtained were then analyzed using a multisequence alignment algorithm from SAGE program (Rogall et al., 1990). This entire process was completed in approximately 2 days. Other nucleic acid targets were analyzed including the *rpoB* gene, encoding the β-subunit of the RNA polymerase, which had the added advantage of detecting rifampin resistance (Kim et al., 1999; Kasai et al., 2000), the 16-23S rDNA internal transcribed spacer (ITS) (Roth et al., 1998), the 32-kDa protein (Soini et al., 1994) and the 65 kDa heat shock protein (Kapur et al., 1995). Each of these targets presented advantages and disadvantages, mainly related to their ability to differentiate closely-related organisms. Today, sequencing of the 16S rDNA has become the gold standard for mycobacteria species identification. The process was eventually automated and commercialized (MicroSeq 500bp and 1500bp 16S rDNA Bacterial Sequencing Kits, Applied Biosystems, Carlsbad, CA), which resulted in standardization of the assay across laboratories. The MicroSeq 16S rDNA bacterial identification assay analyzes a larger portion of the 16S rDNA than the one described earlier by Rogall et al. (Rogall et al., 1990), resulting in increased discriminating power. The introduction of capillary electrophoresis and fluorescent dyes to replace the cumbersome sequencing gels and radioactive labels, the development of genetic analyzer and the National Center for Biotechnology Information (NCBI) tool, BLAST (Basic Local Alignment Sequence Tool), further improved on the use of sequencing for mycobacterial species identification.

DNA sequencing using the MicroSeq system is based on sequencing by capillary electrophoresis and consists of 4 steps: DNA extraction, amplification, sequencing and data analysis. Total genomic DNA extraction is performed simply by lysis of organisms in a chaotropic solution (PrepMan Ultra, Applied Biosystems), followed by heating at 95°C for 10 minutes to kill the organisms. Extraction is followed by 16S rRNA amplification, PCR products clean-up and sequencing PCR and analysis on a genetic analyzer. The sequence obtained is then analyzed against the MicroSeq database library and/or the BLAST database on the NCBI website (http://blast.ncbi.nlm.nih.gov/Blast.cgi).

Studies evaluating the performance of the MicroSeq systems for identification of mycobacteria have repeatedly shown the advantages of using this technique over traditional biochemical tests and with the increase in available and correct sequences in various database, the sensitivity of the assay continues to increase (Patel et al., 2000; Cloud et al., 2002; Hall et al., 2003; Woo et al., 2011). The main limitation of sequencing for identification of mycobacteria as discussed above remains the inability to distinguish several species of mycobacteria based solely on the 16S rRNA including *M. chelonae, M. abscessus,* and *M. immunogenum* and the various members of the *Mtb* complex (Hall et al., 2003; Woo et al., 2011). Alternative sequencing targets (eg., *rpoB*) can often be used to distinguish mycobacterial species which cannot be resolved using the 16S target.

5.7 PCR methods (conventional and real-time)

The pattern of resistance of pyrazinamide (PZA) is often used to distinguish between *Mtb* and *M. bovis/M. bovis* BCG strains (section 5.2.3). Only a few laboratory-developed tests (LDTs) have been designed to differentiate among members of the *Mtb* complex (Parsons et al., 2002; Huard et al., 2003; Pinsky & Banaei, 2008). Pinsky and Banaei (Pinsky & Banaei, 2008) reported a real-time PCR assay, using a series of different primer pairs targeting the RD (region of difference) 9 (present in all *Mtb* complex members), the RD1 (absent in *M. bovis* BCG strains), the RD4 (absent in *M. bovis*). This multiplex real-time PCR uses melt curve analysis from two separate PCRs to identify and distinguish between *Mtb, M. bovis*, and *M. bovis* BCG directly from isolates growing in culture. Similarly, although on a conventional PCR format, the RD1 sequence was used as a target for the differentiation of *Mtb, M. bovis*, and *M. bovis* BCG from culture isolates (Lee et al., 2010).

5.8 Immunoassay methods

There are several commercially-available immunoassay methods which allow the identification of *Mtb* complex from culture by detection of *Mtb*-specific antigens. These tests are rapid requiring only minutes to perform after growth of the organism but literature reports indicate variable performance (Martin et al., 2011; Said et al., 2011; Steingart et al., 2011; Yu et al., 2011)

6. Direct identification of *M. tuberculosis* from clinical specimens

6.1 Line probe assays

The INNO LiPa Mycobacteria (Innogenetics), described previously in section 5.5, has been evaluated for use directly on clinical specimens without waiting for growth of *Mtb* complex in culture. In a study by Perandin et al. (Perandin et al., 2006), the INNO Lipa Mycobacteria assay was evaluated, with slight modifications, on both pulmonary specimens and extrapulmonary specimens (stools, urines, lymph nodes, gastric fluids and pus). The overall sensitivity and specificity of the test was 79.5% and 84.6% respectively for pulmonary specimens and 71.4% and 100 %, respectively for extrapulmonary specimens. As expected the sensitivity and specificity of the assay was much lower when tested on specimens than culture isolates and the authors suggested this was due to the lower numbers of organisms present in specimens.

The INNO-LiPA Rif TB (Innogenetics) test, designed to detect *Mtb* complex and rifampin susceptibility in culture isolates, has also been tested on clinical specimens in multiple studies (Gamboa et al., 1998; de Oliveira et al., 2003; Johansen et al., 2003; Traore et al., 2006). In one of the largest studies, Traore and colleagues (Traore et al., 2006) evaluated the performance of the INNO-LiPA assay by testing 420 sputum samples from both treated and untreated patients, with 311 smear positive and 109 smear negative specimens. The assay detected *Mtb* complex DNA in 92% of smear positive specimens and 94.5% of smear negative specimens, a higher detection rate than culture which detected *Mtb* complex in 74.3% of all specimens.

An alternative version to the line assay GenoType Mycobacterium (Hain LifeScience), the GenoType Mycobacterium Direct Assay (Hain Lifescience) was designed to detect *Mtb* complex and *M. avium*, *M. intracellulare*, *M. kansasii*, and *M. malmoense* directly from clinical specimens. This assay is performed in three parts consisting of an RNA isolation and capture step, followed by an isothermal amplification of the 23S rRNA, and finally a reverse-hybridization of the amplified products on the membrane strips. Evaluation of this assay showed sensitivity and specificity ranging from 80.5-97% to 75-100% respectively when compared to culture (Franco-Alvarez de Luna et al., 2006; Seagar et al., 2008; Neonakis et al., 2009; Kiraz et al., 2010).

In general, the sensitivity of these line assays is lower when tested directly on clinical specimens as compared to their sensitivity when used on culture isolates. However, with a turn-around time of about 2 days compared to at least 6 weeks to obtain growth in culture, these assays, with their high specificity, provide information that is directly useful for clinical management of patients.

6.2 FDA-approved PCR methods

The first FDA-approved amplification test for diagnosis of *Mtb* complex was the Amplified Mycobacterium Tuberculosis Direct (MTD) test (Gen-Probe Inc, San Diego, CA). This assay was based on the amplification of *Mtb* complex rRNA followed by detection of the amplified rRNA by hybridization of chemiluminescent acridinium ester-labeled DNA probes. The sensitivity and specificity of the assay in earlier studies testing against N-acetyl-L-cysteine treated respiratory samples (smear positive and smear negative), was 91.9-100% and 97.6-100%, respectively when compared to culture (Abe et al., 1993; Pfyffer et al., 1994; Welch et al., 1995). The MTD test presented several advantages over traditional methods including the use of rRNA, which is present in several copies in *Mtb* complex, rapid turn-around time (day vs. weeks), single tube amplification and detection, although culture is still required for susceptibility testing of the organisms (Abe et al., 1993; Pfyffer et al., 1994). The MTD test is only FDA-approved for respiratory specimens; however, the assay performance in extrapulmonary specimens has also been evaluated by several investigators. Vlaspodler et al. (Vlaspolder et al., 1995) showed variable sensitivity for different specimens with detection in pleural fluids being as low as 20% (with specificity of 96%) and sensitivity and specificity in other specimens, including urines, lymph nodes, CSF, gastric fluids and lung biopsies, of 100% and 95% respectively. Similar results were obtained in other studies that included a greater numbers of non-respiratory specimens, with sensitivities ranging from 93-100% and specificities of 100% for both smear-positive and smear negative specimens (Chedore & Jamieson, 1999; Woods et al., 2001).

A second PCR assay approved by the FDA was the AMPLICOR *Mycobacterium tuberculosis* test (AMPLICOR MTB; Roche Diagnostic Systems, Somerville, N.J.). This assay targeted the 16S rRNA gene with colorimetric detection using probe hybridization (Piersimoni & Scarparo, 2003). In a study by D'Amato and colleagues, the sensitivity and specificity of the Amplicor MTB when compared to culture as the gold standard was: 55.3% and 99.6% from smear negative and 94.1% and 100% from smear positive respiratory specimens (D'Amato et al., 1995). Other studies showed sensitivity and specificity for the assay ranging from 70.4% to 79.5% with specificity greater than 98% when compared to culture and conventional microscopy (Schirm et al., 1995; Bergmann & Woods, 1996; Devallois et al., 1996) and sensitivity generally increasing 75-98 % for AFB positive specimens (Schirm et al., 1995; Bergmann & Woods, 1996). Testing of non-respiratory samples by the Amplicor MTB assay supported its use in diagnosis of extrapulmonary tuberculosis as the sensitivity and specificity varied from 76%-100% and 99.9-100%, respectively when compared to clinical diagnosis (Shah et al., 1998). These non-respiratory specimens included various tissue biopsies (lung, lymph nodes, liver) and various body fluids (pleural, ascites, CSF, synovial, gastric, pericardial and peritoneal).

A second version of the Amplicor assay, the Cobas Amplicor MTB-PCR (Roche Diagnostics) was developed as a semi-automated assay that combined the amplification, detection and reporting of results (Bodmer et al., 1997; Levidiotou et al., 2003). Evaluation of the new assay showed increased sensitivity over the manual assay with one study testing >1,000 respiratory specimens reporting a sensitivity and specificity of 91.3% and 99.6% (Bodmer et al., 1997) and the other reporting an overall sensitivity and specificity of 82.5% and 99.8% after testing greater than 7,000 specimens (respiratory and non-respiratory)(Levidiotou et al., 2003).

Both the MTD and the Amplicor assays were evaluated on broth samples including BACTECT 12B bottles (Becton Dickinson, Sparks, MD) and the ESP II (Trek Diagnostics, Westlake, OH), with sensitivity of greater than 90% for both assays in both media and specificity of 100% (Hernandez et al., 1997; Smith et al., 1997; Bergmann & Woods, 1999; Desmond & Loretz, 2001).

6.3 Laboratory-developed PCR methods

Several targets, including the 65-kD antigen of *Mtb* complex (Pao et al., 1990; Brisson-Noel et al., 1991; Totsch et al., 1994), the protein antigen B (Sjobring et al., 1990), the repetitive sequences IS6110 (Brisson-Noel et al., 1991; Eisenach et al., 1991; Sankar et al., 2010) and IS986 (Abe et al., 1993), have been used over the years for the detection of *Mtb* complex by LDTs. Earlier tests were based on conventional PCR, with a multi-step manual extraction process followed by amplification and detection of the amplified target on polyacrylamide gel. Depending on the target used, the sensitivity and specificity of these conventional PCR assays directly from respiratory specimens ranged from 84.2-100% and 62.6-100% with culture and clinical diagnosis used as a gold standard. However, due to limitations inherent with conventional PCR including high potential for cross-contamination, real-time PCRs, combined with automated extraction, have largely replaced these methods in clinical laboratories.

Real-time PCR is faster than conventional PCR and does not require post-amplification manipulation of the amplified DNA, reducing the potential for cross-contamination. Several real-time PCR LDTs have been developed for diagnosis of pulmonary tuberculosis. In one of the earlier studies by Miller et al (Miller et al., 2002), a real-time PCR assay was developed on the LightCycler platform (Roche Diagnostics, Indianapolis, IN) with primers targeting the internal transcribed spacer region of the mycobacterium genome with specific hybridization probes designed for the detection of *Mtb* complex. The sensitivity and specificity of this assay for smear-positive respiratory specimens was 98.1% and 100% respectively with a turn-around time of less than 5 hours (Miller et al., 2002). Other studies, with different targets, have reported similar results (Shrestha et al., 2003) and many have been designed as multiplex assays to differentiate *Mtb* complex from other non-tuberculosis mycobacteria based on melting curve analysis (Shrestha et al., 2003). Furthermore, these assays were often shown to be as sensitive and specific as the available commercial assays such as the Cobas Amplicor (Miller et al., 2002; Shrestha et al., 2003).

Both conventional and real-time PCRs have also been developed for the diagnosis of extrapulmonary tuberculosis using both fresh specimens and paraffin-embedded tissues. Some of the fresh specimens that have been evaluated by various PCR include fine needle aspirates and tissue biopsies of lymph nodes, blood, urines, bone marrow aspirates and skin biopsies with variable sensitivities and specificities (Hsiao et al., 2003; Bruijnesteijn Van Coppenraet et al., 2004; Chakravorty & Tyagi, 2005; Ritis et al., 2005; Torrea et al., 2005; Rebollo et al., 2006). Although paraffin-embedded tissues are not optimal samples for PCR, often, they are the only specimens available to rule out tuberculosis. The sensitivity and specificity of PCR assays, conventional and real-time, on paraffin-embedded tissues varies from 64-100% and 73- 100%, respectively (Beqaj et al., 2007; Baba et al., 2008; Nopvichai et al., 2009; Luo et al., 2010).

Unlike PCR assays previously mentioned for differentiation of members of *Mtb* complex, a real-time PCR assay, developed by Halse and colleagues (Halse et al., 2011) at the New York State Public Health Laboratory, showed the ability to differentiate among members of the *Mtb* complex directly from clinical specimens based on the detection of five targets including RD1, RD4, RD9, RD12 and a region external to RD9. The assay was able to detect 155 of 165 clinical specimens (94%) and 708/727 (97%) of positive BACTEC MGIT-960 bottles. Furthermore, this assay was able to distinguish not only *Mtb*, *M. bovis* and *M. bovis* BCG but also *M. africanum*, *M. microti,* and *M. canettii*.

7. Drug resistance testing for *M. tuberculosis*

The CDC published recommendations that drug susceptibility testing be performed on the first *Mtb* complex isolate from a each patient and also if a patient is failing therapy (based on clinical evidence or positive culture after three months on therapy) (MMWR, 1993). This recommendation was formulated following a resurgence in cases of tuberculosis from the mid-1980s to the early 1990s of up to 18% with resistance strains present in as high as 33% of cases in New York city (MMWR, 1993). Susceptibility testing is currently performed most commonly by traditional methods either agar-based or broth based methods with resistance defined as growth of greater than 1% of organisms tested against a specific drug (Canetti et al., 1963).

7.1 Indirect proportion method

Although patient specimens can be tested directly for drug susceptibility with the advantage of decreased time to results, this method is limited to smear-positive specimens and results may be difficult to interpret if contamination occurs (Woods, 2011). The 1% indirect proportion method is performed on Middlebrook 7H10 agar medium poured in a four-quadrant Petri dish with one quadrant serving as the control quadrant and containing no drug and the other three quadrants containing increasing concentration of the drug being tested. The inoculum is prepared using organisms growing on solid or liquid media adjusted to a 1.0 McFarland and diluted to 10^{-2} and 10^{-4}; 0. 1 mL of each dilution is then added to each quadrant of separate plate and incubated for up to three weeks at $37 \pm 1°C$ in an atmosphere of 5 to 10% CO_2 (CLSI, 2003). The percentage of drug resistance is calculated by dividing the total colony count in a quadrant containing drug by the total colony count in the control quadrant (at least 50 colonies) and multiplying by 100. If the percentage is greater than 1%, then the organism is resistant and therapy with the drug tested is likely to fail (CLSI, 2008; Woods, 2011). This method is used primarily for susceptibility testing of the first line drugs, isoniazid (INH), rifampin (RIF) and ethambutol (EMB), as well as second line drugs, when resistance to RIF or two of the first-line drug is detected (CLSI, 2008).

7.2 Rapid broth methods

In order to circumvent the long turn-around time of the agar proportion methods and provide clinicians with timely drug susceptibility results, rapid broth methods were developed for both growth and susceptibility testing of *Mtb* complex. The first system, the BACTEC 460, was a based on measurement of radioactive $^{14}CO_2$ produced by metabolic breakdown of ^{14}C-labelled palmitic acid contained in a 7H12 liquid medium in the presence or absence of specific drugs (Middlebrook et al., 1977; Siddiqi et al., 1981; Snider et al., 1981; Laszlo et al., 1983). The agreement between the conventional and the radiometric susceptibility testing assays varied from 96.4-98% with most results obtained within 7 days (Siddiqi et al., 1981; Laszlo et al., 1983). Additionally, unlike the 1% indirect agar method, the radiometric method was conducive to testing of *Mtb* complex susceptibility against pyrazinamide (PZA), which requires an acidic environment not easily achievable on solid media. Heifets and Isman modified the radiometric method by lowering the pH with addition of phosphoric acid at the same time as PZA but after the growing culture had reached exponential phase (Heifets & Iseman, 1985). This initial study, with limited number of isolates, showed good correlation between PZA susceptibility as measured by the radiometric method and detection of the pyrazinamidase enzyme as described under biochemical testing (Heifets & Iseman, 1985). The method described by Heifets and Isman was further modified and proved useful in facilitating the measurement of PZA susceptibility of *Mtb* complex by the radiometric method (Tarrand et al., 1986; Salfinger & Heifets, 1988).

The BACTEC 460 radiometric method for susceptibility testing was eventually replaced with the fully automated Mycobacteria Growth Indicator tube (MGIT 960, Becton Dickinson, Sparks, MD), which had been introduced for broth culture of mycobacteria species from clinical specimens without the use of radioactive materials (Chew et al., 1998; Heifets et al., 2000). Each drug-containing MGIT bottle is inoculated with either 0.5 mL of a 1:100 dilution of a MGIT tube positive for 1-2 days, a 1:5 dilution of a MGIT tube positive for 3-5 days or a 0.5 McFarland if the inoculum is prepared from an organism growing on solid media (Siddiqi, 2010). The control, drug-free MGIT bottle is inoculated with a 1:100 dilution of the inoculum used for the drug-containing MGIT bottle. The MGIT 960 system automatically interprets the results of the test based on the growth unit (GU). If the GU is greater than 100 for a drug-containing MGIT bottle, the isolate is resistant and if the GU is less than or equal to 100 then the isolate is susceptible. However, for the test to be valid, the GU of the control bottle cannot reach 400 before 4 days or after 13 days, which suggests that the growth was too heavy or too light respectively (Woods, 2011). The MGIT 960 system is FDA-approved for susceptibility testing of *Mtb* complex against the first-line drugs including RIF (2 µg/ml), INH (0.4 µg/ml and 0.1 µg/ml), and EMB (7.5 µg/ml and 2.5 µg/ml), PYZ (100 µg/ml) and streptomycin (STR, 6.0 µg/ml and 2.0 µg/ml) (CLSI, 2008). Evaluation of the MGIT performance for the primary tuberculosis drugs showed results that were comparable to the BACTEC 460 radiometric methods as well as the agar proportion methods (>90% agreement) (Ardito et al., 2001; Adjers-Koskela & Katila, 2003; Scarparo et al., 2004), except for EMB and STR which had agreement varying from less than 80% to 98% (Adjers-Koskela & Katila, 2003; Scarparo et al., 2004; Hall et al., 2006; Garrigo et al., 2007). More recently, the MGIT 960 was evaluated for susceptibility testing of second-line drugs including levofloxacin, amikacin, capreomycin and ethionamide with overall agreement of 96% at critical concentrations when compared to the agar proportion method (Lin et al., 2009). Similar results were obtained in a study comparing the manual version of the MGIT to the agar method using the second-line drugs ofloxacin, kanamycin, ethionamide, and capreomycin (Martin et al., 2008). In both studies, the agreement between the two methods for ethionamide was markedly lower (86-88%) than for the other drugs (Martin et al., 2008; Lin et al., 2009).

Another fully automated broth system that is FDA-approved for susceptibility testing of *Mtb* complex is the VersaTREK instrument (TREK Diagnostics, Cleveland, OH). The VersaTREK (formerly ESP culture system II) is FDA-approved for susceptibility testing of *Mtb* complex against the first-line drugs including RIF (1 µg/ml), INH (0.4 µg/ml and 0.1 µg/ml), ETH (8 µg/ml and 5 µg/ml), and PZA (100 µg/ml) (CLSI, 2008). Drug susceptibility for each isolate tested is manually determined by comparing the time to detection of growth between the control bottle and the bottle containing the drug. If the difference is greater than three days or if the bottle remains negative, the isolate is considered susceptible. If the difference is less than or equal to 3 days, then the isolate is considered resistant. However, for the test to be valid, the time to growth in the control bottle has to be between 3 and 10 days following inoculation with 0.5 mL of a 1:10 dilution of a 1.0 McFarland inoculum (Bergmann & Woods, 1998; Ruiz et al., 2000). Evaluation of the VersaTREK instrument against the agar proportion method or the BACTEC 460 for susceptibility testing of *Mtb* against INH, RIF, ETB, and STR showed results similar to the MGIT 960, with agreement > than 95% for all drugs except ETB and STR (agreement between 90-95%) for which the VersaTrek generally called susceptible organisms that were resistant (Bergmann & Woods, 1998), although only a few isolates were tested in the study. Similar results were obtained by other investigators, except for STR, which unlike the previous study, had an agreement of 99.7% with the BACTEC 460 method (Ruiz et al., 2000).

7.3 Molecular detection of resistance markers

Although conventional methods described above are still the main-stay in detection of drug resistance in most laboratories, several studies have been conducted to developed more rapid and specific methods of detection of multi-drug resistance markers in *Mtb* complex. These assays are based on the detection of specific mutations in a variety of genes reported to confer resistance to several of the anti-tuberculosis drugs.

The Genotype MTBDR*plus* (Hain Lifescience) is a commercial line probe assay developed for the detection of INH and RIF resistance in *Mtb* complex isolates and smear-positive specimens (Hillemann et al., 2007). Resistance to INH results from mutations in genes whose products are involved in the activation and binding of INH including the *katG*, the *inhA*, the *ahpC-oxyR*, *ahpC* and *ndh* genes, while resistance to RIF is due mainly to mutation in the *rpoB* gene, which encodes the β-subunit of the DNA-dependent RNA polymerase, RIF binding target (Zhang & Yew, 2009).

The Genotype MTBDR*plus* assay detects the most common mutations found in the *rpoB*, *katG* and *inhA* genes, an improvement from other line-probe assays such as the INNO-LiPA Rif (Innogenetics) and the GenoType MTBDR (Hain Lifescience), which only target the *rpoB* mutation (INNO-LiPA Rif) or *rpoB* and *katG* mutations (GenoType MTBDR). Evaluation of the Genotype MTBDR*plus* assay by Hillemann et al (Hillemann et al., 2007) on clinical strains and smear-positive sputa revealed a detection rate of 98.7% (74/75) and 96.8% (30/31) of RIF resistance in clinical isolates and sputa specimens respectively. INH resistance was detected in 92% (69/75) and 90% (36/41) of clinical isolates and sputa specimens respectively. Similar detection rate were obtained by Barnard et al (Barnard et al., 2008) who tested 536 consecutive smear-positive sputum specimens with a sensitivity of 98.9% for detection of RIF resistance and 94.2% for the detection of INH resistance when compared to results obtained with conventional methods. Although the assay is limited to the detection of known mutations of RIF and INH, the high concordance rate with conventional methods and the rapid time to results makes the MTBDR*plus* assay a useful test for the management of multi-drug resistance tuberculosis.

Another version of the line probe assay, the GenoType MTBDR*sl* (second-line) (Hain Lifescience), was recently introduced for the detection of mutations in the *gyrA* gene, the 16S rRNA gene and the *embB* gene which confer resistance to fluoroquinolones, aminoglycosides and capreomycin, and ethambutol respectively (Hillemann et al., 2009). This assay shows variable performance characteristics when compared to phenotypic methods or sequencing, ranging from 75.6-90% for fluoroquinolones, 43-100% for aminoglycosides, 71.4-87.5% for capreomycin and suboptimal rate in all studies for ethambutol (38.5-64.2%) (Hillemann et al., 2009; Kiet et al., 2010; Huang et al., 2011; Kontsevaya et al., 2011).

Multiple home-brew PCR assays have been developed for the detection of the most common gene mutations conferring resistance to *Mtb* complex strains. A recent study reports the development of a multiplex real-time PCR assay to detect all known mutations in the *gyrA* gene responsible for conferring resistance to fluoroquinolones (Chakravorty et al., 2011). This assay is based on an asymmetrical PCR using sloppy molecular beacon probes that extends the entire quinolone resistance determining region (QRDR), a region of the *gyrA* gene containing most of the known mutations responsible for fluoroquinolones resistance (Takiff et al., 1994). This assay was 100% sensitive and 100% specific in detecting fluoroquinolones resistance in 92 clinical isolates of *Mtb* complex, when compared to sequencing.

As many as 21 mutations in the *katG* gene can cause decreased activity of INH against *Mtb* complex (Ando et al., 2010). Although several assays have focused on the S315T mutation of *KatG* (Mokrousov et al., 2002; Zhang et al., 2007; Tho et al., 2011), which is known to confer high-level resistance to INH and be present in as many as 90% of resistant *Mtb* isolates in Russia (Marttila et al., 1998; Mokrousov et al., 2002), the study by Ando and colleagues showed that other mutations in the *KatG* gene can cause high-level resistance and those should be included in molecular assays targeting the *katG* gene (Ando et al., 2010).

The utility of the assays is limited since they often target detection of resistance to one class of antimicrobial, depends on the available knowledge of current mutations conferring resistance, and as such, can only be use in conjunction with other assays. Several investigators have focused their efforts in developing assays similar to the MTBDR*plus* assay to include resistant marker to more than one class of antituberculosis drugs and for more than one mutation per gene target (Sekiguchi et al., 2007; Zhang et al., 2007; Ong et al., 2010; Pholwat et al., 2011).

Other molecular assays that have been developed for the detection of resistance markers have included locked nucleic acid probes (van Doorn et al., 2008) and multiplex PCR amplimer conformation analysis (Cheng et al., 2004), pyrosequencing (Marttila et al., 2009; Garza-Gonzalez et al., 2010; Halse et al., 2010), oligonucleotide microarray (Caoili et al., 2006), and mass spectrometry (Wang et al., 2011).

8. Future directions

Clinical diagnostics for *Mtb* continue to evolve (Wilson, 2011) and in some cases, the future may be at our fingertips (Van Rie et al., 2010). For example, the GeneXpert MTB/RIF PCR assay (Cepheid, Sunnyvale, CA) allows for the automated, direct detection of *Mtb* complex in respiratory specimens and it has been endorsed by the WHO for use in low-income countries (WHO, 2008). The Xpert assay provides excellent sensitivity and specificity from direct specimens while providing a same day turn-around time for results (Helb et al., 2010; Boehme et al., 2011; Marlowe et al., 2011; Rachow et al., 2011; Scott et al., 2011). In addition, the assay provides immediate information on RIF resistance and has recently been successfully evaluated using non-respiratory specimens (Ioannidis et al., 2011; Miller et al., 2011).

Older technologies utilized in new ways are also making inroads in *Mtb* diagnostics. The use of mass spectrometry for the identification of *Mtb* complex from culture isolates may replace current standards such as biochemical analysis, nucleic acid hybridization probes, and DNA sequencing due to the ability of mass spectrometry to rapidly and accurately identify *Mtb* in a cost-effective manner while minimizing technologist hands-on time and effort (Saleeb et al., 2011). Although still in it's infancy in the diagnostic microbiology laboratory, this technology may also have utility in predicting drug resistance patterns and evaluating epidemiologic groups (Bouakaze et al., 2011; Massire et al., 2011; Schurch et al., 2011).

Finally, new technologies such as next generation sequencing are still largely utilized for research purposes in microbiology but some authors have suggested that there may come a time when application of this powerful technology will find a niche in the diagnostic microbiology laboratory (Ansorge, 2009; Rogers & Bruce, 2010; Engelthaler et al., 2011; Pallen & Loman, 2011).

9. References

Abe, C., K. Hirano, et al. (1993). "Detection of Mycobacterium tuberculosis in clinical specimens by polymerase chain reaction and Gen-Probe Amplified Mycobacterium Tuberculosis Direct Test." *J Clin Microbiol* 31(12): 3270-3274.

Adjers-Koskela, K. & M. L. Katila (2003). "Susceptibility testing with the manual mycobacteria growth indicator tube (MGIT) and the MGIT 960 system provides rapid and reliable verification of multidrug-resistant tuberculosis." *J Clin Microbiol* 41(3): 1235-1239.

Ando, H., Y. Kondo, et al. (2010). "Identification of katG mutations associated with high-level isoniazid resistance in Mycobacterium tuberculosis." *Antimicrob Agents Chemother* 54(5): 1793-1799.

Ansorge, W. J. (2009). "Next-generation DNA sequencing techniques." *New biotechnology* 25(4): 195-203.

Ardito, F., B. Posteraro, et al. (2001). "Evaluation of BACTEC Mycobacteria Growth Indicator Tube (MGIT 960) automated system for drug susceptibility testing of Mycobacterium tuberculosis." *J Clin Microbiol* 39(12): 4440-4444.

Attorri, S., S. Dunbar, et al. (2000). "Assessment of morphology for rapid presumptive identification of Mycobacterium tuberculosis and Mycobacterium kansasii." *Journal of clinical microbiology* 38(4): 1426-1429.

Baba, K., S. Pathak, et al. (2008). "Real-time quantitative PCR in the diagnosis of tuberculosis in formalin-fixed paraffin-embedded pleural tissue in patients from a high HIV endemic area." *Diagn Mol Pathol* 17(2): 112-117.

Barnard, M., H. Albert, et al. (2008). "Rapid molecular screening for multidrug-resistant tuberculosis in a high-volume public health laboratory in South Africa." *Am J Respir Crit Care Med* 177(7): 787-792.

Beqaj, S. H., R. Flesher, et al. (2007). "Use of the real-time PCR assay in conjunction with MagNA Pure for the detection of mycobacterial DNA from fixed specimens." *Diagn Mol Pathol* 16(3): 169-173.

Bergmann, J. S. & G. L. Woods (1996). "Clinical evaluation of the Roche AMPLICOR PCR Mycobacterium tuberculosis test for detection of M. tuberculosis in respiratory specimens." *J Clin Microbiol* 34(5): 1083-1085.

Bergmann, J. S. & G. L. Woods (1998). "Evaluation of the ESP culture system II for testing susceptibilities of Mycobacterium tuberculosis isolates to four primary antituberculous drugs." *J Clin Microbiol* 36(10): 2940-2943.

Bergmann, J. S. & G. L. Woods (1999). "Enhanced Amplified Mycobacterium Tuberculosis Direct Test for detection of Mycobacterium tuberculosis complex in positive BACTEC 12B broth cultures of respiratory specimens." *J Clin Microbiol* 37(6): 2099-2101.

Bodmer, T., A. Gurtner, et al. (1997). "Evaluation of the COBAS AMPLICOR MTB system." *J Clin Microbiol* 35(6): 1604-1605.

Boehme, C. C., M. P. Nicol, et al. (2011). "Feasibility, diagnostic accuracy, and effectiveness of decentralised use of the Xpert MTB/RIF test for diagnosis of tuberculosis and multidrug resistance: a multicentre implementation study." *Lancet* 377(9776): 1495-1505.

Bouakaze, C., C. Keyser, et al. (2011). "Matrix-Assisted Laser Desorption Ionization-Time of Flight Mass Spectrometry-Based Single Nucleotide Polymorphism Genotyping Assay Using iPLEX Gold Technology for Identification of Mycobacterium tuberculosis Complex Species and Lineages." *J Clin Microbiol* 49(9): 3292-3299.

Brisson-Noel, A., C. Aznar, et al. (1991). "Diagnosis of tuberculosis by DNA amplification in clinical practice evaluation." *Lancet* 338(8763): 364-366.

Bruijnesteijn Van Coppenraet, E. S., J. A. Lindeboom, et al. (2004). "Real-time PCR assay using fine-needle aspirates and tissue biopsy specimens for rapid diagnosis of mycobacterial lymphadenitis in children." *J Clin Microbiol* 42(6): 2644-2650.

Butler, W. R. & L. S. Guthertz (2001). "Mycolic acid analysis by high-performance liquid chromatography for identification of Mycobacterium species." *Clin Microbiol Rev* 14(4): 704-726.

Butler, W. R., K. C. Jost, Jr., et al. (1991). "Identification of mycobacteria by high-performance liquid chromatography." *J Clin Microbiol* 29(11): 2468-2472.

Canetti, G., S. Froman, et al. (1963). "Mycobacteria: Laboratory Methods for Testing Drug Sensitivity and Resistance." *Bull World Health Organ* 29: 565-578.

Caoili, J. C., A. Mayorova, et al. (2006). "Evaluation of the TB-Biochip oligonucleotide microarray system for rapid detection of rifampin resistance in Mycobacterium tuberculosis." *J Clin Microbiol* 44(7): 2378-2381.

Caviedes, L. & D. A. Moore (2007). "Introducing MODS: a low-cost, low-tech tool for high-performance detection of tuberculosis and multidrug resistant tuberculosis." *Indian J Med Microbiol* 25(2): 87-88.

Chakravorty, S., B. Aladegbami, et al. (2011). "Rapid detection of fluoroquinolone-resistant and heteroresistant Mycobacterium tuberculosis by use of sloppy molecular beacons and dual melting-temperature codes in a real-time PCR assay." *J Clin Microbiol* 49(3): 932-940.

Chakravorty, S. & J. S. Tyagi (2005). "Novel multipurpose methodology for detection of mycobacteria in pulmonary and extrapulmonary specimens by smear microscopy, culture, and PCR." *J Clin Microbiol* 43(6): 2697-2702.

Chedore, P. & F. B. Jamieson (1999). "Routine use of the Gen-Probe MTD2 amplification test for detection of Mycobacterium tuberculosis in clinical specimens in a large public health mycobacteriology laboratory." *Diagn Microbiol Infect Dis* 35(3): 185-191.

Chegou, N. N., K. G. Hoek, et al. (2011). "Tuberculosis assays: past, present and future." *Expert review of anti-infective therapy* 9(4): 457-469.

Cheng, A. F., W. W. Yew, et al. (2004). "Multiplex PCR amplimer conformation analysis for rapid detection of gyrA mutations in fluoroquinolone-resistant Mycobacterium tuberculosis clinical isolates." *Antimicrob Agents Chemother* 48(2): 596-601.

Chew, W. K., R. M. Lasaitis, et al. (1998). "Clinical evaluation of the Mycobacteria Growth Indicator Tube (MGIT) compared with radiometric (Bactec) and solid media for isolation of Mycobacterium species." *J Med Microbiol* 47(9): 821-827.

CLSI (2008). Susceptibility Testing of Mycobacteria, Nocardiae, and Other Aerobic Actinomycetes; M24-A2, Approved Standard. Wayne, PA, Clinical and Laboratory Standards Institute.

Cloud, J. L., H. Neal, et al. (2002). "Identification of Mycobacterium spp. by using a commercial 16S ribosomal DNA sequencing kit and additional sequencing libraries." *J Clin Microbiol* 40(2): 400-406.

Cruciani, M., C. Scarparo, et al. (2004). "Meta-analysis of BACTEC MGIT 960 and BACTEC 460 TB, with or without solid media, for detection of mycobacteria." *J Clin Microbiol* 42(5): 2321-2325.

D'Amato, R. F., A. A. Wallman, et al. (1995). "Rapid diagnosis of pulmonary tuberculosis by using Roche AMPLICOR Mycobacterium tuberculosis PCR test." *J Clin Microbiol* 33(7): 1832-1834.

de Oliveira, M. M., A. da Silva Rocha, et al. (2003). "Rapid detection of resistance against rifampicin in isolates of Mycobacterium tuberculosis from Brazilian patients using a reverse-phase hybridization assay." *J Microbiol Methods* 53(3): 335-342.

Desmond, E. P. & K. Loretz (2001). "Use of the Gen-Probe amplified mycobacterium tuberculosis direct test for early detection of Mycobacterium tuberculosis in BACTEC 12B medium." *J Clin Microbiol* 39(5): 1993-1995.

Devallois, A., E. Legrand, et al. (1996). "Evaluation of Amplicor MTB test as adjunct to smears and culture for direct detection of Mycobacterium tuberculosis in the French Caribbean." *J Clin Microbiol* 34(5): 1065-1068.

Drake, T. A., J. A. Hindler, et al. (1987). "Rapid identification of Mycobacterium avium complex in culture using DNA probes." *J Clin Microbiol* 25(8): 1442-1445.

Durst, H. D., M. Milano, et al. (1975). "Phenacyl esters of fatty acids via crown ether catalysts for enhanced ultraviolet detection in liquid chromatography." *Anal Chem* 47(11): 1797-1801.

Eisenach, K. D., M. D. Sifford, et al. (1991). "Detection of Mycobacterium tuberculosis in sputum samples using a polymerase chain reaction." *Am Rev Respir Dis* 144(5): 1160-1163.

Ellner, P. D., T. E. Kiehn, et al. (1988). "Rapid detection and identification of pathogenic mycobacteria by combining radiometric and nucleic acid probe methods." *J Clin Microbiol* 26(7): 1349-1352.

Engelthaler, D. M., T. Chiller, et al. (2011). "Next-generation sequencing of Coccidioides immitis isolated during cluster investigation." *Emerg Infect Dis* 17(2): 227-232.

Floyd, M. M., V. A. Silcox, et al. (1992). "Separation of Mycobacterium bovis BCG from Mycobacterium tuberculosis and Mycobacterium bovis by using high-performance liquid chromatography of mycolic acids." *J Clin Microbiol* 30(5): 1327-1330.

Ford, E. G., S. J. Snead, et al. (1993). "Strains of Mycobacterium terrae complex which react with DNA probes for M. tuberculosis complex." *J Clin Microbiol* 31(10): 2805-2806.

Franco-Alvarez de Luna, F., P. Ruiz, et al. (2006). "Evaluation of the GenoType Mycobacteria Direct assay for detection of Mycobacterium tuberculosis complex and four atypical mycobacterial species in clinical samples." *J Clin Microbiol* 44(8): 3025-3027.

Gamboa, F., P. J. Cardona, et al. (1998). "Evaluation of a commercial probe assay for detection of rifampin resistance in Mycobacterium tuberculosis directly from respiratory and nonrespiratory clinical samples." *Eur J Clin Microbiol Infect Dis* 17(3): 189-192.

Garrigo, M., L. M. Aragon, et al. (2007). "Multicenter laboratory evaluation of the MB/BacT Mycobacterium detection system and the BACTEC MGIT 960 system in comparison with the BACTEC 460TB system for susceptibility testing of Mycobacterium tuberculosis." *J Clin Microbiol* 45(6): 1766-1770.

Garza-Gonzalez, E., G. M. Gonzalez, et al. (2010). "A pyrosequencing method for molecular monitoring of regions in the inhA, ahpC and rpoB genes of Mycobacterium tuberculosis." *Clin Microbiol Infect* 16(6): 607-612.

Gen-Probe (2011). AccuProbe: Mycobacterium Tuberculosis Complex Culture Identification Test.

Goto, M., S. Oka, et al. (1991). "Evaluation of acridinium-ester-labeled DNA probes for identification of Mycobacterium tuberculosis and Mycobacterium avium-

Mycobacterium intracellulare complex in culture." *J Clin Microbiol* 29(11): 2473-2476.

Guthertz, L. S., S. D. Lim, et al. (1993). "Curvilinear-gradient high-performance liquid chromatography for identification of mycobacteria." *J Clin Microbiol* 31(7): 1876-1881.

Ha, D. T., N. T. Lan, et al. (2009). "Microscopic observation drug susceptibility assay (MODS) for early diagnosis of tuberculosis in children." *PloS one* 4(12): e8341.

Hall, L., K. A. Doerr, et al. (2006). "Verification of antimicrobial susceptibility testing of Mycobacterium tuberculosis." *J Clin Microbiol* 44(5): 1921.

Hall, L., K. A. Doerr, et al. (2003). "Evaluation of the MicroSeq system for identification of mycobacteria by 16S ribosomal DNA sequencing and its integration into a routine clinical mycobacteriology laboratory." *J Clin Microbiol* 41(4): 1447-1453.

Halse, T. A., J. Edwards, et al. (2010). "Combined real-time PCR and rpoB gene pyrosequencing for rapid identification of Mycobacterium tuberculosis and determination of rifampin resistance directly in clinical specimens." *J Clin Microbiol* 48(4): 1182-1188.

Halse, T. A., V. E. Escuyer, et al. (2011). "Evaluation of a single-tube multiplex real-time PCR for differentiation of members of the Mycobacterium tuberculosis complex in clinical specimens." *J Clin Microbiol* 49(7): 2562-2567.

Heifets, L., T. Linder, et al. (2000). "Two liquid medium systems, mycobacteria growth indicator tube and MB redox tube, for Mycobacterium tuberculosis isolation from sputum specimens." *J Clin Microbiol* 38(3): 1227-1230.

Heifets, L. B. & M. D. Iseman (1985). "Radiometric method for testing susceptibility of mycobacteria to pyrazinamide in 7H12 broth." *J Clin Microbiol* 21(2): 200-204.

Helb, D., M. Jones, et al. (2010). "Rapid detection of Mycobacterium tuberculosis and rifampin resistance by use of on-demand, near-patient technology." *J Clin Microbiol* 48(1): 229-237.

Hernandez, A., J. S. Bergmann, et al. (1997). "AMPLICOR MTB polymerase chain reaction test for identification of Mycobacterium tuberculosis in positive Difco ESP II broth cultures." *Diagn Microbiol Infect Dis* 27(1-2): 17-20.

Hillemann, D., S. Rusch-Gerdes, et al. (2007). "Evaluation of the GenoType MTBDRplus assay for rifampin and isoniazid susceptibility testing of Mycobacterium tuberculosis strains and clinical specimens." *J Clin Microbiol* 45(8): 2635-2640.

Hillemann, D., S. Rusch-Gerdes, et al. (2009). "Feasibility of the GenoType MTBDRsl assay for fluoroquinolone, amikacin-capreomycin, and ethambutol resistance testing of Mycobacterium tuberculosis strains and clinical specimens." *J Clin Microbiol* 47(6): 1767-1772.

Hsiao, P. F., C. Y. Tzen, et al. (2003). "Polymerase chain reaction based detection of Mycobacterium tuberculosis in tissues showing granulomatous inflammation without demonstrable acid-fast bacilli." *Int J Dermatol* 42(4): 281-286.

Huang, W. L., T. L. Chi, et al. (2011). "Performance assessment of the GenoType MTBDRsl test and DNA sequencing for detection of second-line and ethambutol drug resistance among patients infected with multidrug-resistant Mycobacterium tuberculosis." *J Clin Microbiol* 49(7): 2502-2508.

Huard, R. C., L. C. Lazzarini, et al. (2003). "PCR-based method to differentiate the subspecies of the Mycobacterium tuberculosis complex on the basis of genomic deletions." *J Clin Microbiol* 41(4): 1637-1650.

Ioannidis, P., D. Papaventsis, et al. (2011). "Cepheid GeneXpert MTB/RIF assay for Mycobacterium tuberculosis detection and rifampin resistance identification in patients with substantial clinical indications of tuberculosis and smear-negative microscopy results." *J Clin Microbiol* 49(8): 3068-3070.

Johansen, I. S., B. Lundgren, et al. (2003). "Direct detection of multidrug-resistant Mycobacterium tuberculosis in clinical specimens in low- and high-incidence countries by line probe assay." *J Clin Microbiol* 41(9): 4454-4456.

Julian, E., M. Roldan, et al. (2010). "Microscopic cords, a virulence-related characteristic of Mycobacterium tuberculosis, are also present in nonpathogenic mycobacteria." *J Bacteriol* 192(7): 1751-1760.

Kapur, V., L. L. Li, et al. (1995). "Rapid Mycobacterium species assignment and unambiguous identification of mutations associated with antimicrobial resistance in Mycobacterium tuberculosis by automated DNA sequencing." *Arch Pathol Lab Med* 119(2): 131-138.

Kasai, H., T. Ezaki, et al. (2000). "Differentiation of phylogenetically related slowly growing mycobacteria by their gyrB sequences." *J Clin Microbiol* 38(1): 301-308.

Kellogg, J. A., D. A. Bankert, et al. (2001). "Application of the Sherlock Mycobacteria Identification System using high-performance liquid chromatography in a clinical laboratory." *J Clin Microbiol* 39(3): 964-970.

Kiehn, T. E. & F. F. Edwards (1987). "Rapid identification using a specific DNA probe of Mycobacterium avium complex from patients with acquired immunodeficiency syndrome." *J Clin Microbiol* 25(8): 1551-1552.

Kiet, V. S., N. T. Lan, et al. (2010). "Evaluation of the MTBDRsl test for detection of second-line-drug resistance in Mycobacterium tuberculosis." *J Clin Microbiol* 48(8): 2934-2939.

Kim, B. J., S. H. Lee, et al. (1999). "Identification of mycobacterial species by comparative sequence analysis of the RNA polymerase gene (rpoB)." *J Clin Microbiol* 37(6): 1714-1720.

Kiraz, N., I. Saglik, et al. (2010). "Evaluation of the GenoType Mycobacteria Direct assay for direct detection of the Mycobacterium tuberculosis complex obtained from sputum samples." *J Med Microbiol* 59(Pt 8): 930-934.

Kirschner, P., B. Springer, et al. (1993). "Genotypic identification of mycobacteria by nucleic acid sequence determination: report of a 2-year experience in a clinical laboratory." *J Clin Microbiol* 31(11): 2882-2889.

Koneman, E. W. (2006). Identification of Mycobacteria using Conventional Methods. *In Color Atlas and Textbook of Diagnostic Microbiology.* E. W. Koneman. Philadelphia, Lippincott: 1085-1090.

Kontsevaya, I., S. Mironova, et al. (2011). "Evaluation of Two Molecular Assays for Rapid Detection of Mycobacterium tuberculosis Resistance to Fluoroquinolones in High-Tuberculosis and -Multidrug-Resistance Settings." *J Clin Microbiol* 49(8): 2832-2837.

LaBombardi, V. J., R. Katariwala, et al. (2006). "The identification of mycobacteria from solid media and directly from VersaTREK Myco bottles using the Sherlock Mycobacteria Identification HPLC system." *Clin Microbiol Infect* 12(5): 478-481.

Laszlo, A., P. Gill, et al. (1983). "Conventional and radiometric drug susceptibility testing of Mycobacterium tuberculosis complex." *J Clin Microbiol* 18(6): 1335-1339.

Lebrun, L., F. Espinasse, et al. (1992). "Evaluation of nonradioactive DNA probes for identification of mycobacteria." *J Clin Microbiol* 30(9): 2476-2478.

Lee, H. R., S. Y. Kim, et al. (2010). "Novel multiplex PCR using dual-priming oligonucleotides for detection and discrimination of the Mycobacterium tuberculosis complex and M. bovis BCG." *J Clin Microbiol* 48(12): 4612-4614.

Lee, L. V. (2010). Convential Biochemicals. *Clinical Microbiology Procedures Handbook*. L. S. Garcia. Washington, D.C, American Society for Microbiology. 2: 7.6.1.1.-7.6.3.3.

Levidiotou, S., G. Vrioni, et al. (2003). "Four-year experience of use of the Cobas Amplicor system for rapid detection of Mycobacterium tuberculosis complex in respiratory and nonrespiratory specimens in Greece." *Eur J Clin Microbiol Infect Dis* 22(6): 349-356.

Lim, S. D., J. Todd, et al. (1991). "Genotypic identification of pathogenic Mycobacterium species by using a nonradioactive oligonucleotide probe." *J Clin Microbiol* 29(6): 1276-1278.

Limaye, K., S. Kanade, et al. (2010). "Utility of Microscopic Observation of Drug Susceptibility (MODS) assay for Mycobacterium tuberculosis in resource constrained settings." *The Indian journal of tuberculosis* 57(4): 207-212.

Lin, S. Y., E. Desmond, et al. (2009). "Multicenter evaluation of Bactec MGIT 960 system for second-line drug susceptibility testing of Mycobacterium tuberculosis complex." *J Clin Microbiol* 47(11): 3630-3634.

Liu, P. I., D. H. McGregor, et al. (1973). "Comparison of three culture media for isolation of Mycobacterium tuberculosis: a 6-year study." *Appl Microbiol* 26(6): 880-883.

Luo, R. F., M. D. Scahill, et al. (2010). "Comparison of single-copy and multicopy real-time PCR targets for detection of Mycobacterium tuberculosis in paraffin-embedded tissue." *J Clin Microbiol* 48(7): 2569-2570.

Makinen, J., M. Marjamaki, et al. (2006). "Evaluation of a novel strip test, GenoType Mycobacterium CM/AS, for species identification of mycobacterial cultures." *Clin Microbiol Infect* 12(5): 481-483.

Marlowe, E. M., S. M. Novak-Weekley, et al. (2011). "Evaluation of the Cepheid Xpert MTB/RIF assay for direct detection of Mycobacterium tuberculosis complex in respiratory specimens." *J Clin Microbiol* 49(4): 1621-1623.

Martin, A., D. Bombeeck, et al. (2011). "Evaluation of the BD MGIT TBc Identification Test (TBc ID), a rapid chromatographic immunoassay for the detection of Mycobacterium tuberculosis complex from liquid culture." *J Microbiol Meth* 84(2): 255-257.

Martin, A., A. von Groll, et al. (2008). "Rapid detection of Mycobacterium tuberculosis resistance to second-line drugs by use of the manual mycobacterium growth indicator tube system." *J Clin Microbiol* 46(12): 3952-3956.

Marttila, H. J., J. Makinen, et al. (2009). "Prospective evaluation of pyrosequencing for the rapid detection of isoniazid and rifampin resistance in clinical Mycobacterium tuberculosis isolates." *Eur J Clin Microbiol Infect Dis* 28(1): 33-38.

Marttila, H. J., H. Soini, et al. (1998). "A Ser315Thr substitution in KatG is predominant in genetically heterogeneous multidrug-resistant Mycobacterium tuberculosis isolates originating from the St. Petersburg area in Russia." *Antimicrob Agents Chemother* 42(9): 2443-2445.

Massire, C., C. A. Ivy, et al. (2011). "Simultaneous identification of mycobacterial isolates to the species level and determination of tuberculosis drug resistance by PCR followed by electrospray ionization mass spectrometry." *J Clin Microbiol* 49(3): 908-917.

Middlebrook, G., Z. Reggiardo, et al. (1977). "Automatable radiometric detection of growth of Mycobacterium tuberculosis in selective media." *Am Rev Respir Dis* 115(6): 1066-1069.

Miliner, R. A., K. D. Stottmeier, et al. (1969). "Formaldehyde: a photothermal activated toxic substance produced in Middlebrook 7H10 medium." *Am Rev Respir Dis* 99(4): 603-607.

Miller, M. B., E. B. Popowitch, et al. (2011). "Performance of Xpert MTB/RIF RUO Assay and IS6110 Real-Time PCR for Mycobacterium tuberculosis Detection in Clinical Samples." *J Clin Microbiol*.

Miller, N., T. Cleary, et al. (2002). "Rapid and specific detection of Mycobacterium tuberculosis from acid-fast bacillus smear-positive respiratory specimens and BacT/ALERT MP culture bottles by using fluorogenic probes and real-time PCR." *J Clin Microbiol* 40(11): 4143-4147.

Miller, N., S. Infante, et al. (2000). "Evaluation of the LiPA MYCOBACTERIA assay for identification of mycobacterial species from BACTEC 12B bottles." *J Clin Microbiol* 38(5): 1915-1919.

MMWR (1993). "Initial therapy for tuberculosis in the era of multidrug resistance. Recommendations of the Advisory Council for the Elimination of Tuberculosis." *MMWR Recomm Rep* 42(RR-7): 1-8.

Mokrousov, I., O. Narvskaya, et al. (2002). "High prevalence of KatG Ser315Thr substitution among isoniazid-resistant Mycobacterium tuberculosis clinical isolates from northwestern Russia, 1996 to 2001." *Antimicrob Agents Chemother* 46(5): 1417-1424.

Mokrousov, I., T. Otten, et al. (2002). "Detection of isoniazid-resistant Mycobacterium tuberculosis strains by a multiplex allele-specific PCR assay targeting katG codon 315 variation." *J Clin Microbiol* 40(7): 2509-2512.

Moore, D. A. (2007). "Future prospects for the MODS assay in multidrug-resistant tuberculosis diagnosis." *Future Microbiol* 2(2): 97-101.

Musial, C. E., L. S. Tice, et al. (1988). "Identification of mycobacteria from culture by using the Gen-Probe Rapid Diagnostic System for Mycobacterium avium complex and Mycobacterium tuberculosis complex." *J Clin Microbiol* 26(10): 2120-2123.

Neonakis, I. K., Z. Gitti, et al. (2009). "Evaluation of GenoType mycobacteria direct assay in comparison with Gen-Probe Mycobacterium tuberculosis amplified direct test and GenoType MTBDRplus for direct detection of Mycobacterium tuberculosis complex in clinical samples." *J Clin Microbiol* 47(8): 2601-2603.

Neonakis, I. K., Z. Gitti, et al. (2007). "Evaluation of the GenoType MTBC assay for differentiating 120 clinical Mycobacterium tuberculosis complex isolates." *Eur J Clin Microbiol Infect Dis* 26(2): 151-152.

Nopvichai, C., A. Sanpavat, et al. (2009). "PCR detection of Mycobacterium tuberculosis in necrotising non-granulomatous lymphadenitis using formalin-fixed paraffin-embedded tissue: a study in Thai patients." *J Clin Pathol* 62(9): 812-815.

Ong, D. C., W. C. Yam, et al. (2010). "Rapid detection of rifampicin- and isoniazid-resistant Mycobacterium tuberculosis by high-resolution melting analysis." *J Clin Microbiol* 48(4): 1047-1054.

Pallen, M. J. & N. J. Loman (2011). "Are diagnostic and public health bacteriology ready to become branches of genomic medicine?" *Genome Med* 3(8): 53.

Pao, C. C., T. S. Yen, et al. (1990). "Detection and identification of Mycobacterium tuberculosis by DNA amplification." *J Clin Microbiol* 28(9): 1877-1880.

Parsons, L. M., R. Brosch, et al. (2002). "Rapid and simple approach for identification of Mycobacterium tuberculosis complex isolates by PCR-based genomic deletion analysis." *J Clin Microbiol* 40(7): 2339-2345.

Patel, J. B., D. G. Leonard, et al. (2000). "Sequence-based identification of Mycobacterium species using the MicroSeq 500 16S rDNA bacterial identification system." *J Clin Microbiol* 38(1): 246-251.

Perandin, F., G. Pinsi, et al. (2006). "Evaluation of INNO-LiPA assay for direct detection of mycobacteria in pulmonary and extrapulmonary specimens." *New Microbiol* 29(2): 133-138.

Peterson, E. M., R. Lu, et al. (1989). "Direct identification of Mycobacterium tuberculosis, Mycobacterium avium, and Mycobacterium intracellulare from amplified primary cultures in BACTEC media using DNA probes." *J Clin Microbiol* 27(7): 1543-1547.

Pfyffer, G. E., P. Kissling, et al. (1994). "Direct detection of Mycobacterium tuberculosis complex in respiratory specimens by a target-amplified test system." *J Clin Microbiol* 32(4): 918-923.

Pfyffer, G. E. & F. Palicova (2011). Mycobacterium: General Characteristics, Laboratory Detection, and Staining Procedures. *Manual of Clinical Microbiology, 10th edition.* J. C. Versalovic, K.C.; Funke, G.; Jorgensen, J.H.; Landry, M.L.; and Warnock, D.W. Washington, DC, ASM Press: 472-502.

Pholwat, S., S. Heysell, et al. (2011). "Rapid first- and second-line drug susceptibility assay for Mycobacterium tuberculosis isolates by use of quantitative PCR." *J Clin Microbiol* 49(1): 69-75.

Piersimoni, C. & C. Scarparo (2003). "Relevance of commercial amplification methods for direct detection of Mycobacterium tuberculosis complex in clinical samples." *J Clin Microbiol* 41(12): 5355-5365.

Pinsky, B. A. & N. Banaei (2008). "Multiplex real-time PCR assay for rapid identification of Mycobacterium tuberculosis complex members to the species level." *J Clin Microbiol* 46(7): 2241-2246.

Rachow, A., A. Zumla, et al. (2011). "Rapid and accurate detection of Mycobacterium tuberculosis in sputum samples by Cepheid Xpert MTB/RIF assay--a clinical validation study." *PloS one* 6(6): e20458.

Rebollo, M. J., R. San Juan Garrido, et al. (2006). "Blood and urine samples as useful sources for the direct detection of tuberculosis by polymerase chain reaction." *Diagn Microbiol Infect Dis* 56(2): 141-146.

Richter, E., S. Rusch-Gerdes, et al. (2006). "Evaluation of the GenoType Mycobacterium Assay for identification of mycobacterial species from cultures." *J Clin Microbiol* 44(5): 1769-1775.

Richter, E., M. Weizenegger, et al. (2003). "Evaluation of genotype MTBC assay for differentiation of clinical Mycobacterium tuberculosis complex isolates." *J Clin Microbiol* 41(6): 2672-2675.

Ritis, K., S. Giaglis, et al. (2005). "Diagnostic usefulness of bone marrow aspiration material for the amplification of IS6110 insertion element in extrapulmonary tuberculosis: comparison of two PCR techniques." *Int J Tuberc Lung Dis* 9(4): 455-460.

Rogall, T., T. Flohr, et al. (1990). "Differentiation of Mycobacterium species by direct sequencing of amplified DNA." *J Gen Microbiol* 136(9): 1915-1920.

Rogers, G. B. & K. D. Bruce (2010). "Next-generation sequencing in the analysis of human microbiota: essential considerations for clinical application."*Mol Diagn Ther* 14(6): 343-350.

Roth, A., M. Fischer, et al. (1998). "Differentiation of phylogenetically related slowly growing mycobacteria based on 16S-23S rRNA gene internal transcribed spacer sequences." *J Clin Microbiol* 36(1): 139-147.

Ruiz, P., F. J. Zerolo, et al. (2000). "Comparison of susceptibility testing of Mycobacterium tuberculosis using the ESP culture system II with that using the BACTEC method." *J Clin Microbiol* 38(12): 4663-4664.

Russo, C., E. Tortoli, et al. (2006). "Evaluation of the new GenoType Mycobacterium assay for identification of mycobacterial species." *J Clin Microbiol* 44(2): 334-339.

Said, H. M., N. Ismail, et al. (2011). "Evaluation of TBc identification immunochromatographic assay for rapid identification of Mycobacterium tuberculosis complex in samples from broth cultures." *J Clin Microbiol* 49(5): 1939-1942.

Saleeb, P. G., S. K. Drake, et al. (2011). "Identification of mycobacteria in solid-culture media by matrix-assisted laser desorption ionization-time of flight mass spectrometry." *J Clin Micobiol* 49(5): 1790-1794.

Salfinger, M. & L. B. Heifets (1988). "Determination of pyrazinamide MICs for Mycobacterium tuberculosis at different pHs by the radiometric method." *Antimicrob Agents Chemother* 32(7): 1002-1004.

Sankar, S., B. Balakrishnan, et al. (2010). "Comparative evaluation of nested PCR and conventional smear methods for the detection of Mycobacterium tuberculosis in sputum samples." *Mol Diagn Ther* 14(4): 223-227.

Scarparo, C., P. Piccoli, et al. (2001). "Direct identification of mycobacteria from MB/BacT alert 3D bottles: comparative evaluation of two commercial probe assays." *J Clin Microbiol* 39(9): 3222-3227.

Scarparo, C., P. Ricordi, et al. (2004). "Evaluation of the fully automated BACTEC MGIT 960 system for testing susceptibility of Mycobacterium tuberculosis to pyrazinamide, streptomycin, isoniazid, rifampin, and ethambutol and comparison with the radiometric BACTEC 460TB method." *J Clin Microbiol* 42(3): 1109-1114.

Schirm, J., L. A. Oostendorp, et al. (1995). "Comparison of Amplicor, in-house PCR, and conventional culture for detection of Mycobacterium tuberculosis in clinical samples." *J Clin Microbiol* 33(12): 3221-3224.

Schurch, A. C., K. Kremer, et al. (2011). "Mutations in the regulatory network underlie the recent clonal expansion of a dominant subclone of the Mycobacterium tuberculosis Beijing genotype." *Infect Genet Evol: journal of molecular epidemiology and evolutionary genetics in infectious diseases* 11(3): 587-597.

Scott, L. E., K. McCarthy, et al. (2011). "Comparison of Xpert MTB/RIF with other nucleic acid technologies for diagnosing pulmonary tuberculosis in a high HIV prevalence setting: a prospective study." *PLoS medicine* 8(7): e1001061.

Seagar, A. L., C. Prendergast, et al. (2008). "Evaluation of the GenoType Mycobacteria Direct assay for the simultaneous detection of the Mycobacterium tuberculosis complex and four atypical mycobacterial species in smear-positive respiratory specimens." *J Med Microbiol* 57(Pt 5): 605-611.

Sekiguchi, J., T. Miyoshi-Akiyama, et al. (2007). "Detection of multidrug resistance in Mycobacterium tuberculosis." *J Clin Microbiol* 45(1): 179-192.

Shah, S., A. Miller, et al. (1998). "Rapid diagnosis of tuberculosis in various biopsy and body fluid specimens by the AMPLICOR Mycobacterium tuberculosis polymerase chain reaction test." *Chest* 113(5): 1190-1194.

Shrestha, N. K., M. J. Tuohy, et al. (2003). "Detection and differentiation of Mycobacterium tuberculosis and nontuberculous mycobacterial isolates by real-time PCR." *J Clin Microbiol* 41(11): 5121-5126.

Siddiqi, S. (2010). BACTEC MGIT 960 SIRE-Nonradiometric Susceptibility Testing for Mycobacterium tuberculosis. *Clinical Microbiology Procedures Handbook*. L. S. Garcia. Washington, D.C, American Society for Microbiology. 2: 7.8.5.1-7.8.5.5.

Siddiqi, S. H., J. P. Libonati, et al. (1981). "Evaluation of rapid radiometric method for drug susceptibility testing of Mycobacterium tuberculosis." *J Clin Microbiol* 13(5): 908-912.

Sjobring, U., M. Mecklenburg, et al. (1990). "Polymerase chain reaction for detection of Mycobacterium tuberculosis." *J Clin Microbiol* 28(10): 2200-2204.

Smith, M. B., J. S. Bergmann, et al. (1997). "Detection of Mycobacterium tuberculosis in BACTEC 12B broth cultures by the Roche Amplicor PCR assay." *J Clin Microbiol* 35(4): 900-902.

Snider, D. E., Jr., R. C. Good, et al. (1981). "Rapid drug-susceptibility testing of Mycobacterium tuberculosis." *Am Rev Respir Dis* 123(4 Pt 1): 402-406.

Soini, H., E. C. Bottger, et al. (1994). "Identification of mycobacteria by PCR-based sequence determination of the 32-kilodalton protein gene." *J Clin Microbiol* 32(12): 2944-2947.

Somoskovi, A., J. E. Hotaling, et al. (2001). "Lessons from a proficiency testing event for acid-fast microscopy." *Chest* 120(1): 250-257.

Springer, B., L. Stockman, et al. (1996). "Two-laboratory collaborative study on identification of mycobacteria: molecular versus phenotypic methods." *J Clin Microbiol* 34(2): 296-303.

Steingart, K. R., L. L. Flores, et al. (2011). "Commercial serological tests for the diagnosis of active pulmonary and extrapulmonary tuberculosis: an updated systematic review and meta-analysis." *PLoS medicine* 8(8): e1001062.

Steingart, K. R., M. Henry, et al. (2006). "Fluorescence versus conventional sputum smear microscopy for tuberculosis: a systematic review." *The Lancet Infect Dis* 6(9): 570-581.

Takiff, H. E., L. Salazar, et al. (1994). "Cloning and nucleotide sequence of Mycobacterium tuberculosis gyrA and gyrB genes and detection of quinolone resistance mutations." *Antimicrob Agents Chemother* 38(4): 773-780.

Tarrand, J. J., A. D. Spicer, et al. (1986). "Evaluation of a radiometric method for pyrazinamide susceptibility testing of Mycobacterium tuberculosis." *Antimicrob Agents Chemother* 30(6): 852-855.

Thibert, L. & S. Lapierre (1993). "Routine application of high-performance liquid chromatography for identification of mycobacteria." *J Clin Microbiol* 31(7): 1759-1763.

Tho, D. Q., N. T. Lan, et al. (2011). "Multiplex allele-specific polymerase chain reaction for detection of isoniazid resistance in Mycobacterium tuberculosis." *Int J Tuberc Lung Dis* 15(6): 799-803.

Torrea, G., P. Van de Perre, et al. (2005). "PCR-based detection of the Mycobacterium tuberculosis complex in urine of HIV-infected and uninfected pulmonary and extrapulmonary tuberculosis patients in Burkina Faso." *J Med Microbiol* 54(Pt 1): 39-44.

Tortoli, E., A. Nanetti, et al. (2001). "Performance assessment of new multiplex probe assay for identification of mycobacteria." *J Clin Microbiol* 39(3): 1079-1084.

Totsch, M., K. W. Schmid, et al. (1994). "Rapid detection of mycobacterial DNA in clinical samples by multiplex PCR." *Diagn Mol Pathol* 3(4): 260-264.

Traore, H., A. van Deun, et al. (2006). "Direct detection of Mycobacterium tuberculosis complex DNA and rifampin resistance in clinical specimens from tuberculosis patients by line probe assay." *J Clin Microbiol* 44(12): 4384-4388.

van Doorn, H. R., D. D. An, et al. (2008). "Fluoroquinolone resistance detection in Mycobacterium tuberculosis with locked nucleic acid probe real-time PCR." *Int J Tuberc Lung Dis* 12(7): 736-742.

Van Rie, A., L. Page-Shipp, et al. (2010). "Xpert((R)) MTB/RIF for point-of-care diagnosis of TB in high-HIV burden, resource-limited countries: hype or hope?" *Expert review of molecular diagnostics* 10(7): 937-946.

Vlaspolder, F., P. Singer, et al. (1995). "Diagnostic value of an amplification method (Gen-Probe) compared with that of culture for diagnosis of tuberculosis." *J Clin Microbiol* 33(10): 2699-2703.

Wang, F., C. Massire, et al. (2011). "Molecular characterization of drug-resistant Mycobacterium tuberculosis isolates circulating in China by multilocus PCR and electrospray ionization mass spectrometry." *J Clin Microbiol* 49(7): 2719-2721.

Welch, K., G. Brown, et al. (1995). "Performance of the Gen-Probe amplified Mycobacterium tuberculosis direct test in a laboratory that infrequently isolates Mycobacterium tuberculosis." *Diagn Microbiol Infect Dis* 22(3): 297-299.

Wetmur, J. G. (1991). "DNA probes: applications of the principles of nucleic acid hybridization." *Crit Rev Biochem Mol Biol* 26(3-4): 227-259.

WHO (2008). New Laboratory Diagnostic Tools for Tuberculosis Control. Geneva, Stop TB Partnership and World Health Organization.

Wilson, M. L. (2011). "Recent advances in the laboratory detection of Mycobacterium tuberculosis complex and drug resistance." *Clin Infect Dis: an official publication of the Infectious Diseases Society of America* 52(11): 1350-1355.

Witebsky, F. G. & P. Kruczak-Filipov (1996). "Identification of mycobacteria by conventional methods." *Clin Lab Med* 16(3): 569-601.

Woo, P. C., J. L. Teng, et al. (2011). "Automated identification of medically important bacteria by 16S rRNA gene sequencing using a novel comprehensive database, 16SpathDB." *J Clin Microbiol* 49(5): 1799-1809.

Woodley, C. L., M. M. Floyd, et al. (1992). "Evaluation of Syngene DNA-DNA probe assays for the identification of the Mycobacterium tuberculosis complex and the Mycobacterium avium complex." *Diagn Microbiol Infect Dis* 15(8): 657-662.

Woods, G. L., J. S. Bergmann, et al. (2001). "Clinical Evaluation of the Gen-Probe amplified mycobacterium tuberculosis direct test for rapid detection of Mycobacterium tuberculosis in select nonrespiratory specimens." *J Clin Microbiol* 39(2): 747-749.

Woods, G. L. L., S-Y. G., Desmond, E.P. (2011). Susceptibility Test Methods: Mycobacteria, Nocardia, and Other Actinomycetes. *Manual of Clinical Microbiology*. J. C. Versalovic, K.C.; Funke, G.; Jorgensen, J.H.; Landry, M.L.; and Warnock, D.W. Washington, D.C., ASM Press. 1: 1215-1238.

Yu, M. C., H. Y. Chen, et al. (2011). "Evaluation of the rapid MGIT TBc identification test for culture confirmation of Mycobacterium tuberculosis complex strain detection." *J Clin Microbiol* 49(3): 802-807.

Zhang, S. L., J. G. Shen, et al. (2007). "A novel genotypic test for rapid detection of multidrug-resistant Mycobacterium tuberculosis isolates by a multiplex probe array." *J Appl Microbiol* 103(4): 1262-1271.

Zhang, Y. & W. W. Yew (2009). "Mechanisms of drug resistance in Mycobacterium tuberculosis." *Int J Tuberc Lung Dis* 13(11): 1320-1330.

3

Tuberculosis in Saudi Arabia

Sahal Al-Hajoj

Biological and Medical Research Department
King Faisal Specialist Hospital and Research Centre
Kingdom of Saudi Arabia

1. Introduction

1.1 Demography of Saudi Arabia

Saudi Arabia is the third-largest country in the Middle East by land area, constituting the bulk of the Arabian Peninsula, and the third-largest Arab country. It is bordered by Jordan and Iraq to the north and northeast, Kuwait, Qatar and the United Arab Emirates to the east, Oman in the southeast, and Yemen in the south. It is also connected to Bahrain by the King Fahad Causeway. The Persian Gulf lies to the northeast and the Red Sea to its west. The size of Saudi Arabia is approximately 2,149,690 square kilometers (830,000 sq mi). The total population is 27,136,977 as of the April 2010 census (18,707,576 Saudi nationals and 8,429,401 non-nationals). Until the 1960s, most of the population was nomadic or semi nomadic; due to rapid economic and urban growth, more than 95% of the population is now settled. Some cities and oases have densities of more than 1,000 people per square kilometer (2,600/mile^2). Saudi Arabia's population is characterized by rapid growth and a large cohort of youth.

2. National Tuberculosis Program (NTP) and Directly Observed Therapy (D.O.T.S)

In 1992, the Ministry of Health established a National Tuberculosis Control Committee to implement a control program throughout Saudi Arabia, and in 1999 the committee decided to implement D.O.T.S. The NTP in Saudi Arabia constitutes a manual, recording and reporting system, training, laboratory and X-ray services. Treatment services, drug and equipment supply is funded by the Ministry of Health. In Saudi Arabia there are several institutions providing healthcare for patients with tuberculosis; National Guard hospitals, Military hospitals, Security Forces hospitals and Ministry of Health hospitals. Patients attending private hospitals suspected of having TB are referred to government hospitals. There is no central system of record keeping, such that a patient currently receiving treatment at one institution may present to another with tuberculosis and be recorded as a new case (Al-Hajoj and Alrabiah). All institutions should report to the Ministry of Health, the body responsible for collecting data on Tuberculosis, but we believe that this is not being adhered to (Al-Hajoj and Alrabiah). Saudi Arabia's D.O.T.S success rate is comparatively well below international levels (Al-Hajoj and Alrabiah).

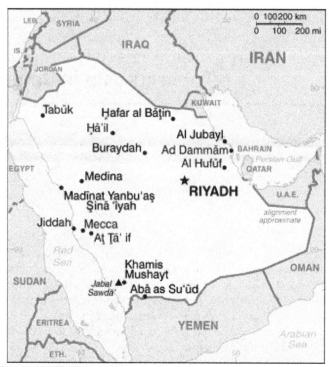

Fig. 1. Map of Saudi Arabia showing the total area, major cities and the borders with other countries.

3. Epidemiology of Tuberculosis world wide

According to a recent report by the World Health Organization (W.H.O); the estimated figure for the global burden of TB in 2009 reached 9.4 million cases and the total deaths hit 1.3 million among HIV-negative people and 0.38 million deaths among HIV-positive people. The report shows that most of the cases were in the South-East Asia, African and Western Pacific regions (35%, 30% and 20%, respectively).

4. Epidemiology of TB in Saudi Arabia

Tuberculosis in Saudi Arabia is still not fully controlled despite the huge efforts exerted by the government, represented by the Ministry of Health. According to the National TB Programs to eradicate the disease, TB continues to cause problems even with the implementation of D.O.T.S. It was anticipated that this program would bring the disease under control, but unfortunately the success has been limited (Al-Hajjaj 2000).

The first nationwide community-based survey of the epidemiology of tuberculosis was conducted by Al-Kassimi et al in 1990. In this study 7,721 subjects were screened in the 5 provinces. Prevalence of positive Mantoux test in non BCG vaccinated subjects and prevalence of bacillary cases on sputum culture were investigated. The authors found that the prevalence of positive Mantoux reaction in children aged 5-14 years was 6% +/- 1.8; higher in urban areas (10%), and lower in rural areas (2%). Yet there were higher prevalence of Mantoux reaction in the urban communities in the Western province (20% +/- 8.7 urban; 1% +/- 1.9 rural). Therefore the authors concluded that Saudi Arabia is among the middle prevalence countries (al-Kassimi, Abdullah et al.). The skin test conversion rate in unvaccinated Saudi Arabian children is about 0.5% per year, lower than in sub-Saharan countries (2%) but higher than in Europe (estimated at 0.1%) (el-Kassimi, Abdullah et al.). Another epidemiological study of tuberculosis infection was carried out between January 1987 and February 1990. In this study a proportional to population size sampling method was used for the whole country. A total of 1,933 subjects were screened and a pre-designed questionnaire was used to collect details of BCG scar, age, sex, residence area, nationality, education, occupation, and a tuberculosis test was done. A number of statistically significant association was found between positive tuberculin test (> 10mm) and age ($p < 0.0001$), sex ($p = 0.018$), nationality ($p = 0.009$), residence area ($p = 0.05$) and occupation ($p = 0.0003$) (Bener and Abdullah). In addition. The W.H.O 2007 estimation of the incidence of TB new cases was 46/100 000 population/year, the incidence of new smear positive cases was 21/100 000 population/year and the estimated prevalence of all forms of TB cases was 65/100 000 population/year. (WHO) report http://www.who.int/tb/country/data/download/en/index1.html. Contrary to W. H. O. report recent data showed that the total cases for the year 2008 was 3,918 in a population of approximately 27,136,977. Therefore according to this report, the incidence of all cases was estimated at 15.8/100 000 and the incidence of smear-positive tuberculosis was 8.2/100 000. However it is believed that the incident rate of TB varies from one region to another and between citizens and expatriates. For instance in Jeddah province (Western Province) Zaman et al studied epidemiology and incidence of Mycobacterium tuberculosis and other mycobacterial species infections in a wide cross-section of population over two (2) years (1987–1989). The study showed that incidence was highest among young adults and varied between Saudi and non-Saudi patients (Zaman). Anther study showed that in Jeddah (Western Province) the rate reached 64 cases per 100,000 compared with 32 per 100,000 in Riyadh (Central Province) (Al-Kassimi 1993; Qari 2002). The childhood and adolescents tuberculosis along with adult tuberculosis are on a rapid increasing phase in the country as per the available published data from the MOH statistics during the last few years (http://www.moh.gov.sa/statistics/index.html) with alarming rate (20%) of high prevalence of MDRTB was reported from Western region of KSA during 2001(M Y Khan 2001).

5. Drug resistance TB in Saudi Arabia

Empirical anti-tuberculosis therapy used in Saudi Arabia usually includes three to four first line drugs including isoniazid, rifampicin, ethambutol, pyrazinamide and streptomycin. Despite the implementation of the D.O.T.S, the number of patients effectively treated in Saudi Arabia has fallen below the WHO target of 85%, (Al-Hajjaj; Alrajhi, Abdulwahab et al.; Samman, Krayem et al.). A retrospective study was conducted which included 147 patients with culture proven diagnosis of tuberculosis seen at the King Khalid National Guard Hospital, Jeddah, between June 1993 and June 1999. One hundred and twenty six patients completed treatment and treatment success was 102/147 (69.4%) and failure 45/147 (30.6%). Noncompliance and drug resistance were considered the main two factors which are significantly associated with treatment failures (Samman, Krayem et al.). Abu-Amero KK reviewed data available for the last 10 years and he showed that the prevalence of single-drug-resistant tuberculosis ranged from 3.4% to 41% for isoniazid, 0% to 23.4% for rifampicin, 0.7% to 22.7% for streptomycin and 0% to 6.9% for ethambutol. However, the prevalence of multi drug-resistant tuberculosis (defined by WHO as resistance to two or more first-line anti tuberculosis drugs) ranged from 1.5% to 44% in different regions (Abu-Amero). Another study on 764 *M. tuberculosis* isolates obtained from 764 patients; resistance was noted in 65 (8.5%). Resistance to isoniazid was the highest, noted in 54 (7.1%); resistance to rifampicin, streptomycin and ethambutol was found to be 21 (2.7%), 29 (3.8%) and 12 (1.6%) isolates respectively. Poly resistance was noted in eight (1%) isolates and mono resistance in 38 (5%) isolates. Multi-drug-resistant *M. tuberculosis* was found in 19 (2.5%) isolates. There were 54 primary resistant isolates (7.6%), and 11 (22%) with acquired resistance. Resistance to at least one agent of the first-line anti-tuberculosis agents was 18.4%. Mono resistance to a single first-line agent was found in 10.9%, while poly resistance was noted in 7.6%. Multi-drug-resistant *tuberculosis* was noted in 5.7% of all isolates. Resistance to isoniazid was most commonly noted in 11% of isolates. Resistance rates to other agents were: rifampin 9.7%, streptomycin 9.1%, pyrazinamide 3.1%, and ethambutol 2.5%. Al-Hajoj et al summarized all available studies as it shown in table-1. However, the author insisted that these studies should be treated with extreme caution as many of them are old, no standardized technique, small and fragmented studies as they were carried out in a single hospital.

City	Drug resistance					MDR-TB	Reference
	RIF	INH	PZA	ETB	STR	%	
Jeddah	20.8	28.7	7.9	6.9	22.8	25	(al-Mazrou, Khoja et al.)
Riyadh	2.8	9.1	5	2.8	1.6	11.8	(Arya)
Jizan (South)	43	80	S	NA	53	44	(Ellis, al-Hajjar et al.)
Dammam	0.2	6	S	S	0.7	7	(Al-Rubaish, Madania et al.)

The above table is a summary of studies from different regions showing the percentage of drug resistance TB for single and multi anti-TB agents. It is not clear which method/s was used in each study. RIF-rifampicin, INH-isoniazid, PZA-pyrazinamide, ETB-ethambutol, STR-streptomycin, MDR-TB multi drug resistant tuberculosis.

Table 1. MDR-TB. Profile cities within the kingdom of Saudi Arabia

Recently, the King Faisal Specialist Hospital and Research Centre (KFSH&RC) TB-research unit undertook the responsibility to study drug resistance rate in the country. This study was planned with the help of W.H.O experts and in collaboration with the Ministry of Health. This study was funded by King Abdulaziz City for Science and Technology (KACST) under project # AT26-110. This study was the first of its type as it covered the whole country and in prospective mannar. The design of the study was to collect all isolates from all regional laboratories for one year. This was in concordance with W.H.O recommendation as there were no data to do cluster collection. All isolates with their epidemiological and clinical data were collected for one year starting from 01 June 2009 until

31 May 2010. A total of 2,842 were collected from 9 regions. 248 and 192 were removed from the total number as we found them to be NTM and repeated cultures respectively. Therefore the DST was carried out for 1904 isolates representing the whole country. A summary of the main findings are in table-2.

Drug	No. of resistant isolates	Rate of resistance
Any drug resistance	537	28.3%
Streptomycin	228	12%
Isoniazid	160	8.42%
Rifampicin	15	0.78%
Ethambutol	58	3.05%
Multi drug resistance	76	4%

Table 2. Summary of finding of an ongoing drug resistance surveillances.

6. Pulmonary and Extra-pulmonary Tuberculosis (EPTB)

11.7%. EPTB was reported in 1991. EPTB rates believed to be varies from one hospital to another and from one region to another (Bukhary and Alrajhi). Between 1979 and 1981 Froude and Kingston reviewed 162 cases diagnosed with EPTB from KFSH&RC. The ratio of pulmonary and extra-pulmonary TB was 1:1 during the 27-month period of the study (Froude and Kingston 1982). In 2001, extra-pulmonary TB was culture-confirmed in 2 out of every 3 cases of TB at KFSH&RC (Alrajhi, Abdulwahab et al. 2002). However, KFSH&RC is known to be a tertiary hospital and may be very selective and as a result this percentage has to be treated with extreme caution. In another hospital in Riyadh TB cases for 9 months between 1981 and 1982 was reviewed by Shanks et al. Out of 47 cases, pulmonary TB was documented in 57% of cases, and 43% were EPTB (Shanks, Khalifa et al. 1983). Mokhtar and Salman studied the details of 125 TB patients. EPTB was found in 15% of all cases identified (Mokhtar and Salman 1983). Onther study showed that EPTB accounted for 59% of all cases between 1987-1989, (Zaman 1991). However, it is worth mentioning that all the above studies may do not reflect the real picture of the incidences of EPTB. All these studies were carried out either at a tertiary hospital or in regional hospital, therefore, we recommend treating these data with extreme caution. For this reason we conducted a nation wide surveillance project to determine the rate of drug resistance in the country. In this project the whole country in a prospective manner was covered. All isolates with their epidemiological and clinical data were collected from all 9 centers where TB specimens are cultured. The total number of isolates collected was 2842. Upon classification of the type of the disease, we found that pulmonary cases form 82.4% while extra-pulmonary cases are at 17.6% (manuscript under preparation).

7. Mycobacteria other than TB

Non-tuberculous mycobacteria (NTM), also known as environmental mycobacteria or atypical mycobacteria or mycobacteria other than tuberculosis (MOTT), are mycobacteria which do not cause tuberculosis or Leprosy. As the incidence of tuberculosis fell slightly, infection by those mycobacteria became more readily recognized around the world. There is a worldwide increase in infections with non-tuberculous mycobacteria due to the emergence of the human immunodeficiency virus (HIV)-epidemic and other factors such as immunosuppressive therapy, malnutrition, and protracted treatment with broad-spectrum antibiotics. Non-tuberculous mycobacteria (NTM) are increasingly recognized as pathogens capable of causing extra-pulmonary disease, especially in immunocompromised individuals. The pathogenecity and clinical relevance of many NTM remain poorly understood. In addition, the optimal treatment of infections caused by many NTM is undefined due to interspecies and intraspecies variabilities, drug resistance, and limited literature describing disease caused by less common organisms.

Nontuberculous mycobacteria (NTM) are common inhabitants of the environment and have been cultured from water, soil, and animal sources worldwide. Human disease is believed to be acquired from environmental exposures, and unlike tuberculosis and leprosy, there has been no evidence of animal-to-human or human-to-human transmission of NTM.

NTM mainly involves the species *M.avium complex [MAC]*, *M. abscessus*, *M.Chelonae M. fortuitum*, *M. scrofulaceum*, *M. marinum and M. kansasii* and there are many other species which is clinically relevant as a pathogen.

However, as tuberculosis declined and modern microbiological methods were developed, the importance of NTM in human disease became increasingly evident. NTM cause four distinct clinical syndromes.

1. Progressive pulmonary disease, especially in older persons caused primarily by *M. avium complex* (MAC) and *M. kansasii*.
2. Superficial lymphadenitis, especially cervical lymphadenitis, in children caused mostly by *MAC*, *M. scrofulaceum*, *M. malmoense* and *M. haemophilum*.
3. Disseminated disease in severely immunocompromised patients.
4. Skin and soft tissue infection usually as a consequence of direct inoculation.

NTM are opportunistic pathogens, mostly affecting patients with preexisting pulmonary disease such as chronic obstructive pulmonary disease [COPD] or tuberculosis (TB), or those with systemic impairment of immunity. The latter group includes those with HIV infection, immunosuppressive drugs users, and leukemia patients. NTM are very common in the environment and resistant to commonly used disinfectants, so they can be present in non-sterile patient material such as sputum and contaminated medical equipment (bronchoscope washers or samples in the laboratory) and consequently cause pseudo infection (Griffith DE 2007). Without evidence of person-to-person transmission of NTM, it is proposed that humans are infected from environmental sources that may include aerosols, soil, food, water and equipment. When NTM are isolated from a usually sterile site (e.g., blood, bone marrow, lymph nodes, synovial fluid), diagnosis of true disease is generally straightforward. However, when NTM are isolated from non-sterile sources, such as sputum or bronchoalveolar lavage samples, the diagnosis is less definitive, especially when the colony numbers are low or NTM are isolated from only one cultured specimen. Therefore, it is a challenge to differentiate true NTM lung disease from contamination and colonization. Thus, finding AFB by microscopy of respiratory specimens or by culture may pose a diagnostic problem for the clinician (Society. 1997).

In recent years, non-tuberculous mycobacteria (NTM) have emerged as an important cause of opportunistic nosocomial infections, but there is little known about the isolation and identification of NTM in Saudi Arabia. Larger, multicenter regional studies or mandatory reporting will be required to better understand the changing epidemiology of NTM in patients with or without HIV infection. There are many cases of NTM infections reported from different regions of Saudi Arabia but the actual numbers of cases are still unknown. However, there are scattered studies about the prevalence of NTM in Saudi Arabia. BaHammam et al showed that NTM is about 9% (BaHammam, Kambal et al.). A nation wide population-based survey however, revealed a much lower figure of 0.004% (Alrajhi and Al-Barrak; Baharoon; Bukhary and Alrajhi; Bukhary and Alrajhi; Sanai and Bzeizi). Recent collection of more than 3000 isolates from all regions in the country revealed that NTM cases are at 10% of total cases. Further study is needed to gain insight into the nature of NTM cases. In year 2010, a new species of NTM which resembled TB in terms of clinical features and response to the treatment was identified in collaboration work between the TB research unit at king Faisal Specialist Hospital and Research Centre and international collaborators. This species was called Riyadhense.

Mycobacterium abscess also was found to cause infection in an immune competent patients (Al-Hajoj et al 2012).

8. Childhood TB

Childhood TB (CHTB) is a neglected aspect of the TB epidemic, despite constituting 20% or more of the TB case-load in many countries with high TB incidence. CHTB is a significant child health problem, but is neglected because it is usually smear-negative and thus it's considered to make a relatively minor contribution to the spread of TB. Perhaps most importantly, there is a real need for prospective epidemiological studies to determine the true burden of TB among children in a wide spectrum of settings worldwide. Recent guidance has already taken a significant step in this direction by recommending NTPs record childhood TB cases by age category and clinical syndrome (WHO 2007).

As children acquire infection with *Mycobacterium tuberculosis* from adults in their environment, the epidemiology of childhood tuberculosis follows TB in adults. While global burden of childhood tuberculosis is unclear, in developing countries the annual risk of tuberculosis infection in children is 2-5 per cent. Nearly 8-20 per cent of the deaths caused by tuberculosis occur in children. It has been suggested that BCG vaccination is responsible for decrease in the occurrence of disseminated and severe disease (S.K. Kabra 2004). Crucially, a definitive microbiological diagnosis of CHTB is achieved in only a minority of cases, as young children rarely develop cavitatory lung disease or expectorate sputum, and a greater proportion of cases are extra-pulmonary. Diagnosis therefore usually relies on poorly validated clinical case definitions, and both under and over-diagnosis of pediatric TB are common, with potentially tragic consequences for children who are not diagnosed (Brent, Anderson et al. 2008). Neonates have the highest risk of progression to disease, and in infancy miliary and meningeal involvement is common. Children from 5 to 10 years of age are less likely to develop disease than other age groups, and adolescent patients can present with progressive primary tuberculosis or cavitary disease (Engelbrecht, Marais et al. 2006). Most children who develop disease do so within 2–12 months of initial infection, with pulmonary TB accounting for 60–80% of all cases. The two most common forms EPTB found in children are Lympho-hematogenous disease with multiple organ involvement and Tuberculous Meningitis [TBM]. The TBM is the most serious complication with involvement of the central nerves system and with a high mortality rate. The TBM is common in children compared to adults and its diagnosis is difficult because signs and symptoms are vague (Anna M M 2005) (Starke JR 2002). The prevalence of MDRTB in children probably reflects the level of primary drug resistance among organisms currently circulating in the community. Comprehensive studies on resistance to anti TB drugs in children are limited. It has been demonstrated that patient with MDRTB cause similar rates of infection and disease among household contacts as do the patients with drug susceptible tuberculosis.(H.Simon Schaaf 2001).

The diagnostic difficulties make to give only a little attention to children with MDRTB or children in contact with it. In controlled studies it has been shown that the rate of infection is even higher in childhood contact as compared to drug sensitive cases. The transmission of MDRTB is higher than that of sensitive TB. Treatment of MDRTB is expensive and associated with lower treatment completion and cure rates. Isoniazid is the effective drug for prophylactic therapy in children with an index case, but Rifampicin is an alternative in cases of Isoniazid resistance. In cases of MDRTB there is no proved regimen of treatment for children. The drug toxicity is much higher with second line and third line drugs regimen when treating MDRTB, multi drug regimen usually necessitating hospitalization and gradual build up of drug dosages and schedules. The treatment for MDRTB is challenging in a child and unfortunately most of the second line drugs do not have pediatric formulations (Ejaz A Khan 2002). Interruption in the transmission of *Mycobacterium tuberculosis* is one of the primary goals of TB control programs. The ability to track specific strains of *M. tuberculosis* improves the understanding of transmission and pathogenesis in a community and helps to control transmission with properly designed strategies (Kathryn DeRiemer 2004). The most common extrathoracic manifestation of TB in children is cervical lymphadenitis. A simple clinical algorithm that identified children with a persistent (longer than 4 weeks) cervical mass of 2×2cm or more, without a visible local cause or response to first-line antibiotics, showed excellent diagnostic accuracy in an area with endemic TB (Marais, Wright et al. 2006). At a global level, the WHO currently reports only smear-positive cases by age. The International Union Against TB and Lung Disease (IUATLD) currently recommends stratifying the reporting of smear-positive cases into two age categories: younger than 15 years of age and 15 years of age and older (D A Enarson 2000).

Reporting of smear-positive cases is considered a practical strategy that complements the Directly Observed Therapy (D.O.T.S) strategy. Nonetheless, an estimated 1.2 cases of smear-negative TB occur for every smear-positive case of TB. Furthermore, approximately 95 percent of cases in children younger than 12 years of age are smear-negative. Thus, the W.H.O policy of reporting only smear-positive cases by age causes a gross underestimation of the burden of TB in children (J.A. Jereb 1993). Childhood TB is a direct reflection of the incidence of adult disease within a community. A case of TB in a child usually represents primary disease transmitted from an infectious adult or adolescent and is considered a sentinel event in public health. In response to a case of childhood TB, local TB control programs ideally will conduct an investigation to identify the potential source of infection and additional cases. Due to limited resources, these investigations are not implemented in many parts of the world (Anna M M 2005). A positive culture is regarded as the 'gold standard test' to establish a definitive diagnosis of TB in a symptomatic child. It is, however, limited by the fact that organisms may be isolated from non-diseased (asymptomatic) children shortly after primary infection, during the initial period of organism multiplication and/or occult dissemination. In addition, traditional culture methods are limited by suboptimal sensitivity, slow turnaround times, excessive cost (automated liquid broth systems) and the low bacteriological yields achieved in children with active TB. It is important to point out that adolescent children (over 10 years of age) frequently develop sputum smear-positive disease that may be diagnosed using traditional methods (B.J. Marais 2005).

As childhood tuberculosis is a sensitive marker for ongoing transmission within a community, control programs should focus on children because they are the reservoirs of future disease (Lalitkanth 2001). Most children with TB in the world are not recorded in the national surveillance systems, even though they are the ones most likely to suffer severe complications of the disease. While there are many challenges in the diagnosis and treatment of TB in children, perhaps the greatest challenge globally is to begin to identify the extent of disease in this forgotten group (Shingadia. 2004). In Saudi Arabia childhood TB is also receiving little attention. However, despite this some cases are getting reported. For instance Peritoneal tuberculosis is relatively rare compared to adults but cases are reported from two regions of Saudi Arabia in children below 12 years (Saleh 1997). Primary tuberculosis of the penis with associated bilateral inguinal lymph node enlargement and a discharging sinus is described in an infant from the Abha Region (Annobil S H 1990). Banjar et al in a controlled study of 151 cases of non cystic fibrosis bronchiectasis conducted in a tertiary care centre in Riyadh among Saudi children, showed TB form 2% of the total cases (Banjar 2007). A case of congenital transmission of tuberculosis is reported from Riyadh region as a cutaneous disease with multiple abscess and resistance to primary antibiotics (Yousef A. Al-Katawee 2007). The central nervous system tuberculosis among children is reported from different regions of the country with considerable mortality rate and diagnostic and treatment problems (Bahemuka M 1989; Al-Deeb SM 1992). In a study of causes of uveitis conducted in an ophthalmology referral centre in Riyadh, it highlighted tubercular uveitis among children during 2002 (Islam and Tabbara).

9.Factors influencing the molecular epidemiology of tuberculosis in Saudi Arabia

9.1 Hajj

Saudi Arabia is a unique place as it is the place for the two holy mosques located in Mecca and Al-Madinah. The two holy mosques are the target for the one billion Muslims from all over the world. Thus every year the two cities Mecca and Al-Madinah receive more than three million for Hajj and visits to the holy mosque in Al-Madinah. The intense congestion of Hajjies, the majority of whom are coming from high endemic places, overcrowds and the close proximity furnish the grounds for infectious diseases transmission including TB. Other factors may influence the transmission including aging pilgrims whom may suffer from underlining disease such as immunological disorders, less hygiene among some of the pilgrims and the physical efforts exerted by pilgrims. As a matter of fact several studies showed that Hajj is an opportunity for TB transmission. Wilder-Smith et al conducted a prospective study to assess the risk of *M. tuberculosis* infection among Hajj pilgrims. He found high risk of *Mycobacterium tuberculosis* infection during the Hajj pilgrimage. In his study he showed that among 357 Singaporean pilgrims; 10% showed a substantial rise in immune response to the QuantiFERON TB assay antigens post-Hajj when compared to a pre-Hajj test (Wilder-Smith, Foo et al. 2005). Alzeer et al studied cases of pneumonia admitted to two hospitals during the 1994 pilgrimage (Hajj) season to Mecca. Sixty-four patients were enrolled in the study, of which 47 (75%) were men with a mean age of 63 years (range 21-91). Nearly all were from developing countries. Diagnosis was established in 46 patients (72%) with *Mycobacterium tuberculosis* being the commonest causative organism (20%) (Alzeer, Mashlah et al. 1998). The main finding of this study is that *Mycobacterium tuberculosis* is a common cause of pneumonia during Hajj season. As a matter of fact the variation of TB incidence among Saudi cities and in favor of Western province was attributed to Pilgrims influx.

9.2 Omra

Omra is another Islamic ritual through which individuals from all over the world target once again Mecca and Al-Madinah. The two holy mosques receive all year long hundreds of thousands whom again do come from endemic places. During the holy month of Ramadan the number of visitors to the two mosques peak again as it reaches up to three million in Mecca and may be another one million at Al-Madinah mosque. During the last 10 days of the holy month of Ramadan the majority of visitors do what is called Etekaf, during which people do not leave the grand mosques. The scene is overwhelming as a person can see individuals are sleeping and sitting next to each others. We believe such circumstances make these places fertile land for transmission of TB.

9.3 Expatriates

Saudi Arabia accommodates 8,429,401 expatriates scattered all over the country. They are in the country for work purposes. In addition considerable unknown numbers are moving around illegally and hide in farms and in houses. Unfortunately the majority of those expatriates are from endemic places; therefore they are forming a source of infection as they do not visit hospitals when they become diseased, fearing deportation after treatment.

9.4 Travelling

The Saudi national nowadays travels around the globe. Also we have a considerable number of students (more than 250 thousand including families members) studying abroad and scattered all over the world including countries where TB is high like India, Philippines and East Europe. We believe that the above mentioned factors are playing a major role in making TB spread and transmitted to the country and to outside of the country. This is supported by our recent finding of molecular epidemiology.

10. Molecular epidemiology of TB in Saudi Arabia

In 2007 we published some data on the molecular epidemiology in Saudi Arabia. A total of 1,505 clinical isolates of *M. tuberculosis*, the isolates were collected over a three year period from seven regions of Saudi Arabia and were genotyped using spoligo and MIRU –VNNTR techniques. A total of 387 individual patterns were obtained (clustering rate of 86.4%, 182 clusters containing between 2 to 130 isolates per cluster). A total of 94% of the strains matched to the spoligotype patterns in an international database. Majority of the isolates (81%) were imported strains including Central Asian-CAS 22.5%, ill-defined T clade 19.5%, East African Indian-EAI 13.5%, Haarlem 7.5%, Latin American Mediterranean-LAM 7.2%, Beijing 4.4%, Manu 2.7%, X 0.9%, and Bovis 0.9%. In addition two clonal complexes with unique spoligotyping signatures (octal codes 703777707770371, and 467777377413771) were specific to Saudi Arabia. Another on going study is taking place in Eastern province, which is a major industrial zone of the country and thus the immigrant population is high (Al-Hajoj et al.). According to the latest census reports, 2.7 million of citizens and 0.8 million of immigrants are living in the Eastern province (Statistics Department 2010). In this study a total of 533 TB isolates were collected with their epidemiological data. All the isolates were genotyped and lineages were assigned by using the online databasewww.miruvntrplus.org. There were 14 lineages identified among the study groups and 24 (4.5%) cases belonged either to undefined lineage or *M. bovis*. Among the total cases, Delhi/CAS (32%) and EAI (21.3%) are dominating, followed by Ghana (9.9%) and Haarlem (9.3%). TB population of the Saudi patients showed a higher predominance of Delhi/CAS (71/33.3%), followed by EAI (32/15%) and Ghana (24/11.3%). On the other hand, the non-Saudi isolates showed the domination of Delhi/CAS (100/31%) and EAI (82/25.5%), followed by Ghana (29/9%). The total numbers of undefined lineages were 17, and *M. bovis* (7 cases) was circulating only among Saudis. Cluster analysis showed 28 clusters of 148 isolates with a size of 2-18. Major clustering was found among the lineages Delhi/CAS (7 clusters) and EAI (6 clusters).

The study showed that some clades are circulating among Saudi only, others circulating among non-Saudi, and the rest circulating among both Saudi and non-Saudi (manuscript under preparation).

11. BCG vaccination

In Saudi Arabia BCG vaccine is given to every born baby as mandatory policy trying to protect the population against TB infection. It is believed that BCG is protecting against TB infection and may protect against Miliary Tuberculosis. BCG vaccination is being debated nowadays in Saudi Arabia as whether to continue to give the vaccine, delay it or stop it all together. Three years ago King Faisal Specialist Hospital and Research Centre held a conference on "Infections in Immunocompromised host" (18-19 November 2008). In this symposium, many specialists expressed their reservations about administering tuberculosis vaccine (BCG vaccine) to newborn children. They pointed out that in some cases of pediatrics with immune deficiencies, it is very important to delay the vaccination plan until the possibility of genetic immune deficiency has been ruled out. This is due to the complication of the vaccine and the dissemination of the disease. In addition, the country lacks data regarding the efficiency of BCG vaccination. In other words, we do not know whether BCG vaccine is protecting or not. Therefore the question is can we stop giving BCG vaccine to our babies? The philosophy behind this question is that BCG vaccine may not protect against TB; otherwise, why do we have up to 4000 cases yearly (according to a recent report by the Ministry of Health) despite the fact that all our babies are vaccinated at birth? BCG vaccination may cause confusion when skin test is carried out. Interpretation of skin test is extremely difficult in light of the fact that the protein used in skin test is shared by many species of mycobacteria. Shared protein is the main cause of the confusion (Mittrucker, Steinhoff et al.). Therefore positive skin test means i) exposure to real infection, ii) exposure to environmental mycobacterium or iii) reaction due to BCG vaccine itself. BCG vaccination causes a particular problem when it comes to diagnosing dormant TB using TST. It is for this reason that the BCG vaccine is not given in many countries such as The Netherlands, UK, and recently France; yet these countries have better control over tuberculosis when compared to many countries, including Saudi Arabia, where BCG vaccine is mandatory.

To role out the confusion caused by BCG vaccination we either have to stop BCG vaccination all together or introduce Interferon-γ tests (interferon gamma release assays, IGRAs) as additional diagnostic tools. IGRAs are based on the ability of the *Mycobacterium tuberculosis* antigens for early secretory antigen target 6 (ESAT-6) and culture filtrate protein 10 (CFP-10) to stimulate host production of interferon-gamma. Because these antigens are not present in nontuberculous mycobacteria or in BCG vaccine, these tests can distinguish between latent tuberculosis infection in asymptomatic patients and exposure to BCG or nontuberculous mycobacteria. The test is approved for diagnosis of latent tuberculosis and has also been used in patients with pulmonary tuberculosis (Al-Orainey; Stephan, Wolf et al.). We fully approve of the establishment of such diagnostic tools everywhere in the country. It is an expensive test at this particular stage but it is worth using, as delay in diagnosing difficult cases such as extra-pulmonary is more costly to the patients (as it might cost them their lives). In addition treating dormant tuberculosis, particularly when it comes to close contact individuals, is far cheaper than treating patients after they show full symptoms of the disease. On the other hand, it is a very bad practice to give prophylaxis to treat dormant tuberculosis based on skin test results as the test has proved its inability to distinguish real infection from exposure to environment tuberculosis or BCG vaccine. Also, giving a prophylaxis indiscriminately based on skin test gives a chance for drug resistance to develop. We believe it is the right time now to review our policy of giving BCG vaccine to our newly born babies as it is creating more confusion rather than providing protection: It causes diseases in immunocompromised patients. BCG vaccine causes confusion when it comes to interpretation of skin test results. Also, it gives false-positive and false-negative results.

12. HIV and TB in Saudi Arabia

Saudi Arabia started surveillance for HIV in 1984. Clinical suspicion, screening of contacts of HIV infected patients, routine screening of blood and organ donors, prisoners ,intravenous drug users, patients with other sexually transmitted infections, expatriates pre-employment testing are among reasons for HIV testing. All cases from 1984 through 2001 were reviewed. A total of 6,046 HIV infections were diagnosed, of which 1,285 (21.3%) of cases were Saudi citizens. HIV infections among Saudi citizens gradually increased over 18 year period, and jumped from 84 to 142 cases per year. The number of cases per 100,000 populations varied widely between regions. The infection was most common in the age group 20-40 years. The modes of transmission among Saudi citizens and expatriates were heterosexual contact, blood transfusion, perinatal transmission, homosexual contact, intravenous drugs, and bisexual contact. A total of 514/1285 (40%) Saudi patients died by year 2001.

TB infection is found to be associating with HIV infection like anywhere in the world. Alrajhi et al reviewed retrospectively medical charts of 437 patients diagnosed with tuberculosis from 1995-2000 in Riyadh. He found that screening was done for 178 (41%) patients: 2 (1.1%) of these were found to be HIV positive.In Saudi Arabia, screening for HIV in tuberculosis patients remains underutilized (Omair, Al-Ghamdi et al.).

217 new adult patients joined the HIV program between 1997 and 2007. TB was diagnosed in 16 patients (7.4%), all of whom had acquired immune-deficiency syndrome at the time of TB diagnosis. Seven developed extra-pulmonary disease (44%), six had pulmonary TB (37%), while three had both (19%). The TB incidence rate was 1,354 per 100,000 among the HIV-infected cohort. The incidence rate of pulmonary TB was 762/100,000 and for extra-pulmonary TB it was 592/100,000. Among pulmonary TB with HIV infection in Saudi Arabia, TB incidence is 30 times higher than in the general population, with significant mortality despite early diagnosis, treatment and tertiary care support (Al-Mazrou, Al-Jeffri et al.; Alrajhi; Alrajhi, Halim et al.; Alrajhi, Halim et al.; Alrajhi, Nematallah et al.; Edathodu, Halim et al.; Kordy, Al-Hajjar et al.; Madani; Madani, Al-Mazrou et al.; Memish and Osoba).

13. References

"Saudi Gazette: Nov. 24, 2010 - Census shows Kingdom's population at more than 27 million" [1]

Siraj Wahab (30 July 2009). "It's another kind of Saudization". Arab News. http://archive.arabnews.com/?page=1&section=0&article=124999&d=30&m=7&y =2009. Retrieved 13 January 2011.

Seok, Hyunho (1991). "Korean migrant workers to the Middle East". In Gunatilleke, Godfrey (ed.). Migration to the Arab World:

Abu-Amero, K. K. "Status of antituberculosis drug resistance in Saudi Arabia 1979-98." East Mediterr Health J 2002 Jul-Sep;8(4-5):664-70.

Al-Deeb SM, Y. B., Sharif HS, Motaery KR. (1992). "Neurotuberculosis: a review." Clin Neurol Neurosurg. 94: S30-3.

Al-Hajjaj, M. S. "The outcome of tuberculosis treatment after implementation of the national tuberculosis control program in Saudi Arabia." Ann Saudi Med. 2000 Mar;20(2):125-8.

Al-Hajjaj, M. S., and I.M Al-Khatim (2000). "High rate of non-compliance with anti-tuberculosis treatment despite a retrieval system:a call for implementation of directly observed therapy in Saudi Arabia." Int J Tuberc Lung Dis 4(4): 345-349.

Al-Hajoj, S. A. "Can we change the way we look at BCG vaccine?" Ann Thorac Med. 2009 Apr;4(2):92-3; author reply 93-4.

Al-Hajoj, S. A. and F. A. Alrabiah "Role of tuberculosis laboratories in Saudi Arabia. A call to implement standardized procedures." Saudi Med J. 2004 Nov;25(11):1545-8.

Al-Hajoj, S. A. and F. A. Alrabiah "Role of tuberculosis laboratories in Saudi Arabia. A call to implement standardized procedures." Saudi Med J 2004 Nov;25(11):1545-8.

Al-Hajoj Sa Fau - Zozio, T., F. Zozio T Fau - Al-Rabiah, et al. "First insight into the population structure of Mycobacterium tuberculosis in Saudi Arabia

Mycobacterium tuberculosis complex genetic diversity: mining the fourth international spoligotyping database (SpolDB4) for classification, population genetics and epidemiology." (0095-1137 (Print)).

Al-Kassimi, A. K. A., MS Al-Hajjaj, IO Al-Orainey, EA Bamgboye and MN Chowdhury (1993). "Nationwide community survey of tuberculosis epidemiology in Saudi Arabia." Tuber.Lung.Dis 74: 254-260.

al-Kassimi, F. A., A. K. Abdullah, et al. "Nationwide community survey of tuberculosis epidemiology in Saudi Arabia." Tuber Lung Dis 1993 Aug;74(4):254-60.

Al-Mazrou, Y. Y., M. H. Al-Jeffri, et al. "HIV/AIDS epidemic features and trends in Saudi Arabia." Ann Saudi Med. 2005 Mar-Apr;25(2):100-4.

al-Mazrou, Y. Y., T. A. Khoja, et al. "High proportion of multi-drug resistant Mycobacterium tuberculosis in Saudi Arabia." Scand J Infect Dis 1997;29(3):323.

Al-Orainey, I. O. "Diagnosis of latent tuberculosis: Can we do better?" Ann Thorac Med. 2009 Jan;4(1):5-9.

Al-Rubaish, A. M., A. A. Madania, et al. "Drug resistance pulmonary tuberculosis in the Eastern Province of Saudi Arabia." Saudi Med J 2001 Sep;22(9):776-9.

Alrajhi, A. A. "Human immunodeficiency virus in Saudi Arabia." Saudi Med J. 2004 Nov;25(11):1559-63.

Alrajhi, A. A., S. Abdulwahab, et al. "Risk factors for drug-resistant Mycobacterium tuberculosis in Saudi Arabia." Saudi Med J. 2002 Mar;23(3):305-10.

Alrajhi, A. A., S. Abdulwahab, et al. (2002). "Risk factors for drug-resistant *Mycobacterium tuberculosis* in Saudi Arabia." Saudi Med J 23(3): 305-10.

Alrajhi, A. A., M. A. Halim, et al. "Mode of transmission of HIV-1 in Saudi Arabia." AIDS. 2004 Jul 2;18(10):1478-80.

Alrajhi, A. A., M. A. Halim, et al. "Presentation and reasons for HIV-1 testing in Saudi Arabia." Int J STD AIDS. 2006 Dec;17(12):806-9.

Alrajhi, A. A., A. Nematallah, et al. "Human immunodeficiency virus and tuberculosis co-infection in Saudi Arabia." East Mediterr Health J. 2002 Nov;8(6):749-53.

Alzeer, A., A. Mashlah, et al. (1998). "Tuberculosis is the commonest cause of pneumonia requiring hospitalization during Hajj (pilgrimage to Makkah)." J Infect 36(3): 303-6.

Anna M M, J. R. S. (2005). "Current concepts of childhood tuberculosis." Seminars in pediatric infectious diseases. 16: 93-104.

Annobil S H , A.-H., Kazi T (1990). "Primary tuberculosis of the penis in an infant." Tubercle 71(3): 229-230.

Arya, S. C. "Drug resistant Mycobacterium tuberculosis in Saudi Arabia." Saudi Med J 2002 Apr;23(4):475.

B.J. Marais, R. P. G., A.C. Hesseling and N. Beyers, (2005). "Adult-type pulmonary tuberculosis in children 10–14 years of age." Pediatr Infect Dis 24: 733-744.

BaHammam, A., A. Kambal, et al. "Comparison of clinico-radiological features of patients with positive cultures of nontuberculous mycobacteria and patients with tuberculosis." Saudi Med J. 2005 May;26(5):754-8.

Bahemuka M, M. J. (1989). "Tuberculosis of the nervous system. A clinical, radiological and pathological study of 39 consecutive cases in Riyadh, Saudi Arabia." J Neurol Sci 90(1): 67-76.

Banjar, H. H. (2007). "Clinical profile of Saudi children with Bronchiectasis." inddian J of Pediatrics. 74(2): 149-152.

Bener, A. and A. K. Abdullah "Reaction to tuberculin testing in Saudi Arabia." Indian J Public Health. 1993 Oct-Dec;37(4):105-10.

Brent, A. J., S. T. Anderson, et al. (2008). "Childhood tuberculosis: out of sight, out of mind?" Transactions of the Royal Society of Tropical Medicine and Hygiene 102(3): 217-218.

Bukhary, Z. A. and A. A. Alrajhi "Extrapulmonary tuberculosis, clinical presentation and outcome." Saudi Med J. 2004 Jul;25(7):881-5.

D A Enarson, H. L. R., T Amadotir (2000). "Management of tuberculosis: a guide for low-income countries." International Union Against Tuberculosis and Lung Disease, Paris, France

Edathodu, J., M. M. Halim, et al. "Mother-to-child transmission of HIV: experience at a referral hospital in Saudi Arabia." Ann Saudi Med. 2010 Jan-Feb;30(1):15-7.

Ejaz A Khan, M. H. (2002). "Recognition and management of tuberculosis in children." Current Pediatrics(12): 545-550.

el-Kassimi, F. A., A. K. Abdullah, et al. "Tuberculin survey in the Eastern Province of Saudi Arabia." Respir Med. 1991 Mar;85(2):111-6.

Ellis, M. E., S. al-Hajjar, et al. "High proportion of multi-drug resistant Mycobacterium tuberculosis in Saudi Arabia." Scand J Infect Dis 1996;28(6):591-5.

Engelbrecht, A. L., B. J. Marais, et al. (2006). "A critical look at the diagnostic value of culture-confirmation in childhood tuberculosis." Journal of Infection 53(6): 364-369.

Froude, J. R. and M. Kingston (1982). "Extrapulmonary tuberculosis in Saudi Arabia, a review of 162 cases." King Faisal Specialist Hospital Medical Journal 2: 85-95.

Griffith DE, A. T., Brown-Elliot BA, Catanzaro A, Daley C, Gordin F, et al. (2007). "An official ATS/IDSA statement: diagnosis, treatment, and prevention of nontuberculous mycobacterial diseases." Am J Respir Crit Care Med. 175: 367-416.

H.Simon Schaaf, R. P. G., Magdalene Kennedy, Nulda Beyers, Peter B Hesseling and Peter R Donald (2001). "Evaluation of young children in contact with adult multi-drug resistant pulmonary tuberculosis: A 30-month follow-up. ." Pediatrics 109(5): 765-771. http://www.moh.gov.sa/statistics/index.html.

Islam, S. M. and K. F. Tabbara "Causes of uveitis at The Eye Center in Saudi Arabia: a retrospective review." Ophthalmic Epidemiol. 2002 Oct;9(4):239-49.

J.A. Jereb, G. D. K. a. D. S. P. (1993). "The epidemiology of tuberculosis in Children." Pediatr Infect Dis 1993(4): 220-231.

Kathryn DeRiemer, C. L. D. (2004). "Tuberculosis transmission based on molecular epidemiologic research. ." Seminars in respiratory and critical care medicine 25(3): 297-306.

Kordy, F., S. Al-Hajjar, et al. "Human immunodeficiency virus infection in Saudi Arabian children: transmission, clinical manifestations and outcome." Ann Saudi Med. 2006 Mar-Apr;26(2):92-9.

Lalitkanth (2001). "Childhood Tuberculosis increasing: But neglected. ." Indian Journal of Tuberculosis. 48(1): 1-2.

M Y Khan, A. J. K., A O Osoba, S WAli, Y Samman, Z Memish (2001). "Increasing resistance of M.tuberculosis to anti-TB drugs in Saudi Arabia. ." Int.journal of Antimicrobial Agents(17): 415-418.

Madani, T. A. "Sexually transmitted infections in Saudi Arabia." BMC Infect Dis. 2006 Jan 10;6:3.

Madani, T. A., Y. Y. Al-Mazrou, et al. "Epidemiology of the human immunodeficiency virus in Saudi Arabia; 18-year surveillance results and prevention from an Islamic perspective." BMC Infect Dis. 2004 Aug 6;4:25.

Marais, B. J. M. F. C. P. M., C. A. M. F. F. F. Wright, et al. (2006). "Tuberculous Lymphadenitis as a Cause of Persistent Cervical Lymphadenopathy in Children From a Tuberculosis-Endemic Area." Pediatric Infectious Disease Journal 25(2): 142-146.

Memish, Z. A. and A. O. Osoba "International travel and sexually transmitted diseases." Travel Med Infect Dis(2005 Aug 18): 2006 Mar;4(2):86-93.

Mittrucker, H. W., U. Steinhoff, et al. "Poor correlation between BCG vaccination-induced T cell responses and protection against tuberculosis." Proc Natl Acad Sci U S A(2007 Jul 18): 2007 Jul 24;104(30):12434-9.

Mokhtar, A. and K. Salman (1983). "Extrapulmonary tuberculosis." Saudi Med J 4: 317-322.

Omair, M. A., A. A. Al-Ghamdi, et al. "Incidence of tuberculosis in people living with the human immunodeficiency virus in Saudi Arabia." Int J Tuberc Lung Dis. 2010 May;14(5):600-3.

Qari, F. A. (2002). "The spectrum of tuberculosis among patients of the King Abdul Aziz University Hospital, Jeddah, Saudi Arabia." Southeast Asian J Trop Med Public Health 33(2): 331-337.

S.K. Kabra, R. L. V. S. (2004). "Some current concepts on childhood tuberculosis." Indian J Med Res 120(October 2004): pp 387-397.

Saleh, M. A.-F. A.-Q., Abdulaziz; Larbi, Emmanuel; Al-Fawaz, Ibrahim; Taha, Omar; Satti, Mohammed B. (1997). "Tuberculous Peritonitis in Children: Report of Two Cases and Literature Review." Journal of Pediatric Gastroenterology & Nutrition 24(2): 222-225.

Samman, Y., A. Krayem, et al. "Treatment outcome of tuberculosis among Saudi nationals: role of drug resistance and compliance." Clin Microbiol Infect. 2003 Apr;9(4):289-94.

Shanks, N. J., I. Khalifa, et al. (1983). "Tuberculosis in Saudi Arabia." Saudi Med J 4: 151-156.

Shingadia., T. W. a. D. (2004). "Global epidemiology of Paediatric tuberculosis." Journal of Infection. 48: 13-22.

Society., A. T. (1997). "Diagnosis and treatment of disease caused by nontuberculous mycobacteria." Am J Respir Crit Care Med. 156: s21-25.

Starke JR, J. H., Baltimore RS, Ed. (2002). Tuberculosis Infection. Pediatric diseases: Principles and practice. . Philadelphia, WB Saunders.

Statistics Department, M. (2010). Health Statistical Year book., Ministry of Health, Saudi Arabia.: 52-53.

Stephan, C., T. Wolf, et al. "Comparing QuantiFERON-tuberculosis gold, T-SPOT tuberculosis and tuberculin skin test in HIV-infected individuals from a low prevalence tuberculosis country." AIDS. 2008 Nov 30;22(18):2471-9.

WHO (2007). "A research agenda for childhood tuberculosis." World Health Organization WHO/HTM/TB/2007.381.

Wilder-Smith, A., W. Foo, et al. (2005). "High risk of Mycobacterium tuberculosis infection during the Hajj pilgrimage." Trop Med Int Health 10(4): 336-9.

Yousef A. Al-Katawee, L. A. A.-M., Abdulrahman S. Al-Showaier (2007). "Congenital tuberculosis presenting as cutaneous disease in a premature infant." Saudi Med. J 28(11): 1739-1740.

Zaman, R. "Tuberculosis in Saudi Arabia: epidemiology and incidence of Mycobacterium tuberculosis and other mycobacterial species." Tubercle 1991 Mar;72(1):43-9.

Zaman, R. (1991). "Tuberculosis in Saudi Arabia: epidemiology and incidence of Mycobacterium tuberculosis and other mycobacterial species." Tubercle 72(1): 43-9.

4

Tuberculosis is Still a Major Challenge in Africa

Simeon I.B. Cadmus[1], Osman El Tayeb[2] and Dick van Soolingen[3,4]
1Department of Veterinary Public Health and Preventive Medicine,
University of Ibadan, Ibadan,
2Damien Foundation,
3Departments of Pulmonary Diseases and Medical Microbiology,
Radboud University of Nijmegen Medical Centre, Nijmegen
4National Tuberculosis Reference Laboratory,
National Institute for Public Health and the Environment (RIVM), Bilthoven,
1Nigeria
2Belgium
3,4Netherlands

1. Introduction

Africa is constituted of 53 independent countries (taking both South and North Sudan as one), has a one billion population and provides home to about 11% of the world's population. The human population in Africa was projected to grow at the rate of 2.6% from the 770 million people in 2005 to 2 billion in 2050 (Shapley, 2008). It currently carries a huge burden of tuberculosis (TB), estimated at 30% of the total global number of cases in 2009, coming second only after Asia (50%). In the same vein, in 2009, approximately 41% (9/22) of the highest burdened countries (HBCs) with TB worldwide were found in Africa (WHO, 2010a). Similarly, the World Health Organization (WHO) in 2007 estimated that the average incidence of TB in African countries more than doubled between 1995 and 2005 (WHO, 2007).

Generally, the burden of TB in Africa is driven by a generalized HIV epidemic; and the African region accounted for approximately 80% of the estimated 11–13% of the TB deaths which were HIV-positive in 2009 (WHO, 2010a). This problem is compounded by the general weak health care systems, inadequate laboratories, and conditions that promote transmission of infection, resulting in the emergence of drug-resistant *Mycobacterium tuberculosis* strains (Chaisson and Martinson, 2008). Other compounding factors, apart from HIV, that have resulted in the increasing trend of TB in Africa are poverty, which is closely related to malnutrition, crowded living conditions, lack of access to free or affordable health care services, and dependence on traditional healers that can facilitate the transmission of tuberculosis (Parson *et al.*, 2011). Occasional wars and civil disturbances worsen this situation and this is even complicated by droughts and regular natural disasters. Other self inflicted problems are poor government funding of health care services, occasioned by massive corruption and leading to diversion of meager local and foreign resources.

Despite these gloomy outlooks, some African countries have achieved commendable landmarks in reversing the frightening global trend of TB. For example, Kenya and the

United Republic of Tanzania were among the 13 countries listed from the HBCs that achieved treatment success rate target of 85% set by WHO for new sputum smear-positive cases of pulmonary TB (WHO, 2010a). Therefore, with concerted efforts and co-ordination within the African continent, greater achievements can be recorded to curtail the scourge of TB which has inflicted so much pain in Africans. Finally, intensified efforts to reduce deaths among HIV/+ TB co-infected cases are needed, especially in sub-Saharan Africa.

2. Surveillance system

The bane of TB diagnosis in Africa has been attributed to poorly coordinated national tuberculosis programs (NTPs), culminating in weak health systems. As a result of this, individuals co-infected with TB/HIV are made to steer through the complicated, harrowing and weak local health systems in order to get medical care. Many shuffle between health clinics for TB medications and district hospitals for antiretroviral drugs in a system where TB and HIV treatment and care are disjointed and therefore disintegrated. While services and drugs are generally free or highly subsidized, patients still complain about the cost of laboratory examinations, hospitalization, and transportation. This arises because patients still have to pay for several other services like X-ray and hospitalization which are really exorbitantly expensive and out of reach for some of the patients. Since most patients have to visit clinics far from their homes, the cost of transportation is often unbearable and the distress of travel further discourages them. Furthermore, TB control relies on passive case finding among individuals self-presenting to health care facilities, followed by either diagnosis based on clinical symptoms or laboratory diagnosis using insensitive sputum smear microscopy. Since repeated visits have to be made because presentations of serial sputum specimens are required (one taken on the spot and the second brought in the following morning), there are generally high default rates due to cost of visits and logistics. As a result of the bottlenecks encountered, patients are reluctant to visit these health facilities, therefore resulting in poor case finding and ability to achieve effective diagnosis and accurate treatment.

Health seeking behavior and non-adherence to therapy has been cited as a major barrier to the control of TB control globally (Gopi et al., 2007). There are reports from Nigeria and other developing countries that delay in TB diagnosis and treatment initiation is common (Salami and Oluboyo, 2002; Gopi et al., 2007; Odusanya and Babafemi, 2004), and this has been ascribed to negligence's from both the patients and doctors. Delay in diagnosis may aggravate the disease, augment the risk of death and enhance person to person transmission in the community (Odusanya and Babafemi, 2004). In Tanzania, 15% of patients were found to report to a health facility within 30 days of the onset of symptoms (Wandwalo and Morkve, 2000) while studies from Nigeria reported 81% (Enwuru et al., 2002) and 83% (Odusanya and Babafemi, 2004) patients delay for more than one month. Reasons for this are patients visiting local and poorly equipped private medical facilities, chemists, prayer houses and traditional healers; coupled with these, are poor knowledge and awareness about the disease among Africans in general (Odusanya and Babafemi, 2004; Enwuru et al., 2007; Okeibunor et al., 2007).

3. Infrastructural facilities and laboratory services

"Lack of new diagnostic tools and inadequate laboratory capacity hinders timely detection and management of drug resistance, with catastrophic consequences when dealing with lethal forms of TB", says Bert Voetberg, a lead health specialist in the World Bank's Africa region. In most African countries, smear microscopy laboratories consist of single rooms and are understaffed. In addition, they generally possess poorly maintained microscopes, and some of these laboratories lack consistent sources of electricity and clean water (Parsons *et al.*, 2011). Thus, the critical factor in TB control regarding early diagnosis and treatment that should limit the spread of the disease and reduce mortality is still an enormous problem in Africa. According to Chaisson and Martinson (2008), throughout Africa, the vast majority of the diagnosis of TB rests on the microscopic detection of acid-fast bacilli in sputum; an insensitive technique that is particularly ill suited for the detection of TB in HIV-infected patients, who have fewer bacilli in their sputum and more frequently suffer from extra-pulmonary TB than HIV negative patients. In patients with active pulmonary TB, only an estimated 45% of infections are detected by sputum microscopy when compared to culture (Dye *et al.*, 2005). This test, first developed in the 1880s and basically unchanged today, has the advantage of being simple, but has very low sensitivity (especially among HIV-coinfected patients). It is also very dependent on the skills of the technician, and a single technician can only process a relatively small number of slides per day (Perkins *et al.*, 2006). In addition, this method cannot differentiate between drug-sensitive and drug resistant TB, nontuberculous mycobacteria, and other Ziehl-Neelsen positive micro-organisms like Nocardia and Rhodocossus species. Due to these limitations, a staggering three million people who present annually with suspected TB may not be properly and timely diagnosed, because their infection (so-called smear-negative disease) cannot be detected by sputum microscopy (Onyebujoh *et al.*, 2006). Moreover, a significant over and misdiagnosis is expected because a part of the ZN positives do not represent tuberculosis. Therefore, the timely introduction of the use of light-emitting diode (LED) fluorescence microscopes (FM) will go a long way in improving the shortcomings of the conventional smear diagnosis of TB (Cuevas *et al.*, 2011; Hung *et al.*, 2007). "The fact that LED microscopes are more affordable than conventional fluorescent microscopes, and can be powered by battery in some cases, makes fluorescent microscopy potentially more widely available, and this should result in a better diagnostic for TB," said lead author Dr. Andrew Whitelaw from the University of Cape Town based on a study carried out in South Africa. It is also believed that other high HIV and TB burden countries in Africa would benefit a lot from the LED microscopy.

Again, laboratories with the capacity to provide culture and (molecular) drug sensitivity test (DST) services are essential for the diagnosis of drug-resistant TB; culture services are also important for diagnosis of smear negative TB, especially in African countries where the prevalence of HIV is high. However, capacity to perform culture and DST is seriously limited in African countries (WHO, 2009). Since the standard of care for TB diagnosis recommended by WHO (2010a) is (i) sputum smear microscopy for all cases and (ii) expansion of the use of culture to diagnose all bacteriologically-positive (not just smear-positive) cases towards the ultimate goal of using culture (or equivalents such as molecular tests) in the diagnosis of all cases, it becomes obvious that most countries in Africa will never achieve this goal because of the serious deficits in both human and infrastructural capacities. This is apparent especially when the demands for a biosafety level 3 facility for culture of *M. tuberculosis* (MTB) is introduced which is out of reach in almost all settings. Currently, very few countries in Africa can effectively carry out culture to confirm cases of TB. As a result of limitation in *Mycobacterium* culture capability, barely 5% countries in Africa can independently carry out drug susceptibility testing for infected TB patients (Table 1). Consequently, accurate diagnosis for effective treatment of TB patients is heavily compromised.

Countries	Population (Million)	Burden of TB incidence (no. of cases /100,000 individuals/ yr)	% of TB patients that are HIV positive (%)	Mortality due to TB/100,000 population	Smear micro-scopy labora-tories per 100,000 population	Culture labs per 5 million popu-lation	Drug susce-ptibility test (DST) labs/ 10 million popu-lation	Second line DST Available	Local TB Funding	National Reference TB Laboratory
Algeria	35	59	NA	2.4	0.7	3.7	0.9	In country	Poor	Yes
Angola	18	298	15	30	0.8	0.3	0.5	No	Fair	Yes
Benin	9	93	16	17	0.6	0.6	0.6	In country	Poor	Yes
Botswana	2	694	66	57	2.3	2.6	5.1	Outside	Poor	Yes
Burkina Faso	16	215	20	55	0.7	0	0	Outside	Poor	Yes
Burundi	8	348	46	77	2.0	0.6	0	No	Poor	Yes
Cameroon	20	182	40	17	NA	NA	NA	In and outside	Poor	Yes
Cape Verde	<1	148	20	27	3.2	0	0	Outside	Poor	Yes
Central African Republic	4	327	33	44	1.6	1.1	2.3	No	Very poor	Yes
Chad	11	283	-	63	0.5	0	0	No	Very poor	Yes
Comoros	<1	39	-	7.8	NA	NA	NA	No	Very poor	Yes
Congo,* Democratic Republic (DRC)	66	372	20	76	2.2	<0.1	0.2	No	Poor	Yes
Congo, Republic	4	382	48	43	0.7	0	0	Outside	Very poor	Yes
Cote d'Ivoire	21	399	30	85	0.5	0.2	0.5	No	Poor	Yes
Djiboutu	<1	620	10	77	1.9	5.8	0	Outside	Very poor	Yes
Egypt	83	19	0	1.1	0.3	1.1	0.1	In country	Fair/ Good	Yes
Equitorial Guinea	<1	117	17	5	4.3	0	0	No	Very Good	No
Eritrea	5	99	-	14	1.5	1.0	2.0	Outside	Poor	Yes
Ethiopia*	83	359	20	64	1.4	0.1	0.2	Outside	Good	Yes
Gabon	1	501	59	62	0.9	3.4	6.8	Outside	Poor	No
Gambia, The	2	269	16	48	1.9	2.9	5.9	No	Poor	Yes
Ghana	24	201	22	46	1.0	0.6	0.8	No	Fair	Yes
Guinea	10	3	24	72	0.5	0.5	1.0	In country	Poor	Yes
Guinea-Bissau	2	229	-	30	3.3	NA	NA	No	Poor	Yes
Kenya*	40	305	44	15	3.0	0.8	1.0	Outside	Poor	Yes
Lesotho	2	634	77	14 (9.5)	0.9	2.4	4.8	Outside	NA	No
Liberia	4	28	1	59	3.7	0	0	In country	Poor	No
Libya	6	40	15	4.1	0.4	2.3	3.1	No	Poor	Yes
Madagascar	20	261	-	57	1.3	0.3	0.5	In country	Poor	Yes
Malawi	15	304	64	25	1.3	0.7	0.7	Outside	Poor	Yes
Mali	13	324	16	88	0.6	0.8	1.5	Outside	Poor	Yes
Mauritania	3	330	12	90	2.2	1.5	3.0	No	Poor	Yes
Mauritius	1	22	6	<1	NA	NA	NA	Outside	NA	Yes
Morocco	32	92	NA	5.8	0.5	2.2	0.6	Outside	Poor	Yes
Mozam-bique*	23	409	66	38	1.9	0.2	0.4	Outside	Poor	Yes
Namibia	2	727	58	31	1.4	2.3	4.6	Outside country	Good	Yes

Countries	Population (Million)	Burden of TB incidence (no. of cases /100,000 individuals/ yr)	% of TB patients that are HIV positive (%)	Mortality due to TB/100,000 popu-lation	Smear micro-scopy labora-tories per 100,000 popu-lation	Culture labs per 5 million popu-lation	Drug susce-ptibility test (DST) labs/ 10 million popu-lation	Second line DST Available	Local TB Funding	National Reference TB Laboratory
Niger	15	181	12	41	0.3	0	0	Outside country	Very poor	No
Nigeria*	155	295	26	73	0.7	0.1	0.2	Outside country	Fair	Yes
Rwanda	10	376	34	76	1.9	0.5	1.0	No	Poor	Yes
Sao Tome & Principe	<1	98	13	19	1.2	0	0	No	Poor	Yes
Senegal	13	282	7	72	0.7	1.2	2.4	In country	Poor	Yes
Seychelles	<1	31	-	2.6	NA	NA	NA	In and outside	Poor	No
Sierra Leone	6	644	11	158	2.0	NA	NA	No	Very poor	Yes
Somalia	9	285	NA	58	0.6	0	0	Non	Very poor	No
South Africa*	50	971	58	45	0.5	1.6	3.2	In and outside country	Excellent	Yes
Sudan	42	119	4	24	0.9	0.1	0.2	Non	Poor	Yes
Swaziland	1	1257	13	64	NA	NA	NA	Outside country	Good	Yes
Tanzania*	44	183	37	9	1.6	0.1	0.2	Outside country	Poor	Yes
Togo	7	446	25	113	1.7	0.8	1.5	Non	Very poor	Yes
Tunisia	10	24	2	1.8	0.6	3.4	4.9	In country	Excellent	Yes
Uganda*	33	293	54	29	2.5	0.9	1.2	In country	Poor	Yes
Zambia	13	433	67	27	1.7	NA	2.3	Non	Poor	Yes
Zimbabwe*	13	742	78	82	1.0	0.4	0.8	Non	Poor	Yes

*African countries listed among the 22 high TB burdened nations in the world

Table 1. Showing the burden and challenges of TB in African countries

To respond to the urgent need for simple and rapid diagnostic tools at the point of treatment in HBCs, the Xpert MTB/RIF assay (GeneXpert, Cephied), a rapid molecular test for TB and rifampicin (RIF) resistance was recently developed. Though relatively new, this molecular assay has been described as one of the most promising in routine diagnosis in developing countries owing to its high sensitivity (98.2%), specificity (99.2%) and short turn-around time (2 hours) (Van Rie et al., 2010). With regards to the detection of RIF resistance, the assay was reported to be highly sensitive (≥97.6%) and specific (≥98.1%), with performance characteristics which are superior to drug susceptibility testing by conventional culture-based assays and line probe assays (Boehme et al., 2010). The rapid detection of MTB in sputum and RIF- resistance allows the physician to make critical patient management decisions regarding therapy during the same medical encounter. As conventional sputum smear microscopy has limited sensitivity and culture takes at least 4–6 weeks to produce result, the Xpert MTB/RIF assay seems a major improvement in African countries where proper facilities are scarce and rates of loss to follow-up are high. The additional advantage of the Xpert MTB/RIF assay is that when performed correctly, it is not associated with a measurable infection risk and results in a lower biohazard compared with conventional smear microscopy, making the assay suitable for point-of-care (POC) use in the typical African setting where bio-containment facilities are not readily available (Banada *et al.*, 2010).

4. Co-morbidities of TB and HIV/AIDS

Globally, an estimated 11-13% of the newly diagnosed TB patients are HIV positive and approximately 80% of these cases are in Africa (WHO, 2010a). The HIV infection is an established epidemiological factor causing additional challenges to the diagnosis of TB; hence, a major contributor to the increased incidence of TB across the world. Infection with HIV-1 increases the risk of reactivating latent TB infection by 80- to 100-fold, and HIV patients who acquire new TB infections also have higher rates of disease progression (Parson *et al.*, 2011). Tuberculosis can occur at all points in the immunosuppressive spectrum of HIV disease, with variable presentations, and, particularly in African countries, where TB is always a major indicator of HIV. Multiple studies have shown that fatality rates are higher for HIV-TB-co-infected patients who are on anti-TB treatment but not antiretroviral therapy (16 to 35%) than for treated TB patients who are HIV negative (4 to 9%) (Mukardi *et al.*, 2001). The study carried out by Ackah *et al*, (1995), in Abidjan, Coˆte d'Ivoire, indicated that the highest death rates occurred in co-infected patients with the lowest CD4 cell counts. This is the same picture in most areas in Africa where HIV is prevalent. Unfortunately, despite the scale up of TB treatment in South Africa, the epidemic of HIV in that country has grievously compromised TB care and control. This scenario has manifested in increased incidence of multidrug resistance TB (MDR-TB) and extensively drug-resistant TB (XDR-TB). The sequel of all these compounding scenarios is a situation in which TB and HIV synergistically potentiates each other in the affected patients leading to difficulties in the accurate diagnosis of TB and eventually in increased rate of mortalities in the region.

Notwithstanding the huge funds expended to fight AIDS, TB and Malaria by the Global Fund and PEPFAR in Africa, the bulk of these funds have been spent on AIDS, therefore leaving a huge deficit in the area of TB. Consequently, most attention in the past was diverted at building both human and infrastructural capacities for AIDS prevention; while that for TB was scarcely given the needed support. This has led to limited diagnostic capacity for TB despite the prompt diagnosis of HIV in some cases; hence, leading to most patients dying of TB. Therefore, the parlance "living with HIV, dying of TB" has become a recurrent decimal in most African countries where TB and HIV are endemic (Parson *et al.*, 2011; Dorman and Chaisson, 2007; Gandhi *et al.*, 2006).

5. Newer diagnostics

In the face of various diagnostic challenges of TB due to compounding factors like poverty, HIV/AIDS and lately, the MDR-TB and XDR-TB infections in some African countries like South Africa, an urgent need has arisen for newer technologies to facilitate prompt diagnosis of TB. Clinical management of TB in African countries is hampered by the lack of rapid, simple and effective diagnostic tests. Correct diagnosis of TB is needed to improve treatment, reduce transmission, and control development of drug resistance.

6. Public-private collaborations

The internationally recommended DOTS strategy has been successfully implemented in the public sector by many National Tuberculosis Programs (NTPs), but in the private sector the quality of care is generally very poor (Uplekar and Rangan, 1993; Uplekar *et al.*, 1998). Since the situation of the NTPs in Africa is far from perfect, the problem has been further complicated by the poor operation of the DOTS program in the expanding private sector that is supposed to be a major TB care provider. Resulting from the weak link between the public and private practitioners in terms of complementary activities, funding and operational researches, several TB programs that are of immense benefits to the patients are denied. This is particularly worrisome in the area of TB diagnosis were limited facilities are available for patient care. Because of the very weak interactions, only few private practitioners in the urban settings provide quality diagnostic services that can support patient care. Moreover, only few of these private care givers are accessible to foreign agencies that can support in the scale up TB diagnosis. The resultant effect of this is a huge gap in TB diagnosis and therefore increased burden of the disease especially among rural dwellers that rely mostly on traditional healers who are not normally integrated into healthcare systems by government establishments. Obviously, these practitioners usually do not work according to the national guidelines for the treatment of TB.

Since traditional practices are common place in Africa and majority of Africans still live in rural settings with low literacy rate, many patients patronize local herbalists and quacks who pretend to be physicians and health givers. Traditionally, since herbal centers are not as expensive as most government health clinics, they are the first point of call for patients. Here, local herbs and other ritual concoctions are given, which in some cases worsen the patients health and this could be on for several weeks to years. Sadly, some of these patients die and some infect their relatives before recourse to government clinics/hospitals when complications would have set in. However, recent findings in the area of ethno-medicine have shown that some of the herbal medications have promising anti-tuberculosis activities. A lot therefore needs to be done by government and private research agencies to look into these assertions and see how traditional health care providers can be integrated into supporting TB care in rural settings in Africa.

Both formal and informal private practitioners comprise the health sector, working on voluntary basis or for profit. The number of professional societies, private hospitals, corporate health providers as well as community and traditional healing homes is fast growing. Therefore, mechanisms for collaboration between the public and private health sectors should be established. In order to promote compliance with treatment guidelines, private care providers should be involved in their development, or checks on the adherence to treatment and cure should be organized by the public sector. They should also be empowered to facilitate training within the sector. Improved program coverage, patient access to diagnostic and treatment services, increased case detection and treatment outcomes, and improved overall quality of care are some of the potential benefits of involving private health providers in delivery of services (Uplekar and Shepards, 1991; Pathania *et al.*, 1997). A model of successful public-private sector collaboration in TB control that is commendable in Africa is exemplified by the activities of the Damien Foundation, Belgium, a voluntary non-profit private TB support agency in Nigeria. This collaboration has over the years led to the achievement of about 85% TB active case finding and establishment of the first MDR-TB treatment Center in Nigeria. Though such other agencies abound in other African countries, however, more demonstrable milestones in terms of TB control coverage has to be set and seen to be achieved to justify the huge money said to be expended by these agencies in Africa.

7. Funding of TB control programs

With the gross domestic product (GDP) of the entire African continent valued at $2.2 million (World Bank, 2011) as against that of the US which is estimated at between $14.6-14.7 trillion (World Bank 2011; BEA, 2011), it is obvious that the continent will be unable to effectively finance and take care of its huge health burden. This is more obvious since the highest placed economy in Africa, Egypt is rated 25 globally with GDP of $467, 000 and the lowest country, Sao Tome and Principe rated 177 globally with GDP of $300. With the myriad of diseases, wars natural disasters and massive corruption in the continent, it will be difficult to fund TB care and especially the diagnostic component given the huge resources required both in human and infrastructural capacities. From the recently released WHO 2010 TB report, nearly all countries in the region relied on external funding and support for its DOTS program (WHO, 2010a). Consequently, TB program across the continent is poorly funded; with only about 5-15% barely in a situation to fund their program domestically (Table 1). Unfortunately, due to the recent global recession seriously having its unprecedented effects on the economy of western nations, the budgets of most donor agencies are grossly reduced, leaving great deficits and reduction in TB control support in Africa.

8. Political commitment

Most African countries are politically unstable and bereft of governments that can provide long term policies to sustain the health system. Given these political challenges, and problems of incessant wars, it is difficult to implement and sustain successful DOTS programs. Of particular reference is Somalia that has been deprived of stable government for almost two decades; therefore, it has no political commitment that will help facilitate any national TB control program. This is evident from the absence of a national TB reference laboratory and a non-existent platform (either local or foreign) to screen for drug resistant TB (WHO, 2010a). Unfortunately however, due to ignorance and lack of political will, some African countries fail to acknowledge the burden of MDR-TB despite the overwhelming evidence that points at this. Fortunately though, after so much foot dragging, some countries in Africa have finally set up mechanisms to carry out national MDR-TB surveys in collaboration with Global fund, Center for Disease Control (CDC) and WHO. One of such countries is Nigeria, and preliminary findings from the survey conducted indicate a high rate of MDR-TB (unpublished personal communication).

In other African countries with apparently stable governments, they are faced with self made problems like corruption, civil unrest that discourage full implementation of the TB control programs. Of particular importance again is the epidemic of HIV/AIDS which has incapacitated Africa, and leaving most governments with no option than to tackle the greater evil and leaving others like TB and Malaria for later days.

Despite the challenges African governments are responsible for; it is most unfortunate that most have only paid lips service to tackling the problem of TB. Sadly enough, they are only gored on by the carrot and stick approaches of the western nations and agencies before they made the little commitment seen so far. It is obvious that a larger role of the African Union (AU) is needed to tackle the challenges of TB. In this direction, there is a need for an AU Blue Print on the policy, mechanism, funding and achievable milestones within a practicable timeframe to reduce the burden of TB comparable to rates seen in Europe and other areas of the world with low burden of the disease.

9. Operational research

The fact that new technologies regarding TB diagnosis and control have been successful in western nations and regions of the world, does not necessarily translate to its success in Africa. In theory, biosafety level 3 laboratories are needed to conduct culture of MTB, however, so far such highly expensive and technically demanding facilities are very scarce in Africa. But also the recently developed molecular techniques that in principle do not need such expensive facilities are not as simple to implement in Africa as some assume. For example, despite the promise of the Xpert MTB/RIF assay in clinical trials, evidence has shown that knowledge to support the broader dissemination and implementation of those interventions (e.g., cost and financing of the intervention, provider training, availability of resources, monitoring the quality of intervention delivery) has limited the successful implementation of such innovations. Our previous experience has shown that substantial barriers have existed to limit prior attempts at implementing new technologies, such as the microscopic observation drug susceptibility assay (MODS) and the nitrate reductase assay (NRA). Accordingly, none of these techniques have been successfully integrated into the diagnostic algorithm for TB in Africa. Since no empirically-supported models exist to guide the dissemination and implementation of some of these technologies, sound operational feasibility projects are required before they are integrated into TB programs in Africa. Failure to carry out these assessments in the past, have lead to serious dire consequences in TB diagnosis despite huge resources that has been expended.

In order to make adequate use of promising pilot research findings, especially translational researches are required in African countries before new techniques are rolled out on a large scale. Of great importance here are translational researches bothering on the use of stool for prompt diagnosis of pediatric TB (Cadmus et al., 2009), adaptation of the front loading smear microscopy (Ramsay et al., 2009), and the use of light emitting diode (LED) microscopes (Cuevas et al., 2011) to mention a few. These translational researches are urgently needed giving the advantages they may offer in combating TB in the continent.

10. Role of international agencies

International agencies have played leading roles in the prevention and control of TB in most African countries in the past 50 years. Therefore, most diagnostic improvements experienced in Africa are driven by foreign donors and expertise. For example, the United States Government through its President's Emergency Plan for AIDS Relief (PEPFAR) spent about $307 million in 15 African countries between 2005 and 2008 for TB/HIV co-infected persons covering 367,000 patients (TTGHC, USA, 2009). Principally, the cost covered among other things routine TB screening in HIV infected people and improving laboratory surveillance systems in order to detect outbreaks of MDR- and XDR-TB. However, judging from the enormity of the burden of TB in the continent, it is obvious that the funds from the US and agencies from other western nations are not sufficient; hence, more needs to be done. This is particularly important in the areas of massive laboratory scale up and quality personnel that will operate the various laboratories since all these are grossly inadequate.

Currently, in Nigeria with the support of the PEPFAR program sponsored by the US government, the University of Maryland, through its Institute of Human Virology (IHV), center in Nigeria is supporting the Nigerian TB program in setting up a TB training school with a biosafety level 3 facility in northern Nigeria. The center has the capacity to carry out

LED fluorescence microscopy, culture and molecular techniques like the Hain assays as well as ancillary HIV diagnostic tests. Though similar sophisticated facilities abound in other African countries like Gambia, Mali, South Africa and Tanzania, they remain highly inadequate. Unfortunately, some of these facilities are merely for research and information gathering, rather than large scale use for TB control in such countries. However, since each program is handled by specific interest, there is limited coverage and sometimes no coordination even at the national level.

In other to facilitate effective TB care in African countries, there is a need for coalition of foreign donors to achieve optimal TB control platform for diagnosis and treatment. A step towards this direction is the formation of "The Tuberculosis Coalition for Technical Assistance (TBCTA). The coalition is guiding TB CARE I which is a USAID five year cooperative agreement (2010-2015) that has been awarded to TBCTA with KNCV Tuberculosis Foundation of the Netherlands as the lead partner. TBCTA is a unique coalition of the major international organizations in TB control. The coalition includes American Thoracic Society (ATS), FHI 360, International Union Against Tuberculosis and Lung Disease (The Union), Japan Anti-Tuberculosis Association (JATA), KNCV Tuberculosis Foundation, Management Sciences for Health (MSH), World Health Organization (WHO). The aim of TB CARE is to contribute to reaching the following specific USAID goals in the TB CARE countries (some African countries inclusive) with significant investment. It aims at (1) Sustaining or exceeding 84% case detection rate and 87% treatment success rate; (2). Treat successfully 2. 55 million new sputum-positive TB cases; (3). Diagnose and treat 57,200 new cases of multi-drug resistant (MDR) TB. Finally, TB CARE focuses on five priority areas that are needed for TB control in Africa namely: increasing political commitment for DOTS; strengthening and expanding DOTS Programs; increasing public and private sector partnerships; strengthening TB and HIV/AIDS collaboration; improving human and institutional capacity. With this anticipated initiative getting fully implemented in Africa, it is envisaged, that there will be a major turn-around in TB care through accurate diagnosis and treatment of patients.

11. Recommendations

To optimize TB control in the African continent, major changes are needed. The local political engagement needs to be enforced, not only to regulate the delicate relationship between the weak public Health care system and the expanding private sector, but also to stimulate international involvement in addressing the challenges faced. If more funding would be available, the implementation of new approaches in the diagnosis and treatment of TB should be considered a scientific discipline in itself; with serious considerations given to the integration of new methods and technologies before they are rolled out in Africa.

12. References

Ackah AN, Digbeu H, Daillo K, Greenberg AE, Coulibaly D, Coulibaly IM, Vetter KM, de Cock KM (1995). Response to treatment, mortality, and CD4 lymphocyte counts in HIV-infected persons with tuberculosis in Abidjan, Coˆte d'Ivoire. Lancet 345:607–610.

Banada PP, Sivasubramani SK, Blakemore R, Boehme C, Perkins MD, Fennelly K, Alland D. (2010). Containment of bioaerosol infection risk by the Xpert MTB/RIF assay and its applicability to point-of-care settings. Journal of Clinical Microbiology, 48: 3551-3557.

Boehme CC, Nabeta P, Hillermen D, Nicol MP, Shenai S, Krapp F, Allen J, Tahirli R, Blakemore R, Rustomjee R, Milovic A, Jones M, O'Brien SM, Persing DH, Ruesch-Gerdes S, Gotuzzo E, Rodrigues C, Alland D, Perkins MD (2010). Rapid Molecular Detection of Tuberculosis and Rifampin Resistance. New England Journal of Medicine 363;11: 1005-1015.

Bureau of Economic Analysis, US. Department of Commerce (2010). Gross Domestic Product Fourth Quarter and Annual 2010 (Advance Estimate) (Accessed August, 6 2011
http://www.bea.gov/newsreleases/national/gdp/2011/pdf/gdp4q10_adv.pdf

Cadmus SIB, Jenkins AO, Godfroid J, Osinusi K, Adewole IF, Murphy RL, Taiwo BO (2009). *Mycobacterium tuberculosis* and *Mycobacterium africanum* in Stools from Children in an Immunization Clinic in Ibadan, Nigeria. International Journal of Infectious Disease 13: 740-744.

Chaisson RE, Martinson NA (2008). Tuberculosis in Africa — Combating an HIV-Driven Crisis: New England Journal of Medicine 358;11: 1089-1092.

Cuevas LE, Al-Sonboli N, Lawson L, Yassin MA, Arbide I, Al-Aghbarim N, Sherchand JB, Al-Absi A, Emenyonu EN, Merid Y, Okobi MI, Onuoha JO, Aschalew M, Aseffa A, Harper G, Cuevas RMA, Theobald SJ, Nathanson C-M, Joly J, Faragher B, Squire SB, Ramsay A (2011). LED Fluorescence Microscopy for the Diagnosis of Pulmonary Tuberculosis: A Multi-Country Cross-Sectional Evaluation. PLoS Med 8(7): e1001057. doi:10.1371/journal.pmed.1001057

Dye C, Watt CJ, Bleed DM, Hosseini SM, Raviglione MC (2005). Evolution of tuberculosis control and prospects for reducing tuberculosis incidence, prevalence, and deaths globally. JAMA 2005; 293: 2767-2775.

Enwuru, CA., Idigbe, EO., Ezeobi, NV, Otegbeye, AF (2002). Care seeking behavioural patterns, awarness and diagnostic process in patients with smear- and culture-positive pulmonary tuberculosis in Lagos, Nigeria. Transactions of the Royal Society of Tropical Medicine and Hygiene 96, 614-616.

Gandhi NR, Moll A, Sturm AW, Pawinski R, Gavender T, Lalloo U, Zeller K, Andrews J, Friedland G (2006). Extensively drug-resistant tuberculosis as a cause of death in patients co-infected with tuberculosis and HIV in a rural area of South Africa. Lancet 368:1575–1580.

Gopi PG, Vasantha M, Muniyandi M, Chandrasekaran V, Balasubramanian R, Narayanan PR (2007). Risk factors for non-adherence to directly observed treatment (DOT) in a rural tuberculosis unti, Sounth India. Indian Journal of Tuberculosis 54:66-70.

Hung NV, Sy DN, Anthony RM, Cobelens FG, van Soolingen D (2007). Flourescence microscopy for tuberculosis diagnosis. Lancet Infectious Disease 7; 4: 238-239.

Mukadi YD, Maher D, Harries A (2001). Tuberculosis case fatality rates in high HIV prevalence populations in sub-Saharan Africa. AIDS 15:143–152.

Odusanya OO, Babafemi JO (2004). Patterns of delays amongst pulmonary tuberculosis patients in Lagos Nigeria. BMC Public Health 2(18):
http://www.biomedcentral.com/1471-2458/4/18.

Okeibunor JC, Onyneho NG, Chukwu JN, Post E (2007). Where do tuberculosis patients go for treatment before reporting to DOTS clinics in southern Nigeria? Tanzania Health Research Bulletin 9;2: 94-101.

Onyebujoh P, Rodriguez W, Mwaba P (2006). Priorities in tuberculosis research. Lancet 367: 940-942.

Parsons LM, A´kos SA, Gutierrez C, Lee E, Paramasivan CN, Abimiku A, Spector S, Roscigno, G, Nkengasong, J (2011). Laboratory Diagnosis of Tuberculosis in Resource-Poor Countries: Challenges and Opportunities. Clinical Microbiology Reviews, 24: 314–350.

Pathania V, Almeida J, Kochi A (1997). TB patients and for profit health care providers in India.WHO/TB/97.223. 1997. Geneva.

Perkins MD, Roscigno G, Zumla A (2006). Progress towards improved tuberculosis diagnostics for developing countries. Lancet 367: 942-943.

Ramsay A, Yassin MA, Cambanis A, Hirao S, Almotawa A, Gammo M, Lovett Lawson L, Arbide I, Al-Aghbari N, Al-Sonboli N, Sherchand JB, Gauchan P, Cuevas LE (2009) Front-Loading SputumMicroscopy Services: An Opportunity to Optimise Smear-Based Case Detection of Tuberculosis in High Prevalence Countries. Tropical Medicine 2009. doi:10.1155/2009/398767.

Salami AK, Oluboyo PO (2002). Hospital prevalence of pulmonary tuberculosis and co-infection with human immunodeficiency virus in Ilorin; a review of nine years (1991-1999). West Afr J Med 21:24-7.

Shapley D (2008). Africa's population "emergency" Study: continent continuing population boom ((Accessed August 14, 2011 http://thedailygreen.com/environmental-news/latest/a).

Testimony on Tuberculosis before the Subcommittee on Africa and Global Health, Committee on Foreign Affairs, House of Representatives (2009) (Accessed August 1, 2011 http://2006-2009. pepfar.gov/press/101387.htm).

Uplekar M, Juvekar S, Morankar S, Rangan S, Nunn P (1998). Tuberculosis patients and practitioners in private clinics in India. International Journal of Tuberculosis and Lung Disease 2:324–9.

Uplekar MW, Rangan S (1993). Private doctors and tuberculosis control in India. Tuberculosis Lung and Disease. 1993; 74:332–7. doi: 10.1016/0962-8479(93)90108-A.

Uplekar MW, Shepard DS (1991). Treatment of tuberculosis by private general practitioners in India. Tubercle 1991; 72: 695-702.

Van Rie, A., Page-Shipp, L., Scott, L., Sanne, I. and Stevens, W (2010) Xpert® MTB/RIF for point-of care diagnosis of TB in high-HIV burden, resource-limited countries: hype or hope? Expert Review of Molecular Diagnostics 10, 937–946.

Wandwalo ER, Morkve O: Delay in tuberculosis case finding and treatment in Mwanza, Tanzania. International Journal of Tuberculosis and Lung Disease 2000, 4:133-8.

WHO, 2010a. Global tuberculosis control: WHO report 2010.

WHO 2010b. Stop TB Partnership and World Health Organization. Global Plan to Stop TB 2011-2015. WHO, Geneva: 2010

WHO report 2007: global tuberculosis control: surveillance, planning, finances Geneva: World Health Organization, 2007. (WHO/HTM/TB/2007.376.).

WHO. Global tuberculosis control: epidemiology, strategy, financing: WHO report 2009. (Accessed May, 13 2010, at http://www.who.int/tb/publications/global_report/2009/en/index.html

World Bank 2010. World Bank PPP GDP 2009 (Accessed August, 6 2011, at http://siteresources.worldbank.org/DATASTATISTICS/Resources/GDP_PPP.pdf).

5

Diagnosis of *Mycobacterium tuberculosis*

Faten Al-Zamel
King Saud University
Saudi Arabia

1. Introduction

Tuberculosis (TB), caused by the intracellular bacterium, *Mycobacterium tuberculosis* (Mtb), has been a major health concern since it plagued ancient Egypt 5 thousand years ago. TB infects 9 million people every year, most of them children (especially in endemic areas), and it leads to approximately 2 million deaths annually (World Health Organization [WHO], 2008; Kabra & Lodha, 2004; Marais & Pai, 2007). These numbers are expected to increase in the coming years because of (1) the AIDS pandemic—a high percentage of the patients with human immunodeficiency virus (HIV) are co-infected with Mtb, and (2) the emergence of drug-resistant strains of the TB organisms (Corbett et al., 2003; Raviglione, 2003; WHO, 1994). This alarming increase in morbidity and mortality highlights the need to strengthen control measures. Accurate and rapid diagnosis is essential for controlling the disease, yet the traditional tests for TB produce results that are either inaccurate or take too long to be definitive. A fast and reliable diagnostic method that could differentiate between active and latent TB infection is lacking as well.

The current routine diagnostic tests for TB: sputum smear microscopy, chest X-ray, Mtb culture, tuberculin skin test, acid-fast staining, and serological tests—all have their limitations. Sputum smear microscopy can produce false negative results, whereas the acid-fast staining requires a large number of bacteria in the sputum to give an accurate reading; a chest X-ray alone is inconclusive; Mtb culture takes too long to produce a result; the tuberculin skin test lacks specificity and reliability; and serological tests, which use different TB antigens to detect Mtb infection, are fast but they lack the necessary sensitivity.

The only available TB vaccine is the bacille Calmette Géurin (BCG) vaccine, which is uneven in its efficacy. Various reports have indicated variable levels of protection ranging from 0 percent to 80 percent in different populations (Fine, 1995; Tuberculosis Research Centre [ICMR], 1999). Therefore, despite the fact that most people in developing countries are vaccinated with BCG at birth, TB is still a major public health problem. The prevalence of TB infection is reported as being as high as 40 percent worldwide, and the annual risk of infection is 2–4 percent worldwide (Anil, 1995).

Clinically, TB has two forms: An active form and a latent form (which is asymptomatic and non-contagious). If undiagnosed and untreated, a patient with active pulmonary TB will transmit the infection to 10–15 people each year (WHO, 2006). However, active TB is also fueled by the vast reservoir of latent TB infections that become reactivated. Immunocompetent individuals latently infected with Mtb have a 10 percent lifetime risk of developing active TB (Syblo, 1980; Harada, 2006). Data show that 5 percent of latently infected individuals will progress to active TB in the first 2 years after acquiring the infection, and an additional 5–10 percent of infected people will develop the active disease later in their lives (Comstock et al., 1974). This risk increases for people co-infected with HIV — especially children, for whom diagnosis of TB is even more challenging (Corbett et al., 2004).

If diagnosed, latent TB infected individuals can be cured with anti-tuberculosis treatment, which prevents progression to the active form of the disease. Because effective TB control can only be achieved with the accurate diagnosis and treatment of both active and latent infections, modern TB control programs require the identification of latent TB infection to the highest clinical standards. Accurate diagnosis and preventive treatment of latently infected individuals can substantially decrease the chance of development into active TB (Cohn, 2000). Delayed diagnosis, because of inaccuracy or the unavailability of diagnostic requirements — including the availability of rapid and accurate diagnostic methods — can preclude timely therapy, which may result in increasing morbidity and mortality, greater lung damage resulting in chronic disability, and higher health care costs (Kehinde et al., 2005; WHO, 2009).

The diagnosis dilemma for clinical TB continues to be a global issue. For pulmonary TB, it can be difficult to obtain robust respiratory specimens from the elderly, the young, and immuno-compromised patients. For those with extra-pulmonary TB, tissue biopsy is essential for histopathological and microbiological diagnosis (Bukhary & Alrajhi, 2004), yet techniques to obtain and examine biopsies are not available in all hospitals and may be associated with complications. A simple, noninvasive, rapid, and accurate method of diagnosis needs to be developed for successful treatment of both active and latent TB; with such a method, person-to person transmission of the disease would be greatly reduced, which would have a major impact on TB morbidity and mortality worldwide (Cambanis et al., 2007).

1.1 Specimen collection

For the detection of pulmonary and/or extrapulmonary TB, tests usually require sputum, gastric lavage, blood, urine, or other bodily fluids (such as cerebrospinal fluid, pleural, or ascetic fluid); in addition, tissue biopsy specimens are collected for the diagnosis of extrapulmonary TB. One of the objectives of developing TB biochemical markers and immunological assays is to replace the need for collecting tissue biopsy specimens from TB patients for diagnosis of the disease. Likewise, the development of immunochromatography tests (ICT), for which urine is used as a specimen, is an attempt to make diagnostic tests less invasive and costly, more rapid, and patient friendly. Up until now, regardless of which test is used, that test is usually accompanied by microbiological tests (smear microscopy and mycobacterial culture of sputum) to diagnose pulmonary TB and to determine the treatment be used. Sputum samples, after being collected, are decontaminated by using normal sodium hydroxide-N-acetyl-L-cystein (NaOH-NALC) and then sometimes centrifuged to get a better yield of the organisms (Kent & Kubica, 1985). Often three sputum samples are collected, including a "spot" specimen collected on the first day (first sputum); a morning (second sputum); and "spot" specimen (third sputum) collected on the second day. However, collecting adequate amount of sputum from patients is not always possible, especially in children younger than 10 years old or in adults who cannot produce enough sputum. In situations like these, procedures to stimulate cough with an aerosol solution and/or bronchoalveolar or gastric lavage can be used (Capelozzi et al., 2011; Mohan et al., 1995; Somu et al.,1995).

2. Traditional TB diagnostic tests and their associated problems

Traditional TB diagnosis usually requires high clinical presentation, laboratory materials, and methods for sputum smear microscopy (acid-fast bacilli), culture on solid and/or liquid media, chest radiography, and the tuberculin skin test. Tissue sampling is usually needed to confirm preliminary results in cases of extra-pulmonary TB. All of these tests have their respective shortcomings.

2.1 Sputum smear microscopy

Sputum-smear microscopy is 100 years old, but it is still the primary, easy to use, and affordable test for the confirmation of pulmonary TB at the lower level of health services. Acid-fast bacilli smear Ziehl-Neelsen (ZN) microscopy, which is prepared from unconcentrated sputum (direct smear), is the main laboratory tool supporting case detection. It is inexpensive and is relatively specific in settings where tuberculosis is endemic. However, direct smear microscopy can produce false-negative results, which have been observed in more than 30–50 percent of adult patients (Miorner et al., 1994; Daniel 1990), particularly in high HIV-prevalent settings (Elliot et al., 1993; Frieden et al., 2003; American Thoracic Society Workshop, 1997), and 85–90 percent of infected children (Newton et al., 2008). The acid-fast bacilli false-negative result rate is attributable, in part, to the low sensitivity of the test, which requires more than 10,000 bacilli per milliliter of sputum for reliable detection (Perkins, 2000). Obtaining good sputum samples can be difficult, and the studious attention of trained and motivated technicians (who are not always available) is necessary.

Many attempts have been made to improve and optimize the performance of smear microscopy, including with new technologies (Mase et al., 2007; Bonnet et al., 2007; Ramsay et al., 2009; Mabaera et al., 2007; Van Deun et al., 2004), such as fluorescence microscopy, which uses inexpensive light-emitting diodes (LED) as an alternative for conventional ZN microscopy. This substitution increases the sensitivity of the test and is easy to use, even in peripheral laboratories where culture facilities are not available (Hooja et al., 2011; Steingart et al., 2006a; Steingart et al., 2006b; Steingart et al., 2007; Van Deun et al., 2008; Trusov et al., 2009; Minion et al., 2009; Bonnet et al., 2011). In fact, the World Health Organization (WHO) Strategic and Technical Advisory Group (STAG) for TB recommended that fluorescence microscopy be phased in as an alternative for ZN (WHO, 2009), because it can be used even in low-income, high TB burden settings. It has been reported that LED fluorescence microscopy, either alone or in combination with single-specimen tests, could increase considerably the identification of smear-positive cases (Cattamanchi et al., 2010).

A wide variety of stains or fluorescence quenchers have been used with the LED fluorescence microscopy; however potassium permanganate at 0.5 percent in water is the stain most frequently used. Although potassium permanganate can produce very good results with the classical fluorescence microscopy systems (using mercury vapor lamps and epifluorecence), the very dark background sometimes makes it difficult to focus. Methylene blue (Mblue) is an alternative to potassium permanganate, which yields comparable results (Van Deun et al., 2010).

In an attempt to improve the performance of smear microscopy, sputum processing methods using household bleach (NaOCl), followed by a specimen concentration step (such as centrifuge or sedimentation, mentioned above), can be done in any laboratory setting before smear microscopy is used (Steingart et al., 2006; Angeby et al., 2004; Annam et al., 2009). However, some reports indicate that NaOCl sedimentation did not improve the performance of LED fluorescence microscopy in the diagnosis of pulmonary TB at low levels of health service in resource-poor countries (Bonnet et al., 2011).

Because the acid-fast bacilli smear is based on sputum, extra-pulmonary TB detection varies with the cytomorphology of inflammation at the site of infection, which is limited and may not exceed 40 percent (Nigussie et al., 2010; Gangane et al., 2008). The sputum smear microscopy test may also identify certain types of bacteria that are not Mtb, thus yielding a false-positive result for TB. The WHO estimates sputum smear microscopy only identifies 35 percent of patients with TB (Harris, 2004; Thornton et al., 1998). Furthermore, the 2010 WHO report indicated that in 2009, 43 percent of the 4.6 million reported new cases of pulmonary TB were diagnosed without microbiological confirmation (WHO, 2010). The failure to confirm TB infection can delay initiation of the appropriate therapy to adequately treat cases, which could prevent the further spreading of the disease (Cambanis et al., 2007).

2.2 Solid or liquid cultures

Solid or liquid cultures are still seen as the gold standard for TB detection because they are sensitive to live Mtb in the sputum sample; they can also provide data on the likely effectiveness of certain chemotherapeutic agents against TB. However, there are serious drawbacks to this test, such as the time needed to obtain the result (3–8 weeks). Clinical and therapeutic decisions are often made before the culture results are available. However, few facilities in low-income settings use culture for the diagnosis of TB; for those facilities the main method of diagnosis is sputum microscopy with acid. When culture *is* used in these settings, the Löwenstein-Jensen solid, egg-based, and agar-based Middlebrook 7H10 media are the ones used to recover mycobacteria from clinical materials (Metchock et al., 1999; Murray et al., 1998); these can take weeks to show results.

2.2.1 Advantages and disadvantages of cultures

A number of manual and automated systems have been developed to reduce the detection time of mycobacteria in clinical specimens. Both the biphasic Septi-chek acid-fast bacilli (Becton Dickinson, Sparks, MD) and the MB-Redox (BiotestAG, Dreieich, Germany) are examples of the manual systems. Advances in technology have led to the development of the automated systems such as radiometric BACTEC 460TB (Becton Dickinson), the fluorometric BACTEC MB9000 and BACTECMGIT (Mycobacteria Growth Indicator Tube), 960 systems (Becton Dickinson), the carbon dioxide–sensing MB/BacT ALERT 3D System (Organon Teknika, Durham, NC), and the pressure-sensing ESP Culture System II (Trek Diagnostic Systems, Westlake, OH). Detection time and isolation of Mtb were considerably improved (7–21 days) with the use of liquid media, such as the radiometric BACTEC 460 TB broth-based system. However, this procedure still requires trained technicians and special attention to safety issues regarding radioisotopes (Salfinger & Pfyffer, 1994; Laszlo et al., 1983). Another disadvantage of the BACTEC 460 TB system is the increased cost of radioactive waste disposal, an issue that encouraged manufacturers to develop a better alternative. The fully automated BACTEC Mycobacteril Growth Indicator Tube (MGIT) liquid medium system with early growth indicators (the BACTEC MGIT 960 system), is faster and more sensitive than both LJ and BACTEC 460 TB for testing the susceptibility of antituberculosis agents, and it is more effective in diagnosing the disease in smear-negative samples; this feature shows great potential to reduce the mortality rate from TB (Lu et al., 2002; Gérôme et al., 2009; Sinirtas et al., 2009; Morcillo et al., 2010).

The BACTEC MGIT 960 system is a high-capacity, fully automated continuous-monitoring system, which can test up to 960 samples for the rapid detection of mycobacteria, making it suitable for those laboratories dealing with a large number of specimens (Somoskovi et al., 2000; Hanna et al., 1999; Tortoli et al., 1999; Lee et al., 2003). In the determination of the early bactericidal activity in the clinical studies of new anti-tuberculosis agents, it has been found that the time of detection of MGIT 960 is better than colony-forming units of Mtb on solid media (Diacon et al., 2010).

Although the WHO recently recommended the expanded use of liquid culture systems, such as MGIT, in resource-constrained settings (WHO, 2007), historically these systems have not been used because of the high cost of the tests and the culture contamination rates (Chihota et al., 2010). The relatively high contamination rates of the MGIT culture has been reported to range from 5.5 to 15 percent in high-income settings, and as high as 29.3 to 33 percent in resource-constrained settings (Chien et al., 2000; Lee et al., 2003; Hanna et al., 1999; Somoskvi et al., 2000; Chihota et al., 2010).

2.2.2 New approaches to cultures

Using simple and inexpensive monoclonal assays, such as the Capilia TB assay (a rapid and low-technology method), which uses monoclonal antibodies to detect a secreted mycobacterial protein (MPB64) during culturing (solid or liquid culture) allows it to differentiate Mtb from non-TB mycobacteria (Muyoyeta et al., 2010; Ngamlert et al., 2009). To shorten the time required for bacterial growth detection, Mtb can be isolated in both liquid- and solid-media cultures (Lu et al., 2002).

Although automated systems such as BACTEC 460 TB, BACTEC 9000, and MGIT can be used to accelerate the growth of the bacteria, they can also produce inaccurate results (Daniel, 1987). Plus, it is not always possible to obtain bacteria in the sputum sample. False-positives, which range from 0.1 percent to 65 percent because of laboratory contamination is another concern with the culture technique (Ruddy et al., 2002). Viable organisms can present additional problems, especially in patients who have started treatment. Therefore, even though culture has thus far been considered the gold standard for TB diagnosis, it still lacks the desired accuracy; it has been estimated that no more than 81 percent of the confirmed TB cases can be detected by culture (API, 2006).

2.3 Tuberculin Skin Test (TST)

Tuberculin skin testing (TST), also known as the Mantoux test or Heaf test, remains in widespread use for both the diagnosis of active TB and the detection of latent TB, and for the identification of TB in health care workers, for whom the incidence of TB is higher than in the general population (Harries et al., 1997; Barrett et al., 1979) and who require routine checkups for accidental acquisition of TB infection and chemoprophylaxis. The TST is a delayed type hypersensitivity skin test: an induration develops and is measured 48 to 72 hours after the intradermal inoculation of purified protein derivatives. It is generally accepted that in adults a TST response greater than or equal to a 10-millimeter induration is indicative of TB infection; however in children, the gauge differs in different settings. Importantly, the TST is still used as an epidemiological tool to screen for TB and to calculate the annual risk of TB through data generated by TST surveys. TST surveys are useful for detection of TB in communities with low case-detection rates, to assess the effect of HIV infection on a TB epidemic, and to better understand the effect of both diseases on children (Farhat et al., 2006).

2.3.1 Limitations of the tuberculin skin test

Although the TST is inexpensive, easily available, and is the preferred test in most TB-prevalent settings, it has a number of limitations. The TST is not patient friendly, in that it requires two visits to the health facility: the first visit is when the test is administered; and the second visit, 2 – 3 days later, is to assess the skin's reaction. It is estimated that one third of the people tested never return after the 48- to 72-hour waiting period to have their tests read (ATS, 2000; Lee & Holzman, 2002).

2.3.2 False positives

Purified protein derivatives contain more than 200 antigens shared with the BCG vaccine and many of the non-TB environmental mycobacteria, which can result in low specificity of the TST (Huebner et al., 1993; Dacso 1990; Diel et al., 2009; Pai et al., 2008). This cross-reactivity results in false-positive reporting for a large percentage of the world's population. Some reports indicate that BCG vaccination can present TST false-positive results for up to 15 years after vaccination (Wang et al., 2002). These variables contribute to the false positive results: (1) the strain and dose of BCG inoculated (Wang et al., 2002; Davids et al., 2006); (2) the method of vaccine administration (Davids et al., 2006); (3) the time since vaccination (Menzies, 2000); (4) the number of BCG scars (Babayigit et al., 2011); and (5) the weight and age at the time of vaccination (Newort et al., 2004). If the BCG vaccine was received in infancy, the impact on TST results is minimal, especially 10 or more years after vaccination. A person's nutrition at the time of vaccination as well as genetic factors can also have an impact on the outcome of the TST results later on (Newport et al., 2004). More frequent, more persistent, and larger TST reactions were observed in individuals who had received the BCG vaccine later in life, ie, after infancy (Pérez-Then et al., 2007; Farhat et al., 2006). Sometimes TST indurations between 5–10 millimeters can still develop for up to 25 years after vaccination (Miret-Cuadras et al., 1996). The TST false positive reaction was not associated with a family history of tuberculosis, with exposure to cigarette smoke, number of household family members, and the presence of respiratory allergic diseases (Babayigit et al., 2011). A number of additional factors can contribute to false-positive results including inaccuracy of reading and documenting the results (Mancuso et al., 2008).

Furthermore, the TST does not distinguish between individuals infected with Mtb, vaccinated with BCG, or infected with environmental non-TB mycobacteria— almost one third of the people who test positive on the TST do not have a TB infection (American Thoracic Society [ATS], 2000; Huebner et al.,1993; von Reyn et al., 2001). Clinically non-TB mycobacteria rarely causes TST false-positives in low-prevalence settings of TB infection, however it does have an effect on the false-positive results of populations with a high prevalence of non-TB mycobacteria (Farhat et al., 2006). This lack of specificity (high rate of false-positive) in diagnosing both active and latent TB (WHO, 1995) is considered the TST's major drawback.

2.3.3 False negatives

The TST can also produce false-negative readings, and these can be product-related (associated with improper storage or handling). The number of tuberculin units inoculated and the type of tuberculin can have an effect on TST reactivity (Farhat et al., 2006). The sensitivity of the test is affected by the immunomodulation of the skin; the DTH response is influenced by illness or immunosuppression, and factors such as HIV infection or a young child's age can result in even lower sensitivity of the test for both latent and active TB (Swaminathan et al., 2008; Selwyn et al., 1992; Pesanti, 1994; Madariaga et al., 2007; Moreno et al., 2001).

2.3.4 The boosting effect

Other disadvantages associated with the TST include the "boosting effect," a phenomenon in which multiple TST administrations over time yield a false positive. The increased tuberculin reaction is seen in some individuals when a second skin test is administered 1 week to 1 year after administration of a first skin test that is nonreactive. This could be explained as an anamnestic recall of immune response that occurs in individuals with remote exposure to mycobacterial antigens. This phenomenon is a problem for people who are regularly screened for TB infection using the TST (for example, health care workers, hemodialysis patients, etc.) and become immunized to purified protein derivatives by the repeated administrations of the test (Dogan et al., 2005; Cengiz & Seker, 2006). Persistent negative TST in latent TB-infected individuals, despite the continued exposure, has been reported. It has been shown that this reaction can be attributed to genetic factors. These genetic factors not only influence the interaction between humans and Mtb but they can affect the outcome of the exposure: exposure but no infection, infection without progression, or progression to disease (Stein et al., 2008). Subjectivity and inter-individual variability, in the administration and reading of the TST can be added to the disadvantages and resultant errors, because it is difficult to administer small amounts of the protein uniformly; that is, the amount of purified protein derivatives delivered in the TST may vary, and this affects the size of the reaction (Chaparas et al., 1985).

Further research is needed to determine the best cut-offs for TST sensitivity, the optimal time for testing candidates, especially for people that need to be tested periodically (such as health care workers), and the cost-effectiveness of the test, given its limitations (Khawcharoenporn et al., 2011).

2.4 Chest X-ray

Chest radiography can be a useful tool to confirm TB when combined with a patient's history, physical exam, and laboratory tests in symptomatic and even smear-negative patients. Pulmonary TB almost always shows abnormalities on the chest radiograph; the pulmonary cavities and lesions are smaller when infected with TB than those caused by other chest health problems.

2.4.1 Disadvantages of chest X-ray

A chest X-ray cannot alone confirm a TB diagnosis. In many cases (40 percent), the infection is not in the lungs; radiography may not detect the early stages of TB disease, because the damage to the lungs may not yet be sufficiently marked to be detectable by a chest X-ray. Also, scarring in the lungs may be detected if previous TB disease has occurred (even if the patient is completely cured), and thus it is difficult to distinguish past cured TB from current TB disease.

2.4.2 Computerized Tomography (CT)

When both chest X-ray and computerized tomography were used to screen for latent TB in pre-transplant patients, abnormal findings were only detected on the chest CT (the chest X-ray results were normal), which indicates that chest CTs can detect latent TB better than chest X-rays (Lyu et al., 2011). Many studies have confirmed that CT has detected pulmonary TB cases that were missed by chest radiographs. Furthermore, high resolution CT alone, or CT together with the TST and INF-γ release assays, were effective in the differentiation between active TB and latent TB (Lee et al., 2010; Boloursaz, 2010). Even in sputum smear–negative sittings, high-resolution CT findings, such as tree-in bud appearance, lobular consolidation, and large nodules, accurately predicted the risk for pulmonary TB with reproducible results (Nakanishi et al., 2009).

2.5 Nucleic acid amplification test

The nucleic acid amplification test detects the nucleic acid specific to Mtb using an amplification technique (Noordhoek et al., 1995; Kadival et al., 1995; Nagi et al., 2007). Nucleic acid amplification is a relatively new assay for TB diagnosis that is available only in specialized, advanced laboratories (ATS, 2000). DNA amplification offers a fairly specific and sensitive diagnostic method in both pulmonary and extra-pulmonary TB, and most studies have shown it to be more sensitive than sputum smear microscopy, but less sensitive than microbial culture (Pfyffer, 1999; Magana-Arachchi et al., 2008). The specificity (ruling in disease) of the nucleic acid amplification test is high when applied to body fluids (extra-pulmonary), such as meningitis and pleural TB).

2.5.1 Limitations of the nucleic acid amplification test

The sensitivity (ruling out disease) can be compromised especially in respiratory specimens, where it can be highly variable and more inconsistent than specific (it is only about 60 percent effective under optimal conditions). This variability can be explained by the use of different cut-off values used in the different studies (Dinnes et al., 2007; Daley & Pai, 2007), in addition to the sequence variation in both commercial and in-house assays (Whilley et al., 2008).

Evaluation of commercial nucleic acid amplification tests in both pulmonary TB and extra-pulmonary TB indicated that nucleic acid amplification tests have high, consistent specificity and positive predictive values in smear-positive patients (Ling et al., 2008; Piersimoni et al., 2002; Reischl et al., 1998; Caruyvels et al., 1996; Coll et al., 2003; Goessens et al., 2005; Miragliotta et al., 2005; Ozkutuk et al., 2006; Guerra et al., 2007; Franco-Alvarez et al., 2006); however, in smear-negative cases, when a rapid diagnostic test is needed, the accuracy of the test is more modest and variable, and the results may be influenced by patient selection and the clinical setting in which the tests are carried out (Brown et al., 1999; Barnes, 1997).

Similar results were obtained when the clinical impact of the nucleic acid amplification test systems were evaluated in low-income countries that have a high burden of TB and HIV. The nucleic acid amplification test assays used in these studies had moderate sensitivity and high specificity for TB in a predominantly HIV-seropositive population with negative sputum-smear (Davis et al., 2011; WHO, 2010).

Different laboratories report significant variability in the reproduction of this test, which can lead to false-positive results (Chedore et al., 2006); this is a major concern because of the DNA contamination of assay reagents. Even though nucleic acid amplification test techniques can amplify a small amount of genetic material, the sample must still contain a certain number of TB bacteria to be effective, and this collection is not always possible, particularly with nonpulmonary TB (Haldar et al., 2007). Therefore, it has been suggested that nucleic acid amplification tests should be combined with other diagnostic tests (for example, tests detecting INF-γ) in order to increase the sensitivity of the test (Dinnes et al., 2007). Another disadvantage of the nucleic acid amplification test is that the assay cannot distinguish dead from viable organisms, so a positive result may indicate active disease even though the TB has been cured (Manjunath et al., 1991).

Although the test itself takes little time to administer, the time required to obtain the results is considerable. Laboratories often culture the sample first, to allow the bacteria to multiply (which takes a few weeks), before carrying out the nucleic acid amplification test. The nucleic acid amplification test method requires some level of technical skill (invasive procedures are sometimes necessary to obtain samples), and is prone to cross contamination. In order to provide valid results, the nucleic acid amplification test must be run in an environment that minimizes and detects cross-contamination and test-appropriate controls. Nucleic acid amplification tests can be expensive, and in underdeveloped countries where the high-burden TB exists, commercial nucleic acid amplification tests are rarely used because of cost and complexity. Although some studies suggest that nucleic acid amplification tests are cost-effective in diagnosing TB even in low-income countries (van Cleeff et al., 2005; Dowdy et al., 2008), their use has been limited. In-house techniques that might be substituted for commercial assays often produce results that can't be validated (Daley et al., 2007). When molecular methods were compared with conventional diagnostic procedures, mostly microscopic detection, it was found that the microscopic method on its own is better than the molecular method, because of the extra care needed to interpret the results (Runa et al., 2011).

2.5.2 New approach to the nucleic acid amplification test

A more recent commercial nucleic acid amplification test (the hyplex TBC test), which meets the demand for a low-cost system, has been introduced. The hyplex test is a qualitative system for the detection of members of the Mtb complex, and it is based on a multiplex polymerase chain reaction followed by reverse hybridization to specific oligonucleotide probes and enzyme-linked immunosorbent assay (ELISA) detection. In comparison to other commercial nucleic acid amplification test systems, the hyplex TBC shows good specificity but lower sensitivity, especially with smear-negative TB specimens; it also gives false-negative results, which puts it in the same class as the other nucleic acid amplification test assays (Hofmann-Thiel et al., 2010).

These observations indicate that commercial nucleic acid amplification tests cannot replace conventional tests and cannot be used alone to confirm TB. Improvement of this technique, especially its sensitivity, is required in order for it to be beneficial for the diagnosis of TB in low-resource countries where the prevalence of disease is higher than in other parts of the world.

3. New, more specific tests

3.1 Antibody-based diagnosis assay (TB ELISA)

Recently, many new serological procedures have been evaluated for diagnosing TB. Enzyme-linked immunosorbent assays (ELISA) theoretically represent attractive serodiagnostic methods, because they are simple, rapid, inexpensive, and do not require much training or sophisticated equipment. Several researchers have tried to develop ELISA tests utilizing different antigens, such as culture filtrate, purified extracts of glycolipid, and mycobacterial sonication antigens, as well as more specific mycobacterial non-recombinant and recombinant antigens of Mtb (Daniel et al., 1986; Escamilla et al., 1996; Laal et al., 1997). Tests using such antigens were designed to detect immunoglobulins IgG, IgM, or IgA against these TB-specific antigens in whole blood, plasma, or serum of both pulmonary and extra-pulmonary TB patients (Imaz et al., 2001; Raja et al., 2002, 2004; Ramalingam et al., 2002; Zheng et al., 1994; Patil et al., 1996). Antigens from mycobacteria other than Mtb (*M. habana*) were also evaluated for their ability to diagnose extra-pulmonary TB using ELISA, and these antigens were found to be effective (Chaturvedi & Gupta 2001). To date, the 38-kDa antigen is the best candidate for the ELISA technique for diagnosing TB in actively infected individuals—but it is not reliable in extra-pulmonary or TB-HIV co-infected patients (Abebe et al., 2007). Because the available ELISA tests cannot achieve a high sensitivity, these tests are unacceptable as single diagnostic tools for TB detection (Chiang et al., 1997; Ravn et al., 2005; Weldingh et al., 2005; Araujo et al., 2004; Raja et al., 2002). The use of relatively low pure Mtb antigens has contributed to the low sensitivity of the test.

Different studies have suggested that a combination of several key antigens (antigen cocktail) may result in better sensitivity. These antigens are presumably the specific, antigens to detect the latent and early stages of the active infection in both pulmonary TB as well as extra-pulmonary TB (Houghton et al., 2002). In order to develop a successful serodiagnostic method for TB, several factors must be considered: antigen recognition by infected individuals varies depending on the stage of the disease; the heterogeneity of human leukocyte antigen in different populations; bacterial load; and the immunological status of the patient (Abebe et al., 2007).

3.1.1 New approaches to ELISA

Recently, an ELISA test (lipoarabinomannan [LAM] antigen-detection assay) that uses urine as a sample has been developed, standardized, and is commercially available (Clearview® TB ELISA) (Boehme et al., 2005; Hamasur et al., 2001; Tessema et al., 2001). This test has many advantages: it is non-invasive, patient friendly, simple (dipstick prototype form of the test is available), rapid (requires 15 minutes to perform), easy to use, and it uses urine, which is a sterile biological fluid that is easier to obtain than sputum, which some patients have difficulties producing. Moreover, the test can be used with other body fluids, including sputum (Dheda, et al., 2010) cerebral-spinal fluid (Patel et al., 2009), and pleural fluid (Dheda K et al., 2009). However, the preliminary data indicate that the sensitivity of the urine LAM, although better than sputum microscopy in HIV-infected patients (Lawn et al., 2009), is still not adequate to replace mycobacterial culture in TB-infected patients, and the diagnostic efficacy is limited and requires further study (Gounder et al., 2011).

A promising, more rapid, and cost-effective form of ELISA has been developed: the Immunochromatographic (ICT) Test Kits; these kits detect serum antibodies against Mtb-specific antigens that are secreted by Mtb during active infection. The high sensitivity, specificity, and positive predictive values suggest that these kits are useful and simple diagnostic tools, especially for resource-poor diagnostic centers (Kumar et al., 2011).

3.2 Interferon-Gamma Release Assays (IGRAs)

Effector T cells of the cell-mediated immune response are normally present as a result of recent host encounters with antigen. T effector cells are short-lived and die off when the antigen is cleared from the host. Due to the short life of the effector T cells, their continued presence indicates that the cellular immune response is fighting a pathogen somewhere in the body. Therefore, diagnosis of an acute infection can be made by noting the presence of the antigen-specific effector T cells in a patient's blood or serum sample and by measuring the release of cytokines by the T effector cells when re-exposed to antigen in vitro. It has been shown recently that TB-specific Th1, Th22, and Th17 cells have an essential role in the immunity against TB infection; this provides a potential target for diagnosis and therapeutic intervention in TB disease (Qiao et al., 2011; Wozniak et al., 2010).

Th1 cells, which secrete INF-γ, are known to protect the body against the Mtb infection. This fact provides a unique way to examine the TB disease for diagnosis, prognosis, and treatment monitoring (Flynn et al., 1993; Boom, 1996; Gallegos et al., 2008). The production of INF-γ is influenced by many external factors, such as TB infection, and internal factors, such as interleukin (IL)-10, IL-12, IL-18, and IL-23 (Yu et al., 2011; Zhang J, et al., 2011; Han et al., 2011; Sahiratmadja et al., 2006). In fact some studies have suggested that some cytokines such as TNF-alpha, IL-2, IL-12, and IL-17 can be used to discriminate between active and latent TB disease (Sutherland et al., 2010; Schauf et al., 1993); however the exact role of each of these cytokines is not fully understood and needs to be investigated further.

Different reports have shown that the peripheral-blood mononuclear cells from patients infected with TB release INF-γ when exposed to Mtb-specific antigens *in vitro* (Ravn et al., 1999; Ulrichs et al., 1998; Lalvani et al., 2001 Mori et al., 2004). Based on these findings, different diagnostic assays have been developed to measure INF-γ released by peripheral-blood mononuclear cells cells in response to Mtb-specific antigens. Two such antigens are the early secreted antigenic target 6-kDa (ESAT-6) protein and culture filtrate protein 10-kDa (CFP-10) (Andersen et al., 2000; Tully et al., 2005). Both antigens have been shown to be important for the growth, survival, and pathogenesis of Mtb (Brodin et al., 2005; Munk et al., 2001). These proteins are secreted by Mtb in great quantities during the infection or when the bacteria are cultured *in vitro* (Andersen et al., 2000; Behr et al., 1999; Pai et al., 2004). Both ESAT-6 and CFP-10 are encoded within the region of deletion 1 (RD1) and are more specific to the organism because they are present in Mtb but are not shared with the BCG vaccine or with most of the environmental mycobacteria (Goletti et al., 2006; Sorensen et al., 1995; Harboe et al., 1996).

3.2.1 The interferon-gamma release assay tests

These discoveries have resulted in the development of two promising, blood-based, commercially available INF-γ release assay tests that have been approved for clinical use for the diagnosis of TB infection, and that use ESAT-6 and CFP-10 antigens: (1) QuantiFERON-TB Gold (QFT-G), which has been replaced in many parts of the world by a safer and simpler test method, QFT-G in-tube assay (QFT-IT) (Cellestis Limited Carnegie, Victoria, Australia) in which an additional Mtb-specific antigen TB7.7 is incorporated into the test (Syed et al., 2009; Stavri et al., 2009); and (2) T-SPOT.TB assay (Oxford Immunotech, Oxford, United Kingdom). Although the two tests share common features, they also have some technical distinctions (Richeldi, 2006). The two INF-γ release assays are designed to measure INF-γ production (INF-γ release assays) in two different ways, from peripheral-blood mononuclear cells of TB patients when exposed *in vitro* to ESAT-6 and CFP-10 proteins. QFT-G measures the quantity of INF-γ secreted by T cells, and T-SPOT.TB assay enumerates the number of TB-specific T cells secreting INF-γ after exposure to TB-specific antigens. Both of the INF-γ release assays require only a single patient visit, and the test results are available within 24 hours (Hill et al., 2004; Richeldi et al., 2004).

Many studies have shown that the QFT-G test is fairly accurate and has modest sensitivity to detect active TB (Kobashi et al., 2006; Kang et al., 2007; Pai et al., 2007). The QFT-G offers specificity of up to 97 percent in clinical trials, sensitivity of up to 89 percent, and provides clinicians with an accurate, reliable, and convenient TB diagnostic tool (Mori et al., 2004; Kobashi et al., 2006).

QFT-G has been useful for the diagnosis and differentiation between pulmonary TB and other pulmonary diseases; however it too has its limitations. Because the results depend on the clinical condition of the patients and the presence of immunosuppressive diseases, patients with localized lesions of TB infection and the elderly can sometimes get false-negative results (Kobashi et al., 2008; Kawabe, 2007).

The T-SPOT.TB test, on the other hand, quantifies the number of the INF-γ-producing TB-specific cells using a technology known as the Enzyme Linked Immunosorbent Spot (ELISPOT) assay, which is widely recognized as the most sensitive technique to measure antigen-specific T cell function. In the T-SPOT.TB assay, recently developed by Lalvani and coworkers, individual T cells specific for the two antigens (ESAT-6 and CFP-10) are enumerated (Lalvani, Pathan et al., 2001; Lalvani, Nagvenkar et al., 2001). With this technique, peripheral-blood mononuclear cells from infected individuals are cultured overnight (16–20 hours) with ESAT-6 and CFP-10 antigens to allow the release of INF-γ by the sensitized T cells (Lalvani & Hill, 1998; Lalvani et al., 1998). A single T cell produces a dark spot, which is the footprint of an individual Mtb-specific T cell, and the number of spots is quantified.

The T-SPOT.TB technique has an estimated pooled specificity of 93 percent and up to 90 percent sensitivity for patients with culture-confirmed TB from low-incidence countries; its sensitivity, therefore, is higher than the TST (Lalvani, Pathan et al., 2001; Lalvani, Nagvenkar et al., 2001), and it has a better performance than the TST in detecting active TB (Ozekinci et al., 2007).

In addition, T-SPOT.TB detects specific T cells at frequencies as low as 1 cell per 300,000 bystander cells (Heeger et al., 2001), making the assay very sensitive for detecting immune responses even in immunosuppressed individuals actively or latently infected, in very young children, in those on anti-TNF-α treatment, in transplant and renal dialysis patients, and in pregnant women (Gebauer et al., 2002; Piana et al., 2007).

Therefore, although QFT-G has some advantages over T-SPOT.TB; for instance, it is relatively easy to perform, requires fewer steps and less-expensive equipment—which makes it more suitable for "on-filed" usage in settings with limited resources—it has been shown in different reports to be less sensitive than the T-SPOT.TB assay (Adetifa et al., 2007). It is notable that the INF-γ release assays may vary in different populations depending on various factors, including genetic background, disease epidemiology, prevalence of HIV infection, exposure to environmental mycobacteria that have similar antigens, malnutrition, and other factors (Pai et al., 2004; Dinnes et al., 2007).

3.2.2 Interferon-gamma release assays: A tool to monitor TB chemotherapy

The response of INF-γ-producing T-cells in INF-γ release assays might be related to bacterial load (Hill et al., 2005); therefore, it could be used as a quantitative surrogate marker to monitor TB chemotherapy and drug efficacy during treatment, progression, or relapses (Komiya et al., 2011; Takayanagi et al., 2011; Ribeiro et al., 2009). In addition, a strong association between the T-SPOT.TB score and the degree of sputum positivity in patients has been reported (Oni et al., 2010).

It has been suggested that INF-γ release assays can provide useful, accurate, and rapid support in the diagnosis of extra-pulmonary TB (Lai et al., 2011; Patel et al., 2010; Lai et al., 2010). Although INF-γ release assays have higher sensitivity and specificity than conventional methods, further studies are needed to evaluate their role in diagnosing children and extra-pulmonary TB infections, especially in high TB-endemic settings (Amdekar et al., 2010).

3.2.3 A comparison of the interferon-gamma release assays with the tuberculin skin test

Both INF-γ release assays (QuantiFERON and T-SPOT.TB)are beginning to replace the TST, and both assays have been approved recently for clinical use in the United States, Europe, and Japan (FDA, 2005; Lalvani, Pathan, 2001). It has been shown that the INF-γ release assays have many advantages over the TSTs in the diagnosis of active as well as latent TB, especially in low-TB-endemic countries (Pai et al., 2004; Dinnes et al., 2007; Fukazawa, 2007; Kang et al., 2007; Ozekinic et al., 2007; Bartu et al., 2008; (Harada et al., 2008; Kabeer et al., 2010; Pia et al., 2008; Diel et al., 2009; Park et al., 2009; Toshiyama et al., 2010; Latorre et al., 2009). Since both assays are specific to Mtb and are not affected by previous exposure to environmental mycobacteria or vaccination with BCG, they have greater specificity and sensitivity than the TST in the diagnosis of latent TB in adults (Ewer et al., 2003; Shams et al., 2005; Kang et al., 2005).

In the majority of studies that compare the performance of INF-γ release assays with TSTs, INF-γ release assays seem to be significantly more accurate than TSTs and have poor agreement with it (I mean the TST), for the diagnosis of active or latent TB, in both immunocompetent or HIV-infected individuals (Rangaka et al., 2007; Mandalakas et al., 2008; Stephan et al., 2008; Jiang et al., 2009; Cağlayan et al., 2011; Cesur et al., 2010). In fact, moderate to poor diagnostic agreement between the different INF-γ release assays tests themselves has been observed (Richeldi et al., 2009; Talati et al., 2009; Latorre et al., 2010).

Nevertheless, determining the accuracy of either one of the INF-γ release assay tests to detect latent infections presents a challenge, because there is no gold standard available (Newton et al., 2008), and the only criteria that can be used is the patient's history of exposure to the disease (if known). Therefore, the accuracy and reliability of the estimated number of the global latent TB cases remains uncertain (Wiker et al., 2010). When INF-γ release assays were compared with TSTs in different longitudinal studies, INF-γ release assays may have a higher predictive value regarding the development of future TB, and unlike the TST, the INF-γ release assays (QFTGIT) results are not affected by gender or age of participants (Bakir et al., 2008; Legesse et al., 2011). Nevertheless, the decision to use INF-γ release assays instead of TSTs is often based on country guidelines and resource and logistics considerations (Cattamanchi et al., 2011).

3.2.4 The indeterminate response of interferon-gamma release assays

All INF-γ release assays are designed to include mitogen stimulation of tested cells as a positive control, along with the different TB-specific antigens used in the tests, to measure the ability of the harvested cells to produce INF-γ; when cells from tested individuals fail to respond sufficiently to either TB-specific antigens or, more specifically to the used mitogen control, the results are considered indeterminate. The indeterminate response can be explained by an error in specimen collection and handling or by the performance of the assay or T-cell anergy, which result in an inadequate response (Papay et al., 2011; Kobashi et al., 2009).

Among the different forms of the INF-γ release assays, QFT-IT has a lower rate of indeterminate results compared with T-Spot.TB, because of the simplicity of the in-tube form, which does not require as many steps as T-Spot.TB, and the fact that there is no storage of blood. T cells interact with antigens as soon as blood is collected into the QFT tubes, minimizing the potential loss of activity during storage of blood specimen.

Differences in indeterminate results have been observed among the different INF-γ release assay tests given to children; with children, both QFT-G and QFT-IT (ELISA-based assays) are significantly more affected by indeterminate results than T-SPOT.TB (ELISPOT-based assay) (Bergamini et al., 2009). These indeterminate results can be minimized by applying the assays after acute inflammation is resolved; this later application also reduces the cost of retesting (Zrinski et al., 2011).

3.2.5 Interferon-gamma release assays and detection of TB in children

Uncertainty about the sensitivity of INF-γ release assays to detect TB in children remains an issue; the use of INF-γ release assays to detect active and latent TB infection in children, seem to perform differently. Some studies have shown that the QFT-IT has a high sensitivity and less indeterminate rates in nonimmunosuppressed children of all age groups (from 1 month to 18 years old) (Zrinski et al., 2011). However, others have shown that both forms of QuantiFERON-TB tests (QFT-G and QFT-IT) were less sensitive and can give more indeterminate results than T-SPOT.TB in children younger than 4 years old (Bergamini et al., 2009; Nicol et al., 2009; Takamatsu, 2008).

It is a priority to detect and contain the disease in this age group. Because young children have a higher chance of developing active TB than older children, as a consequence of an impaired T-cell response (Lewinsohn et al., 2004), the American Academy of Pediatrics has recently recommended that the TST continue to be used to diagnose TB in children younger than 5 years old, and that INF-γ release assays be used for children older than 5 years old (Starke, 2009; Mazurek et al., 2010). However, because of the high risk in the 5-and-under age group, it has been suggested that both tests (QFT and the TST) be used in combination, whenever it is possible. This combination of tests would improve the diagnosis of TB, and the child would be considered infected if either or both are positive (Debord et al., 2011; Pavic et al., 2011). Other studies with children older than five, HIV-infected children, or nonimmunosuppressed children, indicated that indeterminate results with QFT-G, QFT-IT, or T-SPOT.TB—were undetected or uncommon (Bergamini et al., 2009; Mandalakas et al., 2008; Tsiouris et al., 2006).

The variation in the level of cytokines (INF- γ and IL-2) released by cells after stimulation with QFT antigens in children, is age dependent; it can identify those children with latent TB who are younger than 5 years old from those older than 5 years old (Lighter-Fisher et al., 2010).

3.2.6 Interferon-gamma release assays for testing TB in children with cancer

Both the TST and the INF-γ release assays were used to detect TB in children with cancer before their initial chemotherapy. All tests performed suboptimally, and therefore none of them can be used individually to confirm or disprove TB infection (Stefan et al., 2010).

3.2.7 Interferon-gamma release assays and screening for latent TB

In adult patients, latent TB can be detected more effectively with INF-γ release assays than with the TST; QFT-G and QFT-IT can be used for diagnosis and T-SPOT.TB for exclusion (Chang & Leung 2010). However, in some settings, both tests are used to screen for TB (Torres Costa et al., 2011; Katsenos et al., 2011).

Although INF-γ release assays are affected by cellular immune statutes and age, they demonstrate low agreement with the TST and perform better in detecting latent TB in adult patients (Santín Cerezales 2011; Zhao et al., 2011). Both of the INF-γ release assays (T-SPOT.TB and QFT) require only a single patient visit, and the test results are available within 24 hours (Hill et al., 2004; Richeldi et al., 2004).

The Centers for Disease Control and Prevention, USA, recommend that INF-γ release assays can replace the TST (single screening strategy) in all settings (Mazurek et al., 2005). However, recent UK TB guidelines advise screening for latent TB using the TST, followed by INF-γ release assays if the TST is positive (dual screening) (Leyten et al., 2007; Sauzullo et al., 2011; Dosanjh et al., 2008;148: Ritz et al., 2011). The dual screening strategy has been reported to be more cost-effective than the single screening strategy (INF-γ release assay or TST alone) for screening latent TB; however this conclusion and the interpretation of results is relative to the prevalence of TB in the setting as well as the length of contact with the infection (Pooran et al., 2010).

3.2.8 Drawbacks of interferon-gamma release assays

One limitation of the INF-γ release assays is that they are inconsistent in detecting TB in HIV patients. Some reports indicate that they are not the best tools for diagnosing TB among HIV-infected individuals with advanced immunodeficiency diseases, because of low sensitivity resulting from the low T-cell count (Chen et al., 2011). However, other studies reported that the sensitivity of the T-SPOT.TB assay in detecting TB in active HIV disease may be not highly impaired by advanced immunosuppression (Oni et al., 2010).

Another limitation of INF-γ release assays is their inability to distinguish active from past-treated TB infections (Kim et al., 2011; (Kim et al., 2010). The role of INF-γ release assays to distinguish between latent TB and active TB and their predictive ability of the progression of latent TB to active TB infection needs to be studied further, especially in high-burden settings (Dheda et al., 2009). Therefore, although INF-γ release assays have been approved in many countries to diagnose latent TB, especially in adults, this test still has little clinical value in the diagnosis of active TB (Dominguez et al., 2009). Nevertheless, growing evidence supports the idea that recruiting Mtb-specific T cells in active TB from fluids at the "local" sites of infection, such as pleural effusion (Wilkinson et al., 2005; Barnes et al., 1993; Barnes et al., 1989), cerebrospinal fluid (Thomas et al., 2008), ascites (Wilkinson et al., 2005), pericardial fluid (Biglino et al., 2008), and bronchoalveolar lavage (BAL) (Jafari et al., 2006; Jafari et al., 2009) is more effective than blood, in the diagnosis of extra-pulmonary TB. In this way the INF-γ release assays are looking at the "local " site of infection rather than "systemic" Mtb-specific immune response in blood, which may only provide background information about effector memory T-cells in active TB. This provides a promising approach to distinguish active TB from latent TB in routine clinical practice (Jafari et al., 2009).

The cut-off values currently recommended by the manufacturers are being disputed in some studies (Soysal et al., 2008). Consideration of new (low) cut-off values for both T-SPOT.TB and QFT, which may improve the assays' sensitivity, are now recommended, especially in intermediate- and high-endemic areas of TB and HIV (Soysal et al., 2008; Kanunfre et al., 2008; Legesse et al., 2010). The relative complexity of the INF-γ release assays can result in technical errors at many levels, resulting from insufficient cells, reduced cells activated due to prolonged transport or storage of blood, improper handling of specimens, the presence of INF-γ antibodies, and the incorrect addition of mutagen. Any of these technical problems can contribute to the invalidity and inaccuracy (unusual INF-γ measurements) of the test results, adding to its potential disadvantages (Kampmann et al., 2005; Powell et al., 2011).

The level of complexity mentioned above in addition to the requirement for special equipment, skilled laboratory personnel, and the high cost of the INF-γ release assays are among the limitations of the assays, which should be strongly considered, especially in low-resources settings. INF-γ release assays are recommended for use as a confirmation tool when a patient with negative TST is suspected of having TB, or to exclude a positive TST result from BCG vaccination (Sun et al., 2010).

3.2.9 Interferon-gamma release assays and detection of TB in patients with immune-mediated inflammatory diseases

Studies involving immune-mediated inflammatory diseases (such as psoriasis, rheumatoid arthritis, etc.) indicated that INF-γ release assays are superior to the TST for detecting latent TB in both endemic and non-endemic areas (Ponce de Leon et al., 2005; Ponce de Leon et al., 2008; Sellam et al., 2007; Murakami et al., 2009; de Andrade et al., 2011).

Since most of the information on the performance of INF-γ release assays have been gathered from studies done in developed countries, it is important that further research on adults and children be done in developing countries where TB is endemic. These studies should include the presence of additional factors that have been reported to cause false negative results as high as 35.5 percent; these factors include HIV infection, malnutrition, impaired immune status, age, and the different ethnic backgrounds of patients (Pai et al., 2006; Menzies et al., 2007; Im et al., 1991; Landis & Koch, 1977; Legesse et al., 2010; Legesse et al., 2011 Apr 9;11:89).

Despite the progress that has been made in studying the use of INF-γ release assays, additional research is still required to study further the limitations of the assays and the ways to overcome them to improve the best utility of the tests in diagnosing and controlling TB (Lalvani & Pareek 2010; Mazurek et al., 2010).

4. Conclusions

Despite the continued research to identify the key Mtb antigens and biomarkers for developing the ideal diagnostic test, there is not yet a rapid, reliable, and economical method to diagnose both active and latent TB. The importance of diagnosing latent TB is often overshadowed in many parts of the world; however, it is key to controlling the spread of infection. In the last few years, new tests have been developed based on significant advances in understanding the genomic and immunology of Mtb. The new tests include the nucleic acid amplification test, QuantiFERON-TB and T-SPOT.TB, which have the advantages of higher specificity and sensitivity than the conventional tests—important for physicians so that they can avoid the inappropriate treatment of false-positive vaccinated individuals. Yet these new tests have disadvantages as well, including cost, training, and complexity. None of the available microbiological or immunological tests alone can accurately confirm the TB infection, while waiting for the culture results which can take weeks. Given the global burden of this disease, and its potential to spread rapidly, the importance of developing a novel assay or improving the existing methods for TB detection, active and latent, has never been greater.

5. References

Abebe F, Holm-Hansen C, Wiker HG, & Bjune G. (2007). Progress in serodiagnosis of M. tuberculosis infection. *Scand J Immuno*, 66: 176-191

Adams LV, Waddell RD, & Von Reyn CF. T-SPOT. (2008). TB Test(R) results in adults with Mycobacterium avium complex pulmonary disease. *Scand J Infect Dis*, 40(3): 196-203

Adetifa IM, Lugos MD, & Hammond A, et al. (2007). Comparison of two interferon gamma release assays in the diagnosis of Mycobacterium tuberculosis infection and disease in The Gambia. *BMC Infectious Diseases*, 7: 122

Akcay A, Erdem Y, & Altun B, et al. (2003). The booster phenomenon in 2-step tuberculin skin testing of patients receiving long-term hemodialysis. *Am J Infect Control*, 31(6): 371-374

Alonso V, Paul R, Barrera L, & Ritacco V. (2007). False diagnosis of tuberculosis by culture. *Medicina (B Aires)*, 67(3): 287-294

Amdekar YK. (2010). How to optimize current (available) diagnostic tests. *Indian J Pediatr*, Mar; 78(3): 340-4

American Thoracic Society. (2000). Diagnostic standards and classification of tuberculosis in adults and children. *Am J Respir Crit Care Med*, 161: 1376-1395

Andersen P, Munk ME, Pollock JM, & Doherty TM. (2000). Specific immune-based diagnosis of tuberculosis. *Lancet*, 356: 1099-1104

Angeby KA, Hoffner SE, & Diwan VK. (2004). Should the 'bleach microscopy method' be recommended for improved case detection of tuberculosis? Literature review and key person analysis. *Int J Tuberc Lung Dis*, 8: 806–815

Anil P. (1995). Tuberculosis: a snap shot picture. *Health Millions*, 21(1): 8-9

Annam V, Karigoudar MH, & Yelikar BR. (2009). Indian J Pathol Microbiol. Improved microscopical detection of acid-fast bacilli by the modified bleach method in lymphnode aspirates. *Indian J Pathol Microbiol*, Jul-Sep; 52(3): 349-52

API Consensus Expert Committee. (2006). API TB Consensus Guidelines 2006: Management of pulmonary tuberculosis, extra-pulmonary tuberculosis, and tuberculosis in special situations. *J Assoc Physicians India*, 54: 219-234

Araujo Z, Waard JH, & Fernandez de Larrea C, et al. (2004). Study of the antibody response against Mycobacterium tuberculosis antigens in Warao Amerindian children in Venezuela. *Mem Inst Oswaldo Cruz*, 99: 517-524

Aris EA, Bakari M, Chonde TM, Kitinya J, Swai AB. (1999). Diagnosis of tuberculosis in sputum negative patients in Dar es Salaam. *East Afr Med J*, 76(11): 630-634

ATS MMWR Recommendations Report. (2000). Targeted tuberculin testing and treatment of latent tuberculosis infection. *MMWR*, 49 (PR6): 1-51

Attallah AM, Osman S, & Saad A, et al. (2005). Application of a circulating antigen detection immunoassay for laboratory diagnosis of extra-pulmonary and pulmonary tuberculosis. *Clin Chim Acta*, 356(1-2): 58-66

Baba K, Pathak S, & Sviland L, et al. (2008). Real-time quantitative PCR in the diagnosis of tuberculosis in formalin-fixed paraffin-embedded pleural tissue in patients from a high HIV endemic area. *Diagn Mol Pathol*, 17(2), 112-117

Babayiğit Hocaoğlu A, Olmez Erge D, Anal O, Makay B, Uzuner N, & Karaman O. (2011). Characteristics of children with positive tuberculin skin test. *Tuberk Toraks*, Jun; 59(2): 158-63

Bakir M, Millington KA, Soysal A, et al. (2008). Prognostic value of a T-cell-based, interferon-γ biomarker in children with tuberculosis contact. *Ann Intern Med*, 149 (11): 777- 87

Barnes PF, Lu S, Abrams JS, Wang E, Yamamura M, & Modlin RL. (1993). Cytokine production at the site of disease in human tuberculosis. *Infect Immun*, 61: 3482-9

Barnes PF, Mistry SD, Cooper CL, Pirmez C, Rea TH, & Modlin RL. (1989). Compartmentalization of a CD4+ T lymphocyte subpopulation in tuberculous pleuritis. *J Immunol*, 142: 1114-1119

Barnes PF. (1997). Rapid diagnostic tests for tuberculosis: progress but no gold standard. *Am J Respir Crit Care Med*, 155: 1497-8

Barrett-Connor E. (1979). The epidemiology of tuberculosis in physicians. *JAMA*, 241: 33-38

Bartu V, Havelkova M, & Kopecka E. (2008). QuantiFERON-TB Gold in the diagnosis of active tuberculosis. *J Int Med Res*, 36: 434-437

Behr MA, Wilson MA, & Gill WP, et al. (1999). Comparative genomic of BCG vaccines by whole-genome DNA microarrays. *Science*, 284: 1520-3

Bergamini BM, Losi M, Vaienti F, D'Amico R, Meccugni B, Meacci M, De Giovanni D, Rumpianesi F, Fabbri LM, Balli F, & Richeldi L. (2009). Performance of commercial blood tests for the diagnosis of latent tuberculosis infection in children and adolescents. *Pedatrics*, Mar; 123(3): e419-24

Biglino A, Crivelli P, Concialdi E, Bolla C, & Montrucchio G. (2008). Clinical usefulness of elispot assay on pericardial fluid in a case of suspected tuberculous pericarditis. *Infection*, 36:601-604

Boehme C, Molokova E, Minja F, Geis S, & Loscher T, et al. (2005). Detection of mycobacterial lipoarabinomannan with an antigen-capture ELISA in unprocessed urine of Tanzanian patients with suspected tuberculosis. *Trans R Soc Trop Med Hyg*, 99: 893-900

Boloursaz MR, Khalilzadeh S, Baghaie N, Khodayari AA, & Velayati AA. (2010). Radiologic manifestation of pulmonary tuberculosis in children admitted in pediatric ward-Massih Daneshvari Hospital: a 5-year retrospective study. *Acta Med Iran*, Jul-Aug; 48(4): 244-9

Bonnet M, Gagnidze L, Githui W, Guérin PJ, Bonte L, Varaine F, Ramsay A. (2011). Performance of LED-based fluorescence microscopy to diagnose tuberculosis in a peripheral health centre in Nairobi. *Int J Tuberc Lung Dis*, Jan; 15(1): 14-23

Bonnet M, Gagnidze L, Guerin PJ, Bonte L, Ramsay A, Githui W, & Varaine F. (2011). Evaluation of Combined LED-Fluorescence Microscopy and Bleach Sedimentation for Diagnosis of Tuberculosis at Peripheral Health Service Level. PLoS One. 2011;6(5):e20175. Epub 2011 May 31

Bonnet M, Ramsay A, Varaine F, Githui W, & Gagnidze L, et al. (2007). Reducing the number of sputa examined, and thresholds for positivity: an opportunity to optimize smear microscopy. *Int J Tuber Lung Dis*, 11: 953–958

Boom WH. (1996). The role of T-cell subsets in mycobacterium tuberculosis infection. *Infect Agents Dis*, 5(2): 73-81

Brock I, Ruhwald M, Lundgren B, Westh H, Mathiesen LR, & Ravn P. Latent tuberculosis in HIV positive, diagnosed by the M. tuberculosis specific interferon-gamma test. *Respir Res*, 7:56

Brodin P, de Jonge MI, & Majlessi L, et al. (2005). Functional analysis of early secreted antigenic target 6, the dominant T-cell antigen of M. tuberculosis, reveals key residues involved in secretion, complex formation, virulence and immunogenicity. *J Biol Chem*, 280(40): 33953-9

Brown TJ, Power EG, & French GL. (1999). Evaluation of three commercial detection systems for Mycobacterium tuberculosis where clinical diagnosis is difficult. *J Clin Pathol*, 52: 193-7

Bukhary ZA, & Alrajhi AA. (2004). Extrapulmonary tuberculosis, clinical presentation and outcome. *Saudi Med J*, 25: 881-885

Cağlayan V, Ak O, Dabak G, Damadoğlu E, Ketenci B, Ozdemir M, Ozer S, & Saygı A. (2011). Comparison of tuberculin skin testing and QuantiFERON-TB Gold-In Tube test in health care workers. *Tuberk Toraks*, 59(1): 43-7

Cambanis A, Ramsay A, Wirkom V, Tata E, & Cuevas LE. (2007). Investing time inmicroscopy: an opportunity to optimise smear-based case detection of tuberculosis. *Int J Tuberc Lung Dis*, 11: 40–45

Capelozzi VL, Faludi EP, Balthazar AB, Fernezlian SD, Filho JV, & Parra ER. (2011). Bronchoalveolar lavage improves diagnostic accuracy in patients with diffuse lung disease. *Diagn Cytopathol*, Jun 14; doi: 10.1002/dc.21743. [Epub ahead of print]

Cartuyvels R, de Ridder C, Jonckheere S, Verbist L, & van Eldere J. (1996). Prospective clinical evaluation of Amplicor Mycobacterium tuberculosis PCR test as a screening method in a low-prevalence population. *J Clin Microbiol*, 34: 2001-2003

Cashmore TJ, Peter JG, van Zyl-Smit RN, Semple PL, Maredza A, Meldau R, Zumla A, Nurse B, & Dheda K. (2010). Feasibility and diagnostic utility of antigen-specific interferon-gamma responses for rapid immunodiagnosis of tuberculosis using induced sputum. *PLoS One*, Apr 28; 5(4): e10389

Cattamanchi A, Huang L, Worodria W, den Boon S, Kalema N, Katagira W, Byanyima P, Yoo S, Matovu J, Hopewell PC, & Davis JL. (2011). Integrated strategies to optimize sputum smear microscopy: a prospective observational study. *Am J Respir Crit Care Med*, Feb 15; 183(4): 547-51. Epub 2010 Sep 17

Cattamanchi A, Smith R, Steingart KR, Metcalfe JZ, Date A, Coleman C, Marston BJ, Huang L, Hopewell PC, & Pai M. (2011). Interferon-gamma release assays for the diagnosis of latent tuberculosis infection in HIV-infected individuals: a systematic review and meta-analysis. *J Acquir Immune Defic Syndr*, Mar 1; 56(3): 230-8.

Caws M, Tho DQ, & Duy PM, et al. (2007). PCR-restriction fragment length polymorphism for rapid, low-cost identification of isoniazid-resistant Mycobacterium tuberculosis. *J Clin Microbiol*, 45(6): 1789-1793

Cengiz K, Seker A. (2006). Boosted tuberculin skin testing in hemodialysis patients. *Am J Infect Control*, 34(6): 383-387

Cesur S, Hoca NT, Tarhan G, Cimen F, Ceyhan I, Annakkaya AN, Aslan T, & Birengel S. (2010). Evaluation of Quantiferon-TB Gold and tuberculin skin test in patients with tuberculosis, close contact of patients, health care workers and tuberculosis laboratory personnel. *Mikrobiyol Bul*, Oct; 44(4):553-60

Chakravorty S, Sen MK, & Tyagi JS. (2005). Diagnosis of extrapulmonary tuberculosis by smear, culture, and PCR using universal sample processing technology. *J Clin Microbiol*, 43(9): 4357-62

Chang KC, Leung CC. (2010). Systematic review of interferon-gamma release assays in tuberculosis: focus on likelihood ratios. *Thorax*, Mar; 65(3): 271-6

Chaparas SD, Vandiviere HM, Melvin I, Koch G, & Becker C. (1985). Tuberculin test: Variability with the Mantoux procedure. *Am Rev Respir Dis*, 132: 175-177

Chaturvedi V, Gupta HP. (2001). Evaluation of integral membrane antigens of M. habana for serodiagnosis of extrapulmonary tuberculosis: association between levels of antibodies and M. tuberculosis antigens. *FEMS Immunol Med Microbiol*, 33: 1-7

Chedore P, Broukhanski G, Shainhouse Z, & Jamieson F. (2006). False-positive amplified Mycobacterium tuberculosis direct test results for samples containing Mycobacterium leprae. *J Clin Microbiol*, 44(2): 612-3

Chen J, Sun J, Zhang R, Liu L, Zheng Y, Shen Y, Wang Z, Sun F, Li L, & Lu H. (2011). T-SPOT.TB in the diagnosis of active tuberculosis among HIV-infected patients with advanced immunodeficiency. *AIDS Res Human Retroviruses*, Mar; 27(3): 289-94. Epub 2010 Oct 26).

Chiang IH, Suo J, & Bai KJ, et al. (1997). Serodiagnosis of tuberculosis. A study comparing three specific mycobacterial antigens. *Am J Respir Crit Care Med*, 156: 906-911

Chien HP, Yu MC, Wu MH, Lin TP, & Luh KT. (2000). Comparison of the BACTEC MGIT 960 with Lowenstein-Jensen medium for recovery of mycobacteia from clinical specimens. *Int J Tuberc Lung Dis*, 4: 866–870

Chihota VN, Grant AD, Fielding K, Ndibongo B, van Zyl A, Muirhead D, & Churchyard GJ. (2010). Liquid vs. solid culture for tuberculosis: performance and cost in a resource-constrained setting. *Int J Tuberc Lung Dis*, Aug; 14(8): 1024-31

Cho SN, Brennan PJ. (2007). Tuberculosis: diagnostics. *Tuberculosis (Edinb)*, 87(Suppl 1): S14-17

Clark SA, Martin SL, & Pozniak A, et al. (2007). Tuberculosis antigen-specific immune responses can be detected using enzyme-linked immunospot technology in human immunodeficiency virus (HIV)-1 patients with advanced disease. *Clin Exp Immunol*, 150(2): 238-44

Cohn DL. (2000). Treatment of Latent Tuberculosis Infection: Renewed Opportunity for Tuberculosis Control. *Clin Infect Dis*, 31(1): 120-124

Coll P, Garrigó M, Moreno C, & Martí N. (2003). Routine use of Gen-Probe Amplified Mycobacterium Tuberculosis Direct (MTD) test for detection of Mycobacterium tuberculosis with smear-positive and smear-negative specimens. *Int J Tuberc Lung Dis*, 7: 886-891

Comstock GW, Liveasy VT, & Woolpert SF. (1974). The Prognosis of a positive tuberculin reaction in childhood and adolescence. *Am J Epidemiol*, 99: 131-13

Corbett EL, Charalambous S, Moloi VM, Fielding K, Grant AD, Dye C, De Cock KM, Hayes RJ, Williams BG, & Churchyard GJ. (2004). Human immunodeficiency virus and the prevalence of undiagnosed tuberculosis in African gold miners. *Am J Respir Crit Care Med*, 170: 673–679

Corbett EL, Watt CJ, & Walker N, et al. (2003). The growing burden of tuberculosis: global trends and interactions with the HIV epidemic. *Arch Intern Med*, 163: 1009-21

Dacso CC. (1990). Skin Testing for Tuberculosis, In: *Clinical Methods: The history, PHISICAL, AND laboratory Examinations (3rd Edition)*, Walker HK, Hail WD, & Hurst JW, editors. Boston: Butterworths

Daley P, Thomas S, & Pai M. (2007). Nucleic acid amplification tests for the diagnosis of tuberculous lymphadenitis: a systemic review. *Int J Tuberc Lung Dis*, 11(11): 1166-1176

Daniel TM, De Murillo GL, & Sawyer JA, et al. (1986). Field evaluation of enzyme-linked immunosorbent assay for the serodiagnosis of tuberculosis. *Am Rev Respir Dis*, 134: 662-5

Daniel TM. (1987). New approaches to the rapid diagnosis of tuberculosis meningitis. *J Infect Dis*, 155(4): 599-602

Daniel TM. (1990). The rapid diagnosis of tuberculosis: a selective review. *J Lab Clin Med*, 116:277–282

Davids V, HanekomWA, Mansoor N, Gamieldien H, & Gelderbloem SJ, et al. (2006) The effect of bacille Calmette-Guerin vaccine strain and route of administration on induced immune responses in vaccinated infants. *J Infect Dis*, 193: 531–536

Davis JL, Huang L, Worodria W, Masur H, Cattamanchi A, Huber C, Miller C, Conville PS, Murray P, & Kovacs JA. (2011). Nucleic acid amplification tests for diagnosis of smear-negative TB in a high HIV-prevalence setting: a prospective cohort study. *PLoS One*, Jan 27; 6(1): e1632

de Andrade Lima E, de Andrade Lima M, Barros de Lorena VM, de Miranda Gomes Y, Lupi O, & Benard G. (2011). Evaluation of an IFN-gamma Assay in the Diagnosis of Latent Tuberculosis in Patients with Psoriasis in a Highly Endemic Setting. Acta Derm Venereol. 2011 Jun 1. doi: 10.2340/00015555-1151.

Debord C, De Lauzanne A, Gourgouillon N, Guérin-El Khourouj V, Pédron B, Gaudelus J, Faye A, & Sterkers G. (2011). Interferon-gamma Release Assay Performance for Diagnosing Tuberculosis Disease in 0- to 5-year-old Children. *Pediatr Infect Dis J*, Jun 20

Demkow U, Filewska M, & Michalowska-Mitczuk D, et al. (2007). Heterogeneity of antibody response to myobacterial antigens in different clinical manifestations of pulmonary tuberculosis. *J Physiol Pharmacol*, 58(Suppl 5): S117-127

Dheda K, Davids V, Lenders L, Roberts T, Meldau R, Ling D, Brunet L, van Zyl Smit R, Peter J, Green C, Badri M, Sechi L, Sharma S, Hoelscher M, Dawson R, Whitelaw A, Blackburn J, Pai M, & Zumla A. (2010). Clinical utility of a commercial LAM-ELISA assay for TB diagnosis in HIV-infected patients using urine and sputum samples. *PLoS One,* Mar 24; 5(3): e9848

Dheda K, Smit RZ, Badri M, & Pai M. (2009). T-cell interferon-gamma release assays for the rapid immunodiagnosis of tuberculosis: clinical utility in high-burden vs. low-burden settings. *Curr Opin Pulm Med,* 15: 188–200

Dheda K, Van-Zyl Smit RN, Sechi LA, Badri M, & Meldau R, et al. Clinical diagnostic utility of IP-10 and LAM antigen levels for the diagnosis of tuberculous pleural effusions in a high burden setting. *PLoS One,* 4: e4689

Diacon AH, Maritz JS, Venter A, van Helden PD, Andries K, McNeeley DF, & Donald PR. (2010). Time to detection of the growth of Mycobacterium tuberculosis in MGIT 960 for determining the early bactericidal activity of antituberculosis agents. *Eur J Clin Microbiol Infect Dis,* Dec; 29(12): 1561-5. Epub 2010 Sep 4

Diel R, Loddenkemper R, Meywald-Walter K, Gottschalk R, & Nienhaus A. (2009). Comparative performance of tuberculin skin test, QuantiFERON-TB-Gold In Tube assay, and T-Spot.TB test in contact investigations for tuberculosis. *Chest,* 135(4): 1010–1018. doi: 10.1378/chest.08-2048)

Dinnes J, Deeks J, Kunst H, Gibson A, Cummins E, Waugh N, Drobniewski F, & Lalvani A. (2007). A systematic review of rapid diagnostic tests for the detection of tuberculosis. *Health Technol Assess,* 11(3): 1-196

Dogan E, Erkoc R, Sayarlioglu H, & Uzun K. (2005). Tuberculin skin test results and booster phenomenon in two-step tuberculin skin testing in hemodialysis patients. *Ren Fail,* 27(4): 425-8

Dominguez J, De Souza-Galvao M, Ruiz-Manzano J, Latorre I, Prat C, Lacoma A, Mila C, Jimenez MA, Blanco S, & Maldonado J, et al. (2009). T-cell responses to the mycobacterium tuberculosis-specific antigens in active tuberculosis patients at the beginning, during, and after antituberculosis treatment. *Diagn Microbiol Infect Dis,* 63:43–51

Dosanjh DP, Hinks TS, Innes JA, Deeks JJ, & Pasvol G, et al. (2008). Improved diagnostic evaluation of suspected tuberculosis. *Ann Intern Med,* 148:325–336

Dowdy DW, O'Brien MA, & Bishai D. (2008). Cost-effectiveness of novel diagnostic tools for the diagnosis of tuberculosis. *Int J Tuberc Lung Dis,* 12: 1021–1029

El-Masry S, El-Kady I, Zaghloul MH, Al-Badrawey MK. (2008). Rapid and simple detection of a mycobacterium circulating antigen in serum of pulmonary tuberculosis patients by using a monoclonal antibody and Fast-Dot-ELISA. *Clin Biochem,* 41(3): 145-151

Elliott AM, Halwiindi B, Hayes RJ, Luo N, & Tembo G, et al. (1993) The impact of human immunodeficiency virus on presentation and diagnosis of tuberculosis in a cohort study in Zambia. *J Trop Med Hyg,* 96: 1–113

Escamilla L, Mancilla R, Glender W, & López-Marín LM. (1996). Mycobacterium fortuitum glycolipids for the serodiagnosis of pulmonary tuberculosis. *Am J Respir Crit Care Med,* 154: 1864-1867

Ewer K, Deeks J, & Alvarez L, et al. (2003). A comparison of T-cell-based assay with tuberculin skin test for diagnosis of Mycobacterium tuberculosis infection in a school tuberculosis outbreak. *Lancet,* 361:1168-1173

Farhat M, Greenaway C, Pai M, & Menzies D. (2006). False-positive tuberculin skin tests: what is the absolute effect of BCG and non-tuberculous mycobacteria? *Int J Tuberc Lung Dis,* Nov;10(11):1192-204

FDA. 2005. Approval for the use of synthetic peptide antigens used in the QuantiFERON-TB Gold. P10033/S0006 www.fda.gov/cdrh/pma/pmadec04.html

Fine PEM. (1995). Variation in protection by BCG: implications of and for heterologous immunity. *Lancet,* 346: 1339-1345

Flynn JL, Chan J, Triebold KJ, Dalton DK, Stewart TA, & Bloom BR. (1993). An essential role for interferon-gamma resistance to mycobacterium tuberculosis infection. *J Exp Med,* 178: 2249-54

Franco-Álvarez de Luna F, Ruiz P, Gutiérrez J, & Casal M. (2006). Evaluation of the GenoType Mycobacteria Direct assay for detection of Mycobacterium tuberculosis complex and four atypical mycobacterial species in clinical samples. *J Clin Microbiol,* 44:3025-7

Frieden TR, Sterling TR, Munsiff SS, Watt CJ, & Dye C. Tuberculosis. Lancet. 2003;362(9387):887–899. doi: 10.1016/S0140-6736(03)14333-4) (Rapid diagnostic tests for tuberculosis: what is the appropriate use? American Thoracic Society Workshop. Am J Respir Crit Care Med. 1997;155(5):1804–1814),

Fukazawa K. (2007). Application and problems of QuantiFERON TB-2G for tuberculosis control programs: (1) Tuberculosis outbreak in a Cram school. *Kekkaku,* 82(1): 53-59

Gallegos AM, Pamer EG, & Glickman MS. (2008). Delayed protection by ESAT-6-specific effector CD4+ cells after airborne M. tuberculosis infection. *J Exp Med,* 205(10): 2359-2368

Gangane N, Anshu, & Singh R. (2008). Role of modified bleach method in staining of acid-fast bacilli in lymph node aspirates. *Acta Cytol,* May-Jun;52(3):325-8

Gebauer BS, Hricik DE, & Atallah A, et al. (2002). Evolution of the enzyme-linked immunosorbent spot assay for post-transplant alloreactivity as a potentially useful immune monitoring tool. *Am J Transplant,* 2, 857-866

Gérôme P, Fabre M, Soler CP, De Pina JJ, Simon F. (2009). Comparison of the mycobacteria growth indicator tube with solid culture for the detection of tuberculosis complex mycobacteria from blood. *Pathol Biol (Paris),* Feb; 57(1): 44-50. Epub 2008 Jun 30

Goessens WHF, de Man P, Koeleman GM, Luijendijk A, te Witt R, Endtz HP, van & Belkum A. (2005). Comparison of the COBAS AMPLICOR MTB and BDProbeTec ET assays for detection of Mycobacterium tuberculosis in respiratory specimens. *J Clin Microbiol,* 43:2563-6

Goletti D, Butera O, Bizzoni F, Casetti R, Girardi E, & Poccia F. (2006). Region of difference 1 antigen-specific CD4+ memory T cells correlate with a favorable outcome of tuberculosis. *J Infect Dis,* 194(7), 984-92

Gounder CR, Kufa T, Wada NI, Mngomezulu V, Charalambous S, Hanifa Y, Fielding K, Grant A, Dorman S, Chaisson RE, & Churchyard GJ. (2011). Diagnostic accuracy of a urine lipoarabinomannan enzyme-linked immunosorbent assay for screening ambulatory HIV-infected persons for TB. *J Acquir Immune Defic Syndr,* ePub ahead of print on Jul 13

Guerra RL, Hooper NM, Baker JF, Alborz R, Armstrong DT, Maltas G, Kiehlbauch JA, & Dorman SE. (2007).Use of the amplified mycobacterium tuberculosis direct test in a public health laboratory: test performance and impact on clinical care. *Chest*, 132:946-951

Haldar S, Chakravorty S, Bhalla M, De Majumdar S, & Tyagi JS. (2007). Simplified detection of Mycobacterium tuberculosis in sputum using smear microscopy and PCR with molecular beacons. *J Med Microbiol*, 56, 1356-62

Hamasur B, Bruchfeld J, Haile M, Pawlowski A, & Bjorvatn B, et al. (2001). Rapid diagnosis of tuberculosis by detection of mycobacterial lipoarabinomannan in urine. *J Microbiol Methods*, 45:41-52

Han M, Yue J, Lian YY, Zhao YL, Wang HX, & Liu LR. (2011). Relationship between single nucleotide polymorphism of interleukin-18 and susceptibility to pulmonary tuberculosis in the Chinese Han population. *Microbiol Immunol*, Jun; 55(6): 388-93

Han YM, Kim HS, Kim CH, Kang HJ, & Lee KM. Analysis of patients with positive acid-fast bacilli culture and negative T-SPOT.TB results. *Korean J Lab Med*, Aug; 30(4): 414-9

Hanna BA, Ebrahimzadeh A, & Elliott LB, et al. (1999). Multicenter evaluation of the BACTEC MGIT 960 system for recovery of mycobacteria. *J Clin Microbiol*, 37: 748–52

Harada N, Higuchi K, Yoshiyama T, Kawabe Y, & Fujita A, et al. (2008). Comparison of the sensitivity and specificity of two whole blood interferon-gamma assays for M. tuberculosis infection. *J Infect*, 56: 348–353

Harada N. (2006). Characteristics of a diagnostic method for tuberculosis infection based on whole blood interferon-gamma assay. *Kekkaku*, 81(11): 681-6

Harboe M, Oettinger T, Wiker HG, Rosenkrands I, & Andersen P. (1996). Evidence for occurrence of the ESAT-6 protein in Mycobacterium tuberculosis and virulent Mycobacterium bovis and for its absence in Mycobacterium bovis BCG. *Infect Immun*, 64: 16-22

Harries AD, Maher D, & Nunn P. (1997). Practical and affordable measures for the protection of health care workers from tuberculosisin low-income countries. *Bull World Health Organ*, 75: 477–89

Harris A. (2004). What is the additional yield from repeated sputum examinations by microscopy and culture? In: *Tuberculosis Case detection. Treatment and monitoring*. 2nd ed. Frieden TR (Ed.), 46-50, World Health Organization, Geneva.

Heeger PS, Greenspan NS, Kuhlenschmidt S, Dejelo C, Hricik DE, & Schulak JA. (2001). Pretransplant frequency of donor-specific, IFN-gamma-producing lymphocytes is a manifestation of immunologic memory and correlates with the risk of posttransplant rejection episodes. *J Immunol*, 163: 2267-75

Hill PC, Brookes RH, & Fox A, et al. (2004). Large-scale evaluation of enzyme-linked immunospot assay and skin test for diagnosis of Mycobacterium tuberculosis infection against a gradient of exposure in the Gambia. *Clin Infect Dis*, 38(7): 966-73

Hill PC, Fox A, Jeffries DJ, Jackson-Sillah D, Lugos MD, & Owiafe PK, et al. (2005). Quantitative T cell assay reflects infectious load of Mycobacterium tuberculosis in an endemic case contact model. *Clin Infect Dis*, Jan 15; 40(2): 273–8

Hobby GL, Holman AP, Iseman MD, & Jones JM. (1973). Enumeration of tubercle bacilli in sputum of patients with pulmonary tuberculosis. *Antimicrob Agents Chemother*, 4(2), 94-104

Hofmann-Thiel S, Turaev L, & Hoffmann H. 2010. Evaluation of the hyplex TBC PCR test for detection of Mycobacterium tuberculosis complex in clinical samples. *BMC Microbiol,* 2010 Mar 31;10:95

Honscha G, Von Groll A, & Valença M, et al. (2008). The laboratory as a tool to qualify tuberculosis diagnosis. *Int J Tuberc Lung Dis,* 12(2): 218-20

Hooja S, Pal N, Malhotra B, Goyal S, Kumar V, & Vyas L. (2011). Comparison of Ziehl Neelsen & Auramine O staining methods on direct and concentrated smears in clinical specimens. *Indian J Tuberc,* Apr; 58(2): 72-6

Hooper CE, Lee YC, & Maskell NA. (2009). Interferon-gammarelease assays for the diagnosis of TB pleural effusions: hype or real hope? *Curr Opin Pulm Med,* 15 (4): 358-65

Houghton RL, Lodes MJ, & Dillon DC, et al. (2002). Use of multiepitope polyproteins in serodiagnosis of active tuberculosis. *Clin Diagn Lab Immunol,* 9: 883-91

Huebner RE, Schein MF, Bass JB Jr. The tuberculin skin test. Clin Infect Dis. 17(6), 968-975 (1993).

Im JG, Webb WR, Han MC, & Park JH. (1991). Apical opacity associated with pulmonary tuberculosis: high-resolution CT findings. *Radiology,* 178(3): 727–31

Imaz MS, Comini MA, & Zerbini E, et al. (2001). Evaluation of the diagnostic value of measuring IgG, IgM and IgA antibodies to the recombinant 16-kilodalton antigen of M. tuberculosis in childhood tuberculosis. *Int J Tuberc Lung Dis,* 5,1036-43 (2001).

International Union Against Tuberculosis and Lung Disease. (1996). *Tuberculosis Guide for Low Income Countries, 4th ed.* International Union Against Tuberculosis and Lung Disease, Paris.

Jafari C, Ernst M, Kalsdorf B, Greinert U, Diel R, Kirsten D, Marienfeld K, Lalvani A, & Lange C. (2006). Rapid diagnosis of smear-negative tuberculosis by bronchoalveolar lavage enzyme-linked immunospot. *Am J Respir Crit Care,*174:1048-54

Jafari C, Thijsen S, Sotgiu G, Goletti D, Domínguez Benítez JA, Losi M, Eberhardt R, Kirsten D, Kalsdorf B, Bossink A, Latorre I, Migliori GB, Strassburg A, Winteroll S, Greinert U, Richeldi L, Ernst M, & Lange C. (2009). Tuberculosis Network European Trialsgroup. Bronchoalveolar lavage enzyme-linked immunospot for a rapid diagnosis of tuberculosis: a Tuberculosis Network European Trialsgroup study. *Am J Respir Crit Care,* Oct 1; 180(7): 666-73. Epub 2009 Jul 9

Jiang W, Shao L, Zhang Y, Zhang S, Meng C, Xu Y, Huang L, Wang Y, Wang Y, Weng X, & Zhang W. (2009). High-sensitive and rapid detection of Mycobacterium tuberculosis infection by IFN-gamma release assay among HIV-infected individuals in BCG-vaccinated area. *BMC Immunol,* 10: 31

Joh JS, Lee CH, & Lee JE, et al. (2007).The interval between initiation of anti-tuberculosis treatment in patients with culture-positive pulmonary tuberculosis and receipt of drug-susceptibility test results. *J Korean Med Sci,* 22(1): 26-29

Kabeer BSA, Raman B, Thomas A, Perumal V, & Raja A. Role of QuantiFERON-TB Gold, Interferon Gamma Inducible Protein-10 and Tuberculin Skin Test in Active Tuberculosis Diagnosis. PLoS ONE. 2010;5:9051-7) (Pia M, Zwerling A, Menzies D. Systematic review: T-cell-based assays for the diagnosis of latent tuberculosis infections; an update. Ann Intern Med. 2008;149:177-184)

Kabra SK, Lodha R, & Seth V. (2004). Some current concepts on childhood tuberculosis. *Indian J Med Res*, 120(4): 387-97

Kadival GV, D'Souza CD, Kolk AH, & Samuel AM. (1995). Polymerase chain reaction in the diagnosis of tuberculosis. Comparison of two target sequences for amplification. *Zentralbl Bakteriol*, 282(4): 353-61

Kampmann B, Hemingway C, Stephens A, Davidson R, & Goodsall A, et al. (2005). Acquired predisposition to mycobacterial disease due to autoantibodies to IFN-gamma. *J Clin Invest*, 115:2480–8

Kampmann B, Whittaker E, Williams A, Walters S, Gordon A, Martinez-Alier N, Williams B, Crook AM, Hutton AM, & Anderson ST. (2009). Interferon-gamma release assays do not identify more children with active tuberculosis than tuberculin skin test, *Eur Respir J*, 33 (6), 1250-3

Kang YA, Lee HW, & Yoon HI, et al. (2005). Discrepancy between the tuberculin skin test and the whole-blood interferon gamma assay for diagnosis of latent tuberculosis infection in an intermediate tuberculosis-burden country. *JAMA*, 293: 2756-61

Kang YA, Lee, HW, & Hwang SS, et al. (2007). Usefulness of whole-blood interferon-gamma assay and interferon-gamma enzyme-linked immunospot assay in the diagnosis of active pulmonary tuberculosis. *Chest*, 132(3): 959-65

Kanunfre KA, Leite OH, Lopes MI, Litvoc M, & Ferreira AW. (2008). Enhancement of diagnostic efficiency by a gamma interferon release assay for pulmonary tuberculosis. *Clin Vaccine Immunol*,15(6): 1028-30

Katsenos S, Nikolopoulou M, Gartzonika C, Manda-Stachouli C, Gogali A, Grypaiou C, Mavridis A, Constantopoulos SH, & Daskalopoulos G. (2011). Use of interferon-gamma release assay for latent tuberculosis infection screening in older adults exposed to tuberculosis in a nursing home. *J Am Geriatr Soc*, May; 59(5): 858-62

Kawabe Y. (2007). Application and problems of quantiFERON TB-2G for tuberculosis control programs--(2) clinical use of quantiFERON TB-2G. *Kakkaku*, 82(1): 61-66

Kehinde AO, Obaseki FA, Cadmus SI, & Bakare RA. (2005). Diagnosis of tuberculosis: urgent need to strengthen laboratory services. *J Natl Med Assoc*, Mar;97(3):394-6

Kent PT, Kubica GP. (1985). Public health mycobacteriology: a guide for the level III laboratory. Atlanta, GA, USA: Centers for Disease Control, 1985).

Khawcharoenporn T, Apisarnthanarak A, Sungkanuparph S, Woeltje KF, Fraser VJ. (2011). Tuberculin skin test and isoniazid prophylaxis among health care workers in high tuberculosis prevalence areas. *Int J Tuberc Lung Dis*, Jan; 15(1): 14-23

Kibiki GS, Mulder B, & van der Ven AJ, et al. (2007). Laboratory diagnosis of pulmonary tuberculosis in TB and HIV endemic settings and the contribution of real time PCR for M. tuberculosis in bronchoalveolar lavage fluid. *Trop Med Int Health*, 12(10): 1210-7

Kim HJ, Yoon HI, Park KU, Lee CT, & Lee JH. (2011). The impact of previous tuberculosis history on T-SPOT.TB interferon-gamma release assay results. *Int J Tuberc Lung Dis*, Apr; 15(4): 510-6

Kim HS, Kim CH, Hur M, Hyun IG, Park MJ, Song W, Park JY, Kang HJ, & Lee KM. (2010). Clinical usefulness of T-SPOT.TB test for the diagnosis of tuberculosis. *Korean J Lab Med*, Apr; 30(2): 171-7

Kim SH, Choi SJ, Kim HB, Kim NJ, Oh MD, & Choe KW. (2007). Diagnostic usefulness of a T-cell based assay for extrapulmonary tuberculosis. *Arch Intern Med,* 167(20): 2255-9

Kobashi Y, Mouri K, & Yagi S, et al. (2008). Usefulness of the QuantiFERON-TB 2G test for the differential diagnosis of pulmonary tuberculosis. *Intern Med,* 47(4): 237-43

Kobashi Y, Mouri K, Obase Y, Fukuda M, Miyashita N, & Oka M. (2007). Clinical evaluation of QuantiFERON TB-2G test for immunocompromised patients. *Eur Respir J,* 30(5): 945-50

Kobashi Y, Obase Y, Fakuda M, Yoshida K, Miyashita N, Oka M. (2006). Clinical revaluation of the QuantiFERON TB-2G test as a diagnostic methods for differentiating active tuberculosis from nontuberculous mycobacteriosis. Clin Infect Dis, 43: 1540-6

Kobashi Y, Sugiu T, Shimizu H, Ohue Y, Mouri K, Obase Y, Miyashita N, & Oka M. (2009). Clinical evaluation of the T-SPOT.TB test for patients with indeterminate results on the QuantiFERON TB-2G test. *Intern Med,* 48(3): 137-42. Epub 2009 Feb 2

Komiya K, Ariga H, Nagai H, Kurashima A, Shoji S, Ishii H, & Nakajima Y. (2011). Reversion rates of QuantiFERON-TB Gold are related to pre-treatment IFN-gamma levels. *J Infect,* Jul; 63(1): 48-53. Epub 2011 May 17

Kumar VG, Urs TA, & Ranganath RR. (2011). MPT 64 Antigen detection for Rapid confirmation of M.tuberculosis isolates. *BMC Res Notes,* Mar 24; 4: 79

Laal S, Samanich KM, & Sonnenberg MG, et al. (1997). Surrogate marker of preclinical tuberculosis in human immunodeficiency virus infection: antibodies to an 88-kDa secreted antigen of Mycobacterium tuberculosis. *J Infect Dis,* 176: 133-143

Lai CC, Tan CK, Lin SH, Liao CH, Huang YT, Wang CY, Wang JY, Lin HI, & Hsueh PR. (2010). Diagnostic value of an enzyme-linked immunospot assay for interferon-γ in genitourinary tuberculosis. *Diagn Microbiol Infect Dis,* Nov; 68(3): 247-50. Epub 2010 Sep 17).

Lai CC, Tan CK, Lin SH, Liu WL, Liao CH, Huang YT, & Hsueh PR. (2011). Diagnostic value of an enzyme-linked immunospot assay for interferon-γ in cutaneous tuberculosis. *Diagn Microbiol Infect Dis,* May; 70(1): 60-4

Lalvani A, Brookes R, & Wilkinson RJ, et al. (1998). Human cytolytic and interferon gamma-secreting CD8+ T lymphocytes specific for Mycobacterium tuberculosis. *Proc Natl Acad Sci USA,* 95: 270-5

Lalvani A, Hill AV. (1998). Cytotoxic T-lymphocytes against malaria and tuberculosis: from natural immunity to vaccine design. *Clin Sci (Lond),* 95, 531-8

Lalvani A, Nagvenkar P, & Udwadia Z, et al. (2001). Enumeration of T cells specific for RD1-encoded antigens suggests a high prevalence of latent Mycobacterium tuberculosis infection in healthy urban Indians. *J Infect Dis,* 183: 469-77

Lalvani A, Pareek M. (2010). Interferon gamma release assays: principles and practice. *Enferm Infect Microbiol Clin,* Apr;28(4):245-52. Epub 2009 Sep 24

Lalvani A, Pathan AA, & Durkan H, et al. (2001). Enhanced contact tracing and spatial tracing of M. tuberculosis infection by enumeration of antigen-specific T cells. *Lancet,* 357: 2017-21

Lalvani A, Pathan AA, & McShane H, et al. (2001). Rapid detection of M. tuberculosis infection by enumeration of antigen-specific T cells. *Am J Resir Crit Care Med,* 163, 824-8

Lalvani A. (2007). Diagnosing tuberculosis infection in the 21st century: new tools to tackle an old enemy. *Chest*, 131(6): 1898-1906

Landis JR, Koch GG. (1977). The measurement of observer agreement for categorical data. *Biometrics*, 33(1):159–174

Laszlo A, Gill P, Handzel V, Hodgkin MM, & Helbecque DM. (1983). Conventional and radiometric drug susceptibility testing of Mycobacterium tuberculosis complex. *J Clin Microbiol*, 18(6):1335–9

Latorre I, De Souza-Galvao M, Ruiz-Manzano J, Lacoma A, Prat C, Fuenzalida L, Altet N, Ausina V, & Dominguez J. (2009). Quantitative evaluation of T-cell response after specific antigen stimulation in active and latent tuberculosis infection in adults and children. *Diagn Microbiol Infect Dis*, 65:236–246

Latorre I, Martínez-Lacasa X, Font R, Lacoma A, Puig J, Tural C, Lite J, Prat C, Cuchi E, Ausina V, & Domínguez J. (2010). IFN-γ response on T-cell based assays in HIV-infected patients for detection of tuberculosis infection. *BMC Infect Dis*, Dec 10; 10: 348

Lawn SD, Edwards DJ, Kranzer K, Vogt M, Bekker LG, & Wood R. (2009). Urine lipoarabinomannan assay for tuberculosis screening before antiretroviral therapy diagnostic yield and association with immune reconstitution disease. *AIDS*, 2009 Sep 10; 23(14): 1875-80

Lee E, Holzman RS. (2002). Evolution and current use of the tuberculin test. *Clin Infect Dis*, 34: 365-370

Lee JE, Kim HJ, & Lee SW. (2011). The clinical utility of tuberculin skin test and interferon-γ release assay in the diagnosis of active tuberculosis among young adults: a prospective observational study. *BMC Infect Dis*, Apr 18; 11: 96

Lee JJ, Suo J, Lin CB, Wang JD, Lin TY, & Tsai YC. (2003). Comparative evaluation of the Bactec MGIT 960 system with solid medium for isolation of mycobacteria. *Int J Tuberc Lung Dis*, 7: 569–574

Lee JS, Jo EK, & Noh YK, et al. (2008). Diagnosis of pulmonary tuberculosis using MTB12 and 38-kDa antigens. *Respirology*, 13(3): 432-7

Lee SW, Jang YS, Park CM, Kang HY, Koh WJ, Yim JJ, & Jeon K. (2010). The role of chest CT scanning in TB outbreak investigation. *Chest*, May;137(5):1057-64

Legesse M, Ameni G, Mamo G, Medhin G, Bjune G, & Abebe F. (2010). Performance of QuantiFERON-TB Gold In-Tube (QFTGIT) for the diagnosis of Mycobacterium tuberculosis (Mtb) infection in Afar Pastoralists, Ethiopia. *BMC Infect Dis*, Dec 17; 10: 354

Legesse M, Ameni G, Mamo G, Medhin G, Bjune G, & Abebe F. (2011). Community-based cross-sectional survey of latent tuberculosis infection in Afar pastoralists, Ethiopia, using QuantiFERON-TB Gold In-Tube and tuberculin skin test. *BMC Infec Dis*, Apr 9;11:8

Lewinsohn DA, Gennaro ML, Scholvinck L, & Lewinsohn DM. (2004).Tuberculosis immunology in children: diagnostic and therapeutic challenges and opportunities. *Int J Tuberc Lung Dis*, 8(5): 658– 74

Leyten EM, Prins C, & Bossink AW, et al. (2007). Effect of tuberculin skin testing on a Mycobacterium tuberculosis 1212-6s-specific interferon-gamma assay. *Eur Respir J*, 29(6): 1212-6

Lighter-Fisher J, Peng CH, & Tse DB. (2010). Cytokine responses to QuantiFERON® peptides, purified protein derivative and recombinant ESAT-6 in children with tuberculosis. *Int J Tuberc Lung Dis,* Dec; 14(12): 1548-55

Ling DI, Flores LL, & Pai M. (2008). Commercial nucleic-acid amplification tests for diagnosis of pulmonary tuberculosis in respiratory specimens: meta-analysis and meta-regression. *PLoS One,* 3:e1536

Liu KT, Su WJ, & Perng RP. (2007). Clinical utility of polymerase chain reaction for diagnosis of smear-negative pleural tuberculosis. *J Clin Med Assoc,* 70(4): 146-151.

Lu D, Heeren B, & Dunne WM. (2002). Comparison of the Automated Mycobacteria Growth Indicator Tube System (BACTEC 960/MGIT) with Löwenstein-Jensen medium for recovery of mycobacteria from clinical specimens. *Am J Clin Pathol,* Oct;118(4): 542-5

Lyu J, Lee SG, Hwang S, Lee SO, Cho OH, Chae EJ, Lee SD, Kim WS, Kim DS, & Shim TS. (2011). Chest CT is more likely to show latent tuberculosis foci than simple chest radiography in liver transplantation candidates. *Liver Transpl,* Apr 19. doi: 10.1002/lt.22319. [Epub ahead of print

Mabaera B, Lauritsen JM, Katamba A, Laticevschi D, & Naranbat N, et al. (2007) Sputum smear positive tuberculosis: empiric evidence challenges the need for confirmatory smears. *Int J Tuber Lung Dis,* 11: 959–64

Madariaga MG, Jalali Z, & Swindells S. (2007). Clinical Utility of Interferon Gamma Assay in the Diagnosis of Tuberculosis. *J Am Board Fam Med,* 20:540–547. doi: 10.3122/jabfm.2007.06.070109)

Magana-Arachchi D, Perera J, Gamage S, & Chandrasekharan V. (2008). Low cost in-house PCR for the routine diagnosis of extra-pulmonary tuberculosis. *Int J Tuberc Lung Dis,* 12(3): 275-80

Mancuso JD, Tobler SK, Keep LW. (2008). Pseudoepidemics of TST conversions in the U.S. Army after recent deployments. *Am J Respir Crit Care Med.* 177(11):1285-9. (Epub Mar 20, 2008.)

Mandalakas AM, Hesseling AC, & Chegou NN, et al. High level of discordant IGRA results in HIV-infected adults and children. *Int J Tuberc Lung Di,* 12(4):417– 423

Manjunath N, Shankar P, Rajan L, Bhargava A, Saluja S, & Shriniwas. (1991). Evaluation of a polymerase chain reaction for the diagnosis of tuberculosis. *Tubercle,* 72: 21-27

Marais BJ, Pai M. (2007). Recent advances in the diagnosis of childhood tuberculosis. Arch Dis Child. 92(5): 446-452 (2007).

Mase SR, Ramsay A, Henry M, Ng V, & Hopewell PC, et al. (2007). The incremental yield of serial sputum smears in the diagnosis of tuberculosis: asystematic review. *Int J Tuber Lung Dis,* 11: 485–95

Mazurek GH, Jereb J, & Lobue P, et al. (2005). Guidelines for using the QuantiFERON-TB Gold test for detecting Mycobacterium tuberculosis infection, United States. *MMWR Recomm Rep,* 54(RR-15): 49-55

Mazurek GH, Jereb J, Vernon A, LoBue P, Goldberg S, Castro K; IGRA Expert Committee; Centers for Disease Control and Prevention (CDC). (2010). Updated guidelines for using Interferon Gamma Release Assays to detect Mycobacterium tuberculosis infection - United States, 2010. *MMWR Recomm Rep,* Jun 25; 59(RR-5): 1-25

Mazurek M, Jereb J, Vernon A, LoBue P, Goldberg S, & Castro K. Updated guidelines for using interferon gamma release assays to detect Mycobacterium tuberculosis infection – United States, 2010. *MMWR Recomm Rep*, 59(RR-5): 1–25

Menzies D, Pai M, & Comstock G. (2007). Meta-analysis: new tests for the diagnosis of latent tuberculosis infection: areas of uncertainty and recommendations for research. *Ann Intern Med*, 146(5), 340-54

Menzies D. (2000). What does tuberculin reactivity after bacille Calmette-Guerin vaccination tell us? *Clin Infect Dis*, 31 (Suppl 3): S71–74

Metchock BJ, Nolte FS, Wallace RJ Jr. (1999). Mycobacterium. In: *Manual of Clinical Microbiology*, Murray PR, Baron EJ, Pfaller MA, et al, eds. 7th ed. 399-437. ASM Press: Washington, DC.

Mfinanga GS, Ngadaya E, & Mtandu R, et al. The quality of sputum smear microscopy diagnosis of pulmonary tuberculosis in Dar es Salaam, Tanzania. *Tanzan Health Res Bull*, 9(3): 164-8

Middelkoop K, Bekker LG, Myer L, Dawson R, & Wood R. (2008). Rates of tuberculosis transmission to children and adolescents in a community with a high prevalence of HIV infection among adults. *Clin Infect Dis*, Aug 1; 47(3): 349-55

Minion J, Sohn H, & Pai M. (2009). Light-emitting diode technology for TB diagnosis: what is on the market? *Expert Rev Med Devices*,6: 341–5

Miorner H, Gebre N, & Karlsson U, et al. (1994). Diagnosis of pulmonary tuberculosis. *Lancet*, 344: 127

Miragliotta G, Antonetti R, Di Taranto A, Mosca A, & Del Prete R. (2005). Directdetection of Mycobacterium tuberculosis complex in pulmonary andextrapulmonary samples by BDProbeTec ET system. *New Microbiol*, 28: 67-73

Miret-Cuadras P, Pina-Gutierrez JM, & Juncosa S. (1996). Tuberculin reactivity in Bacillus Calmette-Guerin vaccinated subjects. *Tuber Lung Dis*, 77: 52–58

Mohan A, Pande JN, Sharma SK, Rattan A, Guleria R, & Khilnani GC. Bronchoalveolar lavage in pulmonary tuberculosis: a decision analysis approach. *QJM*, Apr;88(4):269-76

Morcillo N, Imperiale B, & Di Giulio B. (2010). Evaluation of MGIT 960 and the colorimetric-based method for tuberculosis drug susceptibility testing. *Int J Tuberc Lung Dis*, Sep; 14(9): 1169-75

Moreno S, Blazquez R, Novoa A, Carpena I, Menasalvas A, Ramirez C, & Guerrero C. (2001). The Effect of BCG Vaccination on Tuberculin Reactivity and the Booster Effect Among Hospital Employees. *Arch Intern Med*, 161:1760–1765. doi: 10.1001/archinte.161.14.1760).

Mori T, Sakatini M, & Yamagishi F, et al. (2004). Specific detection of tuberculosis infection: an interferon-gamma-based assay using new antigens. *Am J Respir Crit Care Med*, 170: 59-64

Munk ME, Arend SM, Brock I, Ottenhoff TH, & Andersen P. (2001). Use of ESAT-6 and CFP 10 antigens for diagnosis of extra-pulmonary tuberculosis. *J Infect Dis*, 183(1): 175-6

Murakami S, Takeno M, Kirino Y, Kobayashi M, Watanabe R, Kudo M, & Ihata A, et al. (2009). Screening of tuberculosis by interferon-gamma assay before biologic therapy for rheumatoid arthritis. *Tuberculosis*, 89: 139–41

Murray PR, Rosenthal KS, Kobayashi GS, et al. (1998). Mycobacterium. In: *Medical Microbiology*, Brown M, ed. 3rd ed. 319-330. Mosby: St Louis, MO

Muyoyeta M, de Haas PE, Mueller DH, van Helden PD, Mwenge L, Schaap A, Kruger C, van Pittius NC, Lawrence K, Beyers N, Godfrey-Faussett P, & Ayles H. (2010). Evaluation of the Capilia TB assay for culture confirmation of Mycobacterium tuberculosis infections in Zambia and South Africa. *J Clin Microbiol*, Oct; 48(10): 3773-5. Epub 2010 Aug 4

Nagi SS, Anand R, & Pasha ST, et al. (2007). Diagnostic potential of IS6110, 38kDa, 65kDa and 85B sequence-based polymerase chain reaction in the diagnosis of Mycobacterium tuberculosis in clinical samples. *Indian J Med Micobiol*, 25(1): 43-49

Nakanishi M, Demura Y, Ameshima S, Kosaka N, Chiba Y, Nishikawa S, Itoh H, & Ishizaki T. (2010). Utility of high-resolution computed tomography for predicting risk of sputum smear-negative pulmonary tuberculosis. *Eur J Radiol*, Mar: 545-50. Epub 2009 Jan 23

Newport MJ, Goetghebuer T, Weiss HA, Whittle H, & Siegrist CA, et al. (2004). Genetic regulation of immune responses to vaccines in early life. *Genes Immun*, 5: 122–129

Newton SM, Brent AJ, Anderson S, Whittaker E, & Kampmann B. (2008). Paediatric tuberculosis. *Lancet Infect Dis*, 8: 498–510

Ngamlert K, Sinthuwattanawibool C, McCarthy KD, Sohn H, Starks A, Kanjanamongkolsiri P, Anek-vorapong R, Tasaneeyapan T, Monkongdee P, Diem L, & Varma JK. (2009). Diagnostic performance and costs of Capilia TB for Mycobacterium tuberculosis complex identification from broth-based culture in Bangkok, Thailand. *Trop Med Int Health*, 2009 Jul;14(7):748-53. Epub 2009 Apr 23

Nicol M P, Davies M A, & Wood K, et al. (2009). Comparison of T-SPOT. TB assay and tuberculin skin test for the evaluation of young children at high risk for tuberculosis in a community setting. *Pediatrics*, 123: 38– 43

Nigussie M, Mamo G. (2010). Detection of acid fast bacilli (AFB) in tuberculous lymphadenitis among adult Ethiopians. *Ethiop Med J*, Oct; 48(4): 277-83

Nishimura T, Hasegawa N, & Mori M, et al. (2008). Accuracy of an interferon-gamma release assay to detect active pulmonary and extra-pulmonary tuberculosis. iInt J Tuberc Lung Dis, 12(3): 269-74

Noordhoek GT, Kaan JA, Mulder S, Wilke H, & Kolk AH. (1995). Routine application of the polymerase chain reaction for detection of Mycobacterium tuberculosis in clinical samples. *J Clin Pathol*, 48(9), 810-4

Oni T, Patel J, Gideon HP, Seldon R, Wood K, Hlombe Y, Wilkinson KA, Rangaka MX, Mendelson M, & Wilkinson RJ. (2010). Enhanced diagnosis of HIV-1-associated tuberculosis by relating T-SPOT.TB and CD4 counts. *Eur Respir J*, 2010 Sep;36(3):594-600. Epub 2010 Jan 14).

Ozekinci T, Ozbek E, & Celik Y. (2007). Comparison of tuberculin skin test and a specific T-cell-based test, T-Spot.TB, for the diagnosis of latent tuberculosis infection. *J Int Med Res*, Sep-Oct; 35(5): 696-703

Ozkutuk A, Kirdar S, Ozden S, & Esen N. (2006). Evaluation of Cobas Amplicor MTB test to detect Mycobacterium tuberculosis in pulmonary and extrapulmonary specimens. *New Microbiol*, 29:269-73

Oztürk N, Sürücüoğlu S, & Ozkütük N, et al. (2007). Comparison of interferon-gamma whole blood assay with tuberculin skin test for the diagnosis of tuberculosis infection in tuberculosis contacts. *Mikrobiyol Bul,* 41(2): 193-202

Pai M, Joshi R, Bandyopadhyay M, Narang P, Dogra S, Taksande B, & Kalantri S. (2007). Sensitivity of a whole-blood Interferon-gamma assay among patients with pulmonary Tuberculosis and variation in T-cell responses during anti-Tuberculosis treatment. *Infection,* 35(2): 98-108

Pai M, Kalantri S, & Dheda K. (2006). New tools and emerging technologies for the diagnosis of tuberculosis: part I. Latent tuberculosis. *Expert Rev Mol Diagn,* 6: 413-22

Pai M, Riley LW, & Colford JM Jr. (2004). Interferon-gamma assays in the immunodiagnosis of tuberculosis: a systemic review. *Lancet Infect Dis,* 4(12): 761-776

Pai M, Zwerling A, & Menzies D. (2008). Systematic review: T-cell-based assays for the diagnosis of latent tuberculosis infection: an update. *Ann Intern Med,* 149(3):177–184

Pai M. (2004). The accuracy and reliability of nucleic acid amplification tests in the diagnosis of tuberculosis. *Natl Med J India,*17(5): 233-236

Papay P, Eser A, Winkler S, Frantal S, Primas C, Miehsler W, Angelberger S, Novacek G, Mikulits A, Vogelsang H, & Reinisch W. (2011). Predictors of indeterminate IFN-γ release assay in screening for latent TB in inflammatory bowel diseases. *Eur J Clin Invest,* Mar 17

Park SY, Park YB, Choi JH, Lee JY, Kim JS, & Mo EK. (2009). The diagnostic value of interferon-γ assay in patients with active tuberculosis. *Tuberc Respir Dis,* 66:13–19

Patel VB, Bhigjee AI, Paruk HF, Singh R, Meldau R, et al. (2009). Utility of a novel lipoarabinomannan assay for the diagnosis of tuberculous meningitis in a resource-poor high-HIV prevalence setting. *Cerebrospinal Fluid Res,* 6:13

Patel VB, Singh R, Connolly C, Coovadia Y, Peer AK, Parag P, Kasprowicz V, Zumla A, Ndung'u T, & Dheda K. (2010). Cerebrospinal T-cell responses aid in the diagnosis of tuberculous meningitis in a human immunodeficiency virus- and tuberculosis-endemic population. *Am J Respir Crit Care Med.* Aug 15;182(4):569-77. Epub 2010 May 4)

Patil SA, Gourie-Devi M, & Anand AR, et al. (1996). Significance of mycobacterial immune-complex (IgG) in the diagnosis of tuberculin meningitis. *Tuber Lung Dis,* 77:164-7

Pavić I, Zrinski Topić R, Raos M, Aberle N, & Dodig S. (2011) May 12. Interferon- γ release assay for the diagnosis of latent tuberculosis in children younger than 5 years of age. *Pediatr Infect Dis J,* May 12 [Epub ahead of print]).

Pepper T, Joseph P, Mwenya C, et al. (2008). Normal chest radiography in pulmonary tuberculosis: implications for obtaining respiratory specimen cultures. *Int J Tuberc Lung Dis,* 12(4): 397-403

Perez-Stable EJ, Slutkin G. (1985). A demonstration of lack of variability among six tuberculin skin test readers. *Am J Public Health,* 75(11): 1341-3

Pérez-Then E, Shor-Posner G, Crandall L, & Wilkinson J. (2007). The relationship between nutritional and sociodemographic factors and the likelihood of children in th e Dominican Republic having a BCG scar. *Rev Panam Salud Publica,* Jun; 21(6): 365-72

Perkins MD. (2000). New diagnostic tools for tuberculosis. *Int J Tuberc Lung Dis,* 4(Suppl 2): S182-8

Pesanti EL. (1994). The negative tuberculin test. Tuberculin, HIV and anergy panels. *Am J Respir Crit Care Med*, 149:1699–709

Pfyffer GE. (1999). Nucleic acid amplification for mycobacterial diagnosis. *J Infect*, 39: 21-26

Piana F, Ruffo Codecasa L, Baldan R, Miotto P, Ferrarese M, & Cirillo DM. (2007). Use of T-SPOT.TB in latent tuberculosis infection diagnosis in general and immunosuppressed populations. *New Microbiol*, 30 (3), 286-90

Piersimoni C, Scarparo C, Piccoli P, Rigon A, Ruggiero G, Nista D, & Bornigia S. (2002). Performance assessment of two commercial amplification assays for direct detection of Mycobacterium tuberculosis complex from respiratory and extrapulmonary specimens. *J Clin Microbiol*, 40: 4138-42

Ponce de Leon D, Acevedo-Vasquez E, Alvizuri S, Gutierrez C, Cucho M, & Alfaro J, et al. (2008). Comparison of an interferon-gamma assay with tuberculin skin testing for detection of tuberculosis (TB) infection in patients with rheumatoid arthritis in a TB-endemic population. *J Rheumatol*, 35: 776–81

Ponce de Leon D, Acevedo-Vasquez E, Sanchez-Torres A, Cucho M, Alfaro J, & Perich R, et al. (2005). Attenuated response to purified protein derivative in patients with rheumatoid arthritis: study in a population with a high prevalence of tuberculosis. *Ann Rheum Dis*, 64: 1360–5

Pooran A, Booth H, Miller RF, Scott G, Badri M, Huggett JF, Rook G, Zumla A, & Dheda K. (2010). Different screening strategies (single or dual) for the diagnosis of suspected latent tuberculosis: a cost effectiveness analysis. *BMC Pulm Med*, Feb 22;10:7).

Powell RD 3rd, Whitworth WC, Bernardo J, Moonan PK, & Mazurek GH. (2011). Unusual interferon gamma measurements with QuantiFERON-TB Gold and QuantiFERON-TB Gold in-tube tests. *PLoS One*, 6(6):e20061. Epub 2011 Jun 8

Qiao D, Yang BY, Li L, Ma JJ, Zhang XL, Lao SH, & Wu CY. (2011). ESAT-6- and CFP-10-specific Th1, Th22 and Th17 cells in tuberculous pleurisy may contribute to the local immune response against Mycobacterium tuberculosis infection. *Scand J Immunol*, Apr; 73(4): 330-7

Raja A, Ranganathan UD, & Bethunaickan R. (2008). Improved diagnosis of pulmonary tuberculosis by detection of antibodies against multiple Mycobacterium tuberculosis antigens. *Diagn Microbiol Infect Dis*, 60(4), 361-8

Raja A, Uma Devi KR, Ramalingam B, & Brennan PJ. (2002). Immunoglobulin G, A and M responses in serum and circulating immune complexes elicited by the 16-kilodalton antigen of M. tuberculosis. *Clin Diag Lab Immunol*, 9(2), 308-12

Raja A, Uma Devi KR, Ramalingam B, & Brennan PJ. (2004). Improved diagnosis of pulmonary tuberculosis by detection of free and immune complex-bound ant -30 kDa antibodies. *Diagn Microbiol Infect Dis*, 50: 523-9

Ramalingam B, Uma DK, Swaminathan S, & Raja A. (2002). Isotype-specific antibody response in childhood tuberculosis against purified 38 kDa antigen of M. tuberculosis. *J Trop Pediatr*, 48: 188-9

Ramsay A, Bonnet M, Gagnidze L, Githui W, & Varaine F, et al. (2009). Sputum, sex and scanty smears: New case-definition may reduce sex disparities in smear-positive tuberculosis. *Int J Tuber Lung Dis*, 13: 613–9

Rangaka MX, Wilkinson KA, Seldon R, Van Cutsem G, Meintjes GA, Morroni C, Mouton P, Diwakar L, Connell TG, Maartens G, & Wilkinson RJ. (2007). Effect of HIV-1 infection on T-Cell-based and skin test detection of tuberculosis infection. *Am J Respir Crit Care Med*, 175: 514-20

Raviglione MC. (2003). The TB epidemic from 1992 to 2002. *Tuberculosis (Edinb)*, 83, 4-14

Ravn P, Demissie A, & Eguale T, et al. (1999). Human T cell responses to the ESAT-6 antigen from M. tuberculosis. *J Infect Dis*, 179(3): 637-45

Ravn P, Munk ME, & Andersen AB, et al. (2005). Prospective evaluation of a whole-blood test using Mycobacterium tuberculosis-specific antigens ESAT-6 and CFP-10 for diagnosis of active tuberculosis. *Clin Diagn Lab Immunol*, 12:491-6

Reischl U, Lehn N, Wolf H, & Naumann L. (1998). Clinical evaluation of automated COBAS AMPLICOR MTB assay for testing respiratory and nonrespiratory specimens. *J Clin Microbiol*, 36:2853-60

Ribeiro S, Dooley K, Hackman J, Loredo C, Efron A, & Chaisson RE, et al. (2009). T-SPOT.TB responses during treatment of pulmonary tuberculosis. *BMC Infect Dis*, 9: 23

Richeldi L, Ewer K, Losi M, et al. (2004). T-cell-based tracking of multidrug resistant tuberculosis infection after brief exposure. *Am J Respir Crit Care Med*, 170(3): 288-95

Richeldi L, Losi M, D'Amico R, Luppi M, Ferrari A, Mussini C, Codeluppi M, Cocchi S, Prati F, & Paci V, et al. (2009). Performance of tests for latent tuberculosis in different groups of immunocompromised patients. *Chest*,136: 198-204

Richeldi L. An update on the diagnosis of tuberculosis infection. (2006). *Am J Respir Crit Care Med*, n.d.: 736-47

Ritz N, Yau C, Connell TG, Tebruegge M, Leslie D, & Curtis N. (2011). Absence of interferon-gamma release assay conversion following tuberculin skin testing. *Int J Tuberc Lung Dis*, Jun;15(6): 767-9

Ruddy M, McHugh TD, & Dale JW, et al. (2002). Estimation of the rate of unrecognized cross-contamination with mycobacterium tuberculosis in London microbiology laboratories. *J Clin Microbiol*, 40(11): 4100-4

Runa F, Yasmin M, Hoq MM, Begum J, Rahman AS, Ahsan CR. (2011) Molecular versus conventional methods: clinical evaluation of different methods for the diagnosis of tuberculosis in Bangladesh. *J Microbiol Immunol Infect*, Apr; 44(2): 101-5. Epub 2011 Jan 14

Sahiratmadja E, Alisjahbana B, de Boer T, Adnan I, Maya A, Danusantoso H, Nelwan RH, Marzuki S, van der Meer JW, van Crevel R, van de Vosse E, & Ottenhoff TH. (2007). Dynamic changes in pro- and anti-inflammatory cytokine profiles and gamma interferon receptor signaling integrity correlate with tuberculosis disease activity and response to curative treatment. *Infect Immun*, Feb; 75(2): 820-9. Epub 2006 Dec 4

Salfinger M, Pfyffer GE. (1994). The new diagnostic Mycobacteriology laboratory. *Eur J Clin Microbiol Infect Dis*,13: 961-79

Santín Cerezales M, Benítez JD. (2011). Diagnosis of tuberculosis infection using interferon-γ-based assays. *Enferm Infecc Microbiol Clin*, Mar;29 Suppl 1:26-33

Sapkota BR, Ranjit C, & Macdonald M. (2007). Rapid differentiation of Mycobacterium tuberculosis and Mycobacterium leprae from sputum by polymerase chain reaction. *Nepal Med Coll J*, 9(1):12-16

Sauzullo I, Massetti AP, Mengoni F, Rossi R, Lichtner M, Ajassa C, Vullo V, & Mastroianni CM. (2011). Influence of previous tuberculin skin test on serial IFN-γ release assays. *Tuberculosis (Edinb)*, Jul; 91(4): 322-6. Epub 2011 Jun 12)

Schauf V, Rom WN, & Smith KA, et al. (1993). Cytokine gene activation and modified responsiveness to interleukin-2 in the blood of tuberculosis patients. *J Infect Dis,* 168: 1056–9

Sekiguchi J, Miyoshi-Akiyama T, & Augustynowicz-Kopeć E, et al. (2007). Detection of multidrug resistance in Mycobacterium tuberculosis. *J Clin Microbiol,* 45(1), 179-192

Sellam J, Hamdi H, Roy C, Baron G, Lemann M, & Puéchal X, et al. (2007). Comparison of in vitro-specific blood tests with tuberculin skin test for diagnosis of latent tuberculosis before anti-TNF therapy. *Ann Rheum Dis,* 66: 1610–5

Selwyn PA, Sckell BM, Alcabes P, Friedland GH, Klein RS, Schoenbaum EE. (1992). High risk of active tuberculosis in HIV-infected drug users with cutaneous anergy. *JAMA,* 268:504–9

Shams H, Weis SE, & Klucar P, et al. (2005). Enzyme-linked immunospot and tuberculin skin testing to detect latent tuberculosis infection. *Am J Respir Crit Care Med,* 172: 1161-8

Sinirtas M, Ozakin C, & Gedikoglu S. (2009). Evaluation of the fully automated BACTEC MGIT 960 system for testing susceptibility of Mycobacterium tuberculosis to front line antituberculosis drugs and comparison with the radiometric BACTEC 460 TB method. *Mikrobiyol Bul,* Jul;43(3):403-9.

Somoskovi A, Kodmon C, Lanstos A, Bártfai Z, Tamási L, & Füzy J, et al. (2000). Comparison of recoveries of Mycobacterium tuberculosis using the automated BACTEC MGIT 960 System, BACTEC 460 TB System and Lowenstein-Jensen Medium. *J Clin Microbiol,* 38:2395-7

Somoskvi A, Kidman C, & Lantos A, et al. (2000). Comparison of recoveries of Mycobacterium tuberculosis using the automated BACTEC MGIT 960 system, the BACTEC 460 TB system and Lowenstein-Jensen medium. *J Clin Microbiol* m 38: 2395–7

Somu N, Swaminathan S, Paramasivan CN, Vijayasekaran D, Chandrabhooshanam A, Vijayan VK, & Prabhakar R. (1995). Value of bronchoalveolar lavage and gastric lavage in the diagnosis of pulmonary tuberculosis in children. *Tuber Lung Dis,* Aug; 76(4): 295-9

Sørensen AL, Nagai S, Houen G, Andersen P, & Andersen AB. (1995). Purification and characterization of a low-molecular-mass T-cell antigen secreted by Mycobacterium tuberculosis. *Infect Immun,* 63: 1710-7

Soysal A, Torun T, Efe S, Gencer H, Tahaoglu K, & Bakir M. (2008). Evaluation of cut-off values of interferon -gamma-based assays in the diagnosis of M.tuberculosis infection. *Int J Tuberc Lung Dis,* 12: 50–6

Spyridis N, Chakraborty R, Sharland M, & Heath PT. (2007). Early diagnosis of tuberculosis using an INF-gamma assay in a child with HIV-1 infection and a very low CD4 count. *Scand J Infect Dis,* 39(10): 919-21

Starke J. (2009). Predictive values of blood tests to diagnose LTBI have not been established in children. *AAP News,* 30: 14

Stavri H, Ene L, Popa GL, Duiculescu D, Murgoci G, marica C, Ulea I, Cus G, & Popa MI. (2009). Comparison of tuberculin skin test with whole-blood interferon gamma assay and ELISA, in HIV positive children and adolescents with TB. *Roum Arch Microbiol Immunol,* 68(1), 14-19

Stefan DC, Dippenaar A, Detjen AK, Schaaf HS, Marais BJ, Kriel B, Loebenberg L, Walzl G, & Hesseling AC. (2010). Interferon-gamma release assays for the detection of Mycobacterium tuberculosis infection in children with cancer. *Int J Tuberc Lung Dis,* Jun; 14(6): 689-94

Stein CM, Zalwango S, Malone LL, Won S, Mayanja-Kizza H, Mugerwa RD, Leontiev DV, Thompson CL, Cartier KC, Elson RC, Iyengar SK, Boom WH, & Whalen CC. (2008). Genome Scan of M. tuberculosis infection and Disease in Ugandans. *PloS ONE,* 3(12), e4094

Steingart K R, Ng V, & Henry M, et al. (2006). Sputum processing methods to improve the sensitivity of smear microscopy for tuberculosis: a systematic review. *Lancet Infect Dis,* 6: 664–74

Steingart KR, Henry M, Ng V, Hopewell PC, & Ramsay A, et al. (2006) .Fluorescence versus conventional sputum smear microscopy for tuberculosis: a systematic review. *Lancet Inf Dis,* 6: 570–81

Steingart KR, Ng V, & Henry M, et al. (2006). Sputum processing methods to improve the sensitivity of smear microscopy for tuberculosis: a systematic review. *Lancet Infect Dis,* 6(10): 664-74

Steingart KR, Ramsay A, & Pai M. (2007). Optimizing sputum smear microscopy for the diagnosis of pulmonary tuberculosis. *Expert Rev Anti Infect Ther,* 5: 327–31

Stephan C, Wolf T, Goetsch U, Bellinger O, Nisius G, Oremek G, Rakus Z, Gottschalk R, Stark S, Brodt HR, & Staszewski S. (2008). Comparing QuantiFERON-tuberculosis gold, T-SPOT tuberculosis and tuberculin skin test in HIV-infected individuals from a low prevalence tuberculosis country. *AIDS,* 22: 2471–9

Sun L, Yan HM, Hu YH, Jiao WW, Gu Y, Xiao J, Li HM, Jiao AX, Guo YJ, & Shen AD. (2010). IFN-γ release assay: a diagnostic assistance tool of tuberculin skin test in pediatric tuberculosis in China. *Chin Med J (Engl),* Oct; 123(20): 2786-91

Sutherland JS, de Jong BC, Jeffries DJ, Adetifa IM, & Ota MO. (2010). Production of TNF-alpha, IL-12(p40) and IL-17 can discriminate between active TB disease and latent infection in a West African cohort. *PLoS One,* Aug 24;5(8):e12365

Swaminathan S, Subbaraman R, & Venkatesan P, et al. (2008).Tuberculin skin test results in HIV-infected patients in India: implications for latent tuberculosis treatment. *Int J Tuberc Lung Dis,* 12(2):168-173

Syblo K. (1980). Recent advances in epidemiological research in tuberculosis. *Adv Tuberc Res,* 20: 1-63

Syed AKB, Sikhamani R, Swaminathan S, Perumal V, Paramasivam P, & Raja A. (2009). Role of Interferon Gamma Release Assay in Active TB Diagnosis among HIV Infected Individuals. *PLoS One,* 4(5): e5718

Takamatsu I. Study Group of QFT in Pediatrics. Multicenter study of QuantiFERON in child tuberculosis. Tokyo, Japan: Ministry of Health, Labour and Welfare, 2008);

Takashima T, Higuchi T. (2008). Mycobacterial tests. *Kekkaku,* 83(1), 43-59

Takayanagi K, Aoki M, Aman K, Mitarai S, Harada N, Higuchi K, Okumura M, Yoshiyama T, Ogata H, & Mori T. (2011). Analysis of an interferon-gamma release assay for monitoring the efficacy of anti-tuberculosis chemotherapy. *Jpn J Infect Dis,* 64(2): 133-8

Talati NJ, Seybold U, Humphrey B, Aina A, Tapia J, Weinfurter P, Albalak R, & Blumberg HM. (2009). Poor concordance between interferon-gamma release assays and tuberculin skin tests in diagnosis of latent tuberculosis infection among HIV-infected individuals. *BMC Infect Dis*, 9:15

Tessema TA, Hamasur B, Bjun G, Svenson S, & Bjorvatn B. (2001). Diagnostic evaluation of urinary lipoarabinomannan at an Ethiopian tuberculosis centre. *Scand J Infect Dis*, 33: 279–284.

Thomas MM, Hinks TS, Raghuraman S, Ramalingam N, Ernst M, Nau R, Lange C, Kosters K, Gnanamuthu C, & John GT, et al. (2008). Rapid diagnosis of mycobacterium tuberculosis meningitis by enumeration of cerebrospinal fluid antigen-specific T-cells. *Int J Tuberc Lung Dis*,12:651–7

Thornton CG, MacLellan KM, Brink TL, Passen S. (1998). In vitro comparison of NALC-NaOH, Tween 80 and C18-Carboxypropylbetaine for processing of specimens for recovery of mycobacteria. *J Clin Microbiol*, 36: 3558-66

Torres Costa J, Silva R, Ringshausen FC, Nienhaus A. (2011). Screening for tuberculosis and prediction of disease in Portuguese healthcare workers. *J Occup Med Toxicol*, Jun 9; 6: 19

Tortoli E, Cichero P, Piersonetti C, Simonetti MT, Gesu G, & Nista D. (1999). Use of BACTEC MGIT 960 for recovery of mycobacteria from clinical specimens: Multicenter study. *J Clin Microbiology*, 37: 3578-82

Toshiyama T, Harada N, Higuchi K, Sekiya Y, & Uchimura K. (2010). Use of the QuantiFERON-TB Gold Test for screening tuberculosis contacts and predicting active disease. *Int J Tuberc Lung Dis*, 14:819–27

Trusov A, Bumgarner R, & Valijev R, et al. (2009). Comparison of L umin™ LED fl uorescent attachment, fl uorescent microscopy and Ziehl-Neelsen for AFB diagnosis. *Int J Tuberc Lung Dis*, 13: 836–841

Tsiouris SJ, Austin J, & Toro P, et al. (2006). Results of a tuberculosis-specific IFN-gamma assay in children at high risk for tuberculosis infection. *Int J Tuberc Lung Dis*, 10 (8):939– 941

Tuberculosis Research Centre (ICMR), Chennai. (1999). Fifteen year follow up of trial of BCG vaccines in south India for tuberculosis prevention. *Indian J Med Res*, 110: 56-69

Tully G, Kortsik C, & Höhn H, et al. (2005). Highly focused T cell responses in latent human pulmonary M. tuberculosis infection. *J Immunol*, 174: 2174-84

Ulrichs T, Munk ME, & Mollenkopf H, et al. (1998). Differential T cell responses to M. tuberculosis ESAT-6 in tuberculosis patients and healthy donors. *Eur J Immunol*, 28: 3949-58

van Cleeff M, Kivihya-Ndugga L, Githui W, Ng'ang'a L, & Kibuga D, et al. (2005). Cost-effectiveness of polymerase chain reaction versus Ziehl-Neelsen smear microscopy for diagnosis of tuberculosis in Kenya. *Int J Tuberc Lung Dis*, 9: 877–883

van Cleeff MR, Kivihya-Ndugga LE, Meme H, Odhiambo JA, & Klatser PR. (2005). The role and performance of chest X-ray for the diagnosis of tuberculosis: a cost-effectiveness analysis in Nairobi, Kenya. *BMC Infect Dis*, 12(5), 111

Van Deun A, Aung KJ, Hamid Salim A, Gumusboga M, Nandi P, & Hossain MA. (2010). Methylene blue is a good background stain for tuberculosis light-emitting diode fluorescence microscopy. *Int J Tuberc Lung Dis*, Dec; 14(12): 1571-5

Van Deun A, Salim AH, Cooreman E, Daru P, & Das AP, et al. (2004). Scanty AFB smears: What's in a name? *Int J Tuber Lung Dis*, 8: 816–823

Van Deun, Chonde T M, Gumusboga M, & Rienthong S. (2008). Performance and acceptability of the FluoLED Easy module for tuberculosis fluorescence microscopy. *Int J Tuberc Lung Dis*, 12:1009–14

von Reyn CF, Horsburgh CR, Olivier KN, Barnes PF, Waddell R, Warren C, Tvaroha S, Jaeger AS, Lein AD, Alexander LN, Weber DJ, & Tosteson AN. (2001). Skin test reactions to Mycobacterium tuberculosis purified protein derivative and Mycobacterium avium sensitin among health care workers and medical students in the United States. *Int J Tuberc Lung Dis*, 2001; 5: 1122–8

Wang L, Turner MO, Elwood RK, Schulzer M, & FitzGerald JM. (2002). A meta-analysis of the effect of Bacille Calmette Guerin vaccination on tuberculin skin test measurements. *Thorax*, 57(9): 804–9

Weldingh K, Rosenkrands I, Okkels LM, Doherty TM, & Andersen P. (2005). Assessing the serodiagnostic potential of 35 Mycobacterium tuberculosis proteins and identification of four novel serological antigens. *J Clin Microbiol*, 43: 57-65

Whilley DM. Lambert SB, Bialasiewicz S, Goire N, Nissen MD, et al. (2008). False-negative results in nucleic acid amplification tests-do we need to routinely use two genetic targets in all assays to overcome problems caused by sequence variation? *Crit Rev Microbiol*, 34(2): 71-6

WHO. (2008). Global Tuberculosis Control: Surveillance, Planning and Financing. WHO, Geneva

WHO. (2006). Global Tuberculosis Control: Surveillance, Planning, and Financing. WHO, Geneva

WHO. (1994). The HIV/AIDS and tuberculosis epidemics: implications for TB control. WHO/TB/CARG (4)/94.4

WHO. (2009). New Diagnostic Working Group of the Stop TB Partnership. Pathways to better diagnostics for tuberculosis- A blueprint for the development of TB diagnostics. WHO, Geneva

WHO. (2010) Global TB control Report 2010. WHO, Geneva

WHO Tuberculosis Research office. (1995). Further studies of geographic variation in naturally acquired tuberculin sensitivity. Bull World Health Organization., 12,63-83

Wiker HG, Mustafa T, Bjune GA, & Harboe M. (2010). Evidence for waning of latency in a cohort study of tuberculosis. *BMC Infect Dis*,10:37

Wilkinson KA, Wilkinson RJ, Pathan A, Ewer K, Prakash M, Klenerman P, Maskell N, Davies R, Pasvol G, & Lalvani A. (2005). Ex vivo characterization of early secretory antigenic target 6-specific T cells at sites of active disease in pleural tuberculosis. *Clin Infect Dis*, 40:184–187

Wozniak TM, Saunders BM, Ryan AA, & Britton WJ. (2010). Mycobacterium bovis BCG-specific Th17 cells confer partial protection against Mycobacterium tuberculosis infection in the absence of gamma interferon. *Infect Immun*, Oct; 78(10): 4187-94. Epub 2010 Aug 2.

Yu CC, Liu YC, Chu CM, Chuang DY, Wu WC, & Wu HP. Factors associated with in vitro interferon-gamma production in tuberculosis. J Formos Med Assoc. 2011 Apr;110(4):239-46)

Zhang J, Chen Y, Nie XB, Wu WH, Zhang H, Zhang M, He XM, & Lu JX. (2011). Interleukin-10 polymorphisms and tuberculosis susceptibility: a meta-analysis. *Int J Tuberc Lung Dis,* May;15(5): 594-601

Zhao J, Wang Y, Wang H, Jiang C, Liu Z, Meng X, Song G, Cheng N, Graviss EA, & Ma X. (2011). Low agreement between the T-SPOT®.TB assay and the tuberculin skin test among college students in China. *Int J Tuberc Lung Dis,* Jan;15(1):134-6

Zheng YJ, Wang RH, Lin YZ, & Daniel TM. (1994). Clinical evaluation of the diagnostic value of measuring IgG antibody to 3 mycobacterial antigenic preparations in the capillary blood of children with tuberculosis and control subjects. *Tuber Lung Dis,* 75(5), 366-70

Zrinski Topić R, Zoričić-Letoja I, Pavić I, & Dodig S. (2011). Indeterminate results of QuantiFERON-TB Gold In-Tube assay in nonimmunosuppressed children. *Arch Med Res,* Feb;42(2):138-43

6

Diagnosis of Smear-Negative Pulmonary Tuberculosis in Low-Income Countries: Current Evidence in Sub-Saharan Africa with Special Focus on HIV Infection or AIDS

Claude Mambo Muvunyi[1,2] and Florence Masaisa[1,3]
*[1]Department of Clinical Chemistry, Microbiology and Immunology,
Ghent University Hospital, De Pintelaan, Ghent,
[2]Department of Clinical Biology, Centre Hospitalier Universitaire-Butare,
National University of Rwanda, Butare, Rwanda;
[3]Department of Internal Medicine, Centre Hospitalier Universitaire-Butare,
National University of Rwanda, Butare,
[1]Belgium
[2,3]Rwanda*

1. Introduction

1.1 Background

Tuberculosis (TB) remains a major global public health problem and it persists as a major cause of human mortality and morbidity, affecting almost a third of the world's population [Sudre et al., 1992; WHO 2002]. There were 9.2 million new cases of tuberculosis worldwide in 2006, with the highest rates of disease in African countries. Despite efforts to control tuberculosis and reduce the rate of infections, the lack of accurate laboratory diagnosis hinders these efforts. The rapid spread of the human immunodeficiency virus (HIV) in sub-Saharan African countries has led to dramatic rises in incidence of TB cases and has been associated with worsening treatment outcomes, even in well functioning TB programmes [Raviglione et al., 1997]. The impact of the HIV epidemic on tuberculosis depends on the degree of overlap between the population infected with HIV and that infected with Mycobacterium tuberculosis. In sub-Saharan Africa the prevalence of both infections is high with considerable overlap between the infected populations, since the age distribution of both infections is concentrated in the 20-50-year age group. In 1994 there were an estimated 4.8 million people worldwide infected with both M. tuberculosis and HIV, of whom over 75% were reported to be living in sub-Saharan Africa (6). Worldwide estimates of the proportions of new tuberculosis cases attributable to HIV infection were 4% in 1990, 8% in 1995, projected to 14% by the year 2000 [WHO 2002]. HIV-related infection thus accounts for a relatively small but increasing proportion of the global tuberculosis burden. In sub-Saharan Africa, however, it accounts for a greater part of the burden: an estimated 30% or more of tuberculosis cases by the year 2000 [WHO 2002]. THE WORLD HEALTH

ORGANIZATION (WHO) estimated that both the number of cases of tuberculosis worldwide and the percentage attributable to coexisting HIV infection would increase substantially during the decade between 1990 and 2000 [WHO 2002]. Furthermore, most of this burden occurs among the low-income countries of the world, particularly those in sub-Saharan Africa, the region most heavily affected since the beginning of the HIV epidemic[Sudre et al., 1992].

Although both culture techniques and the introduction of nucleic acid-based tests can improve laboratory diagnosis [Perkins and Cunningham, 2007], these procedures are not widely available in most low-income countries. Instead, in most low income countries, the diagnosis of pulmonary tuberculosis (PT) still relies on the search for Acid-Fast Bacilli (AFB) in sputum smears, which has sensitivity between 50 and 80% in well-equipped laboratories [Aber et al., 1980]. In low-income countries, poor access to high-quality microscopy services contributes to even lower rates of AFB detection. Furthermore, in countries with high prevalence of both pulmonary tuberculosis and HIV infection, the detection rate is even lower owing to the paucibacillary nature of pulmonary tuberculosis in patients with HIV infection. In fact, HIV changes the presentation of smear-negative pulmonary tuberculosis from a slowly progressive disease with low bacterial load and reasonable prognosis, to one with reduced pulmonary cavity formation and sputum bacillary load, more frequent involvement of the lower lobes, and an exceptionally high mortality rate [Hopewell, 1992; Jones et al., 1993]. This means that there are many cases of PT that are not going to be diagnosed by this test, and they are denominated smear-negative pulmonary tuberculosis (SNPT). Therefore, it is often necessary to make a clinico-radiological diagnosis of smear-negative TB using an algorithm and to initiate empirical TB treatment while awaiting culture results. Therefore, early identification of persons who have TB, whether smear positive or smear negative, is desirable both to enable appropriate isolation procedures and to provide a basis for early institution of therapy. Conversely, correct prediction of persons who are unlikely to have TB is important as well to limit the expense and potential toxicity of empiric therapy. A clinical prediction rule (CPR) is defined as a "decision making tool for clinicians that includes three or more variables obtained from the history, or physical examination of the patient, or from simple diagnostic tests and that either provides the probability of an outcome or suggest a diagnostic or therapeutic course of action. Given the lack of resources to use sophisticated laboratory tests for this problem in most developing countries, we will try to develop a CPR to diagnose Smear-negative pulmonary tuberculosis.

The primary objective of this chapter will be to conduct a systematic review of the literature to gather data on evaluation of various criteria, algorithms, and clinical indicators used in low-income countries in the diagnosis of PT in people with suspected tuberculosis but repeated negative sputum smears with particular consideration of HIV infection or AIDS. This review will be of help therefore to develop it in the format of a score based on simple clinical variables for the diagnosis of Smear-negative pulmonary tuberculosis.

This article will describe the incidence, natural history and differential diagnoses of smear-negative pulmonary TB in HIV negative and HIV-positive patients. The various strategies that have attempted to address smear-negative TB will then be reviewed; highlighting plausible interventions for developing countries and areas for future research.

1.2 Definition of smear-negative pulmonary tuberculosis

Smear-negative tuberculosis is currently defined as symptomatic illness in a patient with at least two sputum smear examinations negative for AFB on different occasions in whom pulmonary tuberculosis is later confirmed by culture, biopsy, or other investigations[WHO 2007]. Guidelines from some developing countries like Malawi through their national Tuberculosis Program recommends that the diagnosis of smear negative TB be based on four criteria of (i) cough for more than 3 weeks, (ii) three sputum smears negative for AFB, (iii) no response to an antibiotic, and (iv) a chest x-ray compatible with TB[Hargreaves et al., 2000].

The following are suggested case definitions for use in HIV-prevalent settings[WHO 2007]

Smear-Positive Pulmonary Tuberculosis

- One sputum smear examination positive for AFB **and**
- Laboratory confirmation of HIV infection **or**
- Strong clinical evidence of HIV infection*

Smear-Negative Pulmonary Tuberculosis

- At least two sputum specimens negative for AFB **and**
- Radiographical abnormalities consistent with active tuberculosis **and**
- Laboratory confirmation of HIV infection **or**
- Strong clinical evidence of HIV infection* **and**
- Decision by a clinician to treat with a full course of antituberculosis chemotherapy

OR

- A patient with AFB smear-negative sputum which is culture-positive for *Mycobacterium tuberculosis*

1.3 Impact of HIV on TB infection

Persons with HIV-1 infection are at increased risk of active TB due to reactivation of latent TB and more rapid progression to disease after TB infection. It is well known that the risk of TB is greatly increased in HIV-infected persons, and some of the underlying mechanisms are being elucidated. Effective immunity to TB involves coordination of responses between the innate and adaptive immune systems, both of which are altered by HIV[Patel and Koziel, 2009]. The strongest risk factor for developing TB disease in HIV lies in helper T-cell type 1 (Th1) adaptive immunity, specifically the progressive decline in CD4 T-cell count associated with advanced HIV [Williams and Dye, 2003]. In patients with prior TB exposure as assessed by a positive Purified protein derivative (PPD) response, the incidence of TB is 2.6%/year for those with a CD4 T-cell count greater than 350/ml, 6.5%/year for those with aCD4 T-cell count from 200 to 350/ml, and 13.3%/year for those with a CD4 T-cell count less than 200/ml [Antonucci et al., 1995]. With decline of the CD4 T-cell count, there is also a higher risk of anergy to skin test reactions, suggesting dysfunction of delayed-type hypersensitivity dependent on Th1-type immunity [Markowitz et al., 1993]. There is also in vitro evidence for qualitative dysfunction of CD4 T cells in HIV. Compared with TB-infected patients without HIV infection, peripheral blood mononuclear cells from patients coinfected with HIV and TB have decreased proliferative T-cell responses and reduced IFN-g production to *Mycobacterium tuberculosis* in vitro, whereas anti-inflammatory IL-10 production is preserved [Zhang et al., 1994]. However, the observation that TB incidence increases shortly after HIV seroconversion, and before reduction in peripheral blood CD4 T-cell counts [Sonnenberg et al., 2005], suggests that HIV confers additional mechanisms of susceptibility to TB infection. Investigations into the progression of primary HIV infection to AIDS suggest that primary HIV infection is associated with a precipitous decrease in mucosal CD4 memory T cells [Brenchley et al., 2006a], which may set the stage for chronic immune activation and CD4 T-cell depletion through mucosal translocation of bacteria through the gut [Brenchley et al., 2006b]. Thus, mucosal CD4 memory T-cell depletion may provide a potential mechanism to account for disrupted T-cell function in early HIV infection, although whether similar events occur in the lung mucosa has not yet been established [Brenchley et al., 2008]. Indeed, primary HIV infection is associated with decreased PPD-specific IFN-secreting T cells [Sutherland et al., 2006; Geldmacher et al., 2008] and ESAT (early secreted antigenic target)-6–specific T cells [Geldmacher et al., 2008] in the blood, suggesting that early depletion of memory T cells may affect specific immunity to TB. Lung lavage enzymelinked immunospot (ELISPOT) studies also suggest decreased bacillus Calmette-Gue´rin (BCG)– or PPD-specific pulmonary CD4 T cells in asymptomatic HIV-infected persons compared with HIV-negative persons [Kalsdorf et al., 2009]. HIV–TB coinfection may also be associated with increased serum levels of IL-4, an anti-Th1 type cytokine that hinders immune response to MTb [Dheda et al., 2005]. Interestingly, alveolar lavage cells from coinfected individuals may have intact ability to secrete IFN-g in response to MTb antigens in vitro [Dheda et al., 2005], although this may not translate to equivalent cell function and cell numbers in vivo.

Independent of CD4 T-cell count, HIV also affects the function of innate immune cells, especially alveolar macrophages (AMs), which serve as the main reservoir for MTb infection [Russell, 2001; Dheda et al., 2009]. MTb has evolved to persist within macrophages in part through prevention of MTb phagosomal fusion with lysosomes, thus preventing intracellular killing of MTb [Brown et al., 1969; Mwandumba et al., 2004]. AMs can combat intracellular parasitization by releasing immune-activating cytokines or chemokines, and by programmed cell death or apoptosis [Oddo et al., 1998; Keane et al., 2000]. Apoptosis benefits the host by promoting intracellular killing of MTb [Oddo et al., 1998; Keane et al., 2000] and improving antigen presentation by additional phagocytes to activate adaptive immunity [Schaible et al., 2003; Winau et al., 2006]. Whereas asymptomatic HIV infection does not affect the intracellular growth of MTb [Day et al., 2004; Kalsdorf et al., 2009], AMs from asymptomatic HIV-infected subjects have increased phagocytosis of MTb [Day et al., 2004; Patel et al., 2007], decreased release of specific cytokines and chemokines [Saukkonen et al., 2002], and similarly impaired MTb phagosomal maturation [Mwandumba et al., 2004] compared with AMs from healthy subjects. AMs from HIV-infected subjects also have decreased apoptosis in response to MTb [Patel et al., 2007]; the mechanism may involve increased lung levels of IL-10 in HIV, which up-regulates BCL-3 (B-cell lymphoma 3–encoded protein), an apoptosis inhibitor [Patel et al., 2009]. HIV infection of macrophages also inhibits autophagy [Kyei et al., 2009], another cellular process that may be critical for macrophage intracellular killing of MTb [Gutierrez et al., 2004].

1.4 Rationale

The focus of this chapter is on sub-Saharan Africa (SSA). Countries in the developing world and especially in sub-Saharan Africa are the most affected by the TB epidemic. Worldwide, in 2008, the estimated global TB incidence rate was 139 cases per 100,000 population, which equates to 9.4 million (range, 8.9–9.9 million) incident TB cases. This represents an 11% increase in TB incidence rate and a 40% increase in the number of TB cases, compared with estimates from 1990[WHO 2009]. This global increase in rates was attributable to increases in the SSA and was mainly driven by the HIV epidemic. Particularly in SSA, mirroring the HIV epidemic, TB incidence and TB-associated death rates have doubled, and the number of TB cases and TB-related deaths has tripled in comparison with estimated figures from 1990[WHO 2009]. The HIV epidemic has fuelled the tuberculosis epidemic in the region. Of the 9.4 million incident cases in 2009, an estimated 1.0–1.2 million (11–13%) were HIV-positive, with a best estimate of 1.1 million (12%). Of these HIV-positive TB cases, approximately 80% were in the African Region (http://www.who.int/tb/publications/global_report/2010/). The relative risk of developing TB in HIV-positive individuals, compared with HIV-negative individuals, is 21 in high HIV prevalence countries and 37 in low HIV prevalence countries[WHO 2009]. Moreover, these co-infected people have at least a 30% lifetime risk of developing active tuberculosis, thus contributing to the increase in the number of tuberculosis cases in the region. In Africa, TB is often the first manifestation of HIV infection, and accounts for a disproportionate burden of morbidity and mortality in co-infected patients [Munyati et al., 2005].

As a consequence, HIV is the single most significant risk factor for the development of TB, and HIV patients are at increased risk for primary and reactivation disease, as well as exogenous reinfection [Sonnenberg et al., 2001]. The risk of death in co-infected patients is two to four times that of HIV individuals without TB, independent of CD4 count [Whalen et al., 1995; Connolly et al., 1999]. In addition, coinfected patients have a markedly greater risk of progression to AIDS compared with HIV patients without TB [Whalen et al., 1997]. The focus of this chapter is therefore sub-Saharan Africa, the region of the world most severely affected by the HIV/TB co-epidemic.

2. Search strategy

We used a combination of systematic review, document analysis, and global expert opinion to prepare this chapter. We identified relevant publications by searches of Medline, PubMed, Embase, HealthSTAR, and Web of Science with the keywords: "tuberculosis", "*Mycobacterium tuberculosis*", "sputum negative", "smear negative", AFB negative", "negative for AFB", "HIV" , "diagnosis" and "treatment" for papers published in English between 1990 and December, 2010. Studies were included in the review if they reported on tuberculous disease in people with HIV infection or AIDS in sub- Saharan Africa and if the disease had been stratified into smear-positive and smear-negative. We reviewed data for smear-negative pulmonary tuberculosis only for patients who were also HIV positive. All retrieved titles and abstracts were scrutinised for the relevance to the topic. Analytical studies that identified demographic, clinical, radiological, or simple laboratory based indicators facilitating the diagnosis of smear-negative tuberculosis were included. An assessment of methodological quality was undertaken for each paper.

We used the WHO definition of a case of smear-negative pulmonary tuberculosis: at least two sputum specimens negative for acid-fast bacilli, abnormalities on radiography consistent with active tuberculosis, no response to broad-spectrum antibiotics, and a decision by a clinician to treat with a full course of antituberculosis chemotherapy.

3. Frequency of smear-negative pulmonary tuberculosis

Given the immunopathological spectrum seen in HIV-infected TB patients, it would be expected that the proportion of patients with smear-negative PT should increase in areas where the prevalence of HIV is high. Initial impressions were that HIV infection in sub-Saharan Africa was associated with a large and predominant increase in smear-negative PT [Harries, 1990]. It is apparent from cross-sectional studies, however, that the majority of HIV-positive PT patients are smear positive, although the proportion of smear-negative patients is greater among those infected with HIV than among those who are HIV-negative [Elliott et al., 1990; Nunn et al., 1992]. Since the advent of HIV, the annual incidence of TB has more than doubled in some African countries [De Cock et al., 1992; Wilkinson and Davies, 1997], and there has been a disproportionate increase in the reported rate of smear-negative disease. A study in Zambia [Elliott et al., 1993] of over 100 patients with culture-positive PT found that 24% of those who were HIV-seronegative had a negative sputum smear, compared with 43% of those who were HIV-seropositive. With good routine reporting systems, the national tuberculosis programmes of countries such as Malawi and the United Republic of Tanzania have reported a larger increase in new cases of smear negative than of smear-positive PT in the last 10 years [Graf 1994].

Other studies showed that the proportion of cases of smear-negative pulmonary tuberculosis in HIV-positive tuberculosis patients ranged from 10% to 61% [Affolabi et al., ; Long et al., 1991; Elliott et al., 1993; Harries et al., 1997; Behr et al., 1999; Bruchfeld et al., 2002; Zachariah et al., 2003; Kang'ombe et al., 2004; Yassin et al., 2004; Chintu and Mwaba, 2005]. The apparent variation in the incidence of negative sputum smear between these studies may be due to differences in the study populations. Some studies were conducted among patients seen at specialist institution-based centres who may be more or less likely to be smear-positive depending on the referral procedure. The level of immunosuppression among the HIV-positive patients in the various studies may also have differed. Less severely immunocompromised HIV-positive patients tend to have classic cavitary TB which is smear-positive [De Cock et al., 1992; Desta et al., 2009]. As the level of immunocompromise increases with advancing HIV disease, atypical pulmonary features predominate and smear examinations prove less sensitive It is not clear at present whether these figures reflect the true pattern of PT or whether there is an over diagnosis or under diagnosis of smear-negative cases. Reports from national tuberculosis programmes of the pattern of PT are influenced by various factors such as the criteria used to diagnose smear-negative PT, the extent to which these criteria are followed in clinical practice, and the number of other respiratory diseases that can resemble and be misdiagnosed as PT. Moreover, access to health services and DOTS in most resource-constrained settings with high HIV infection rates is restricted and services reach only a fraction of the population. If the availability of these services were increased, we expect that a much higher frequency of disease would be seen. Negative smears could also be the result of poor quality smear microscopy from inadequate sputum collection, storage, and staining, reading errors, or poor laboratory services. In children, the diagnosis of pulmonary tuberculosis is especially difficult because the disease is paucibacillary and collection of sufficient sputum for smear microscopy and culture is difficult [Chintu and Mwaba, 2005]. HIV-positive patients with smear-negative tuberculosis are more likely to die during or before diagnosis than HIV-negative patients because of their immunosuppression, which leads to further under estimates of the magnitude of the problem.

4. Transmission of tuberculosis from smear negative patients

TB patients whose sputum smears are AFB negative are generally regarded as less infectious than those whose smears are positive. The relative TB transmission rate among patients with smear-negative, culture-positive pulmonary disease, compared with patients with smear-positive disease, was found to be 0.24 in cohort study in the Netherlands [Tostmann et al., 2008]. Overall, 17% of TB transmission events were attributable to source patients with sputum smear-negative, culture-positive disease [Tostmann et al., 2008]. These important findings are consistent with report from similar studies from San Francisco, California, and Vancouver, British Columbia [Behr et al., 1999; Hernandez-Garduno et al., 2004], collectively showing that in high-income countries, 10%–20% of TB transmission at the population level is attributable to source cases with smear-negative pulmonary TB. Tostmann and co-worker [Tostmann et al., 2008] speculated on the relevance of their data for countries in which HIV infection is endemic and rates of smear-negative TB disease are high. In these countries with a high incidence of TB, microscopic examination of sputum smear samples is often the only available diagnostic test for TB. As a result, patients with smear-negative TB do not receive a diagnosis in a timely manner; thus, disease may further develop, initiation of treatment may be delayed, and further TB transmission may occur [Siddiqi et al., 2003]. In view of these observations, one can conclude that transmission attributable to smear-negative pulmonary TB cases at the community level may be important in these regions.

Whether this is true for HIV-positive patients with pulmonary tuberculosis remains to be established. One study from Zambia concluded that patients with HIV-associated pulmonary tuberculosis were less infectious than seronegative patients [Elliott et al., 1993], whereas results from Zaire showed no difference in rates of infection among household contacts [Klausner et al., 1993]. Moreover, In sub-Saharan Africa, HIV infection has had a devastating impact on TB control [Lawn et al., 2006; WHO 2009]. In a study of a community in a township in Cape Town, South Africa, for example, the antenatal HIV seroprevalence rate is 30%, and the annual TB notification rate has increased to 11500 cases per 100,000 population [Lawn et al., 2006] almost 200-fold higher than TB rates in The Netherlands. This has been associated with a major and disproportionate increase in the rate of smear-negative disease among HIV-infected individuals [Lawn et al., 2006].

5. Diagnosis of smear negative TB in Sub-Saharan African

In the absence of rapid and simple tools to diagnose tuberculosis, health institutions should avail guidelines or algorithms to assist clinical decision-making in HIV-prevalent and resource-constrained settings, to expedite the diagnostic process and minimize incorrect diagnosis and mortality. As much as possible, patients should be correctly diagnosed and treated for smear-negative pulmonary tuberculosis; however, treatment of those without the disease should be avoided. The diagnosis of PT in adults in most African countries is based on simple techniques such as clinical assessment, sputum smear microscopy and chest radiography. Although specificity is high [Hargreaves et al., 2001; van Cleeff et al., 2003; Apers et al., 2004], major concerns include low sensitivity [Harries et al., 1997; Hargreaves et al., 2001] and delayed diagnosis of smear-negative disease [Harries et al., 1997; Colebunders and Bastian, 2000]. The accuracy of both microscopy and radiography is reduced by HIV, and so assessment of diagnostic approaches with existing methods and continuing research into new diagnostics are necessary [Colebunders and Bastian, 2000; Kivihya-Ndugga et al., 2003; Angeby et al., 2004].

Tuberculin skin testing in adults is not useful for individual diagnosis in populations with a high prevalence of M. tuberculosis infection. In addition, for HIV-infected individuals, there is the problem that cutaneous anergy increases as the CD4 lymphocyte count declines. In Zaire, over 50% of HIV-positive PT patients with a CD4 lymphocyte count <200/4l had a negative tuberculin skin test [Mukadi et al., 1993]. Techniques that are widely available in industrialized countries for obtaining pulmonary specimens (such as induced sputum and fibre-optic bronchoscopy with bronchoalveolar lavage) and for analysing them (such as culture, antigen detection and polymerase chain reaction) are beyond the resources of most hospitals in sub-Saharan Africa.

5.1 Criteria used to diagnose smear-negative TB

5.1.1 Clinical criteria

Smear-negative tuberculosis is found to be more common in older than younger patients in a country with low prevalence of HIV infection [Samb et al., 1999]. However, countries with high HIV prevalence have an even age distribution, probably because HIV affects younger age-groups [Parry, 1993]. HIV is also more common in patients with smear-negative tuberculosis than in those with smear-positive disease. As for clinical indicators, pulmonary TB remains the most frequent form of active TB in HIV-1 infected persons, even those with low CD4 counts. Although the clinical presentation of pulmonary TB is different to the presentation of pulmonary TB in HIV-1 uninfected patients, the most common symptoms remain cough, fever, night sweats and significant weight loss [Batungwanayo et al., 1992; Bruchfeld et al., 2002]. Relative to HIV-1 uninfected patients, weight loss and fever are more common, whereas haemoptysis is less common and some studies have reported a decreased proportion of patients with cough [Selwyn et al., 1998; Kassu et al., 2007]. Although HIV-infected persons with TB may have the classic symptoms of TB (eg, productive cough, chest pain, shortness of breath, hemoptysis, fever, night sweats, and/or weight loss), many such patients have few symptoms or have symptoms that are even less specific than those mentioned. Cough persisting for longer than 3 weeks warrants AFB microscopy, according to the current WHO guidance. However, one study, in an area of high HIV and tuberculosis prevalence, confirmed smear-negative tuberculosis in 35% of patients with cough unresponsive to antibiotics of only 1–3 weeks duration [Banda et al., 1998]. Most of these patients had atypical changes on chest radiography. That study suggests that pulmonary tuberculosis should be considered in patients with short duration of cough associated with weight loss and lack of response to antibiotics, particularly those who live in overcrowded places in areas with high prevalence of HIV infection and tuberculosis. It has been noted recently that a small proportion of HIV infected patients with TB are minimally symptomatic or asymptomatic, particularly in developing countries with a high burden of both HIV infection and TB [Bassett et al., 2009; Edwards et al., 2009].

A number of studies in Africa have tried to identify frequently occurring clinical features in smear-negative tuberculosis in areas with high prevalence of HIV infection and tuberculosis. A study, in Tanzania and Burundi, identified four clinical criteria for diagnosis of smear-negative tuberculosis [Samb et al., 1997]: presence of cough for longer than 21 days (odds ratio 5·43[1·95–15·1]); presence of chest pain for longer than 15 days (1·98 [0·77–5·12]); absence of expectoration (odds ratio for expectoration 0·42 [0·15–1·18]); and absence of shortness of breath (odds ratio for breathlessness 0·26 [0·01–0·66]). Diagnosis of smear negative tuberculosis by any two of these criteria exhibited high sensitivity but low specificity (sensitivity 85%, specificity 67%, positive predictive value 43%, and negative predictive value 94%). When three of the criteria were considered, the specificity improved while the sensitivity decreased (sensitivity 49%, specificity 86%, positive predictive value 50%, and negative predictive value 86%). The gold standard against which these clinical indicators were evaluated was Sputum culture, tissue histology, and positive clinical and radiological response to the antituberculosis therapy. However, patients with chronic lung disorders were excluded from the study, which limits the extent to which it can be generalised. The prevalence of HIV was high (71%) in both case and control groups.

In another hospital-based study in Ethiopia, the most frequent symptoms in patients with pulmonary tuberculosis (both smear positive and smear negative) than in those without pulmonary tuberculosis were loss of appetite, weight loss, fever, night sweats, chest pain, haemoptysis, and breathlessness were more common [Tessema et al., 2001]. However, patients with smear-negative tuberculosis had night sweats for a longer time. Smear-positive patients were more likely to have fever and weight loss than the smear negative group (odds ratios 4·1 [1·2–15·0] and 6·4 [2·3–17·8], respectively). The diagnosis by a group of tuberculosis physicians, which may have been due to lack of resources, although the authors do not clarify the reason in the paper, was used as the gold standard for diagnosis of pulmonary tuberculosis. However, in an area with low prevalence of HIV infection and high prevalence of tuberculosis, one study based in Senegal found no clinical features differentiating smear-negative from smear-positive tuberculosis other than the absence of cough (odds ratio 10·0 [1·96–50·0]) [Samb et al., 1997]. Limitations of this study were that it had a small sample size and that the diagnosis was confirmed by means of sputum culture in only 20% of cases. The overall prevalence of HIV in both case and control groups was 8·9%. Our search could only retrieve one study that included subjects from a population with low prevalence of both HIV infection and tuberculosis [Kanaya et al., 2001]. Cough with expectoration was considered as a negative predictor of smear-negative tuberculosis (odds ratio 0·3 [0·1–0·6]). This study could not identify any other differentiating clinical features, possibly owing to the small sample size.

5.1.2 Radiographic criteria

Although the classical radiographic hallmarks of PT are cavitation, apical distribution, bilateral distribution, pulmonary fibrosis, shrinkage and calcification, no pattern is absolutely diagnostic of tuberculosis. Interpretation of chest X-rays of individuals suspected to have PT is difficult. In the pre-HIV era, there was considerable inter- and intra-observer variation in chest X-ray interpretation by radiologists and chest physicians [Thoman 1979].

In sub-Saharan Africa with limited microbiological services, the problem is compounded because there are few trained radiologists or chest physicians, and in most district hospitals chest X-rays are interpreted by relatively inexperienced medical officers or paramedics., survey in Malawi showed that medical officers misdiagnosed a third of clinical vignettes, which described typical radiographic signs of tuberculosis [Nyirenda et al., 1999]. The nonspecific findings of pulmonary infiltrates, in the middle or lower lobes, in HIV positive PT patients adds to the difficulties of correct radiographic diagnosis. It is now well recognized in industrialized countries [Pedro-Botet et al., 1992; Greenberg et al., 1994] and countries in sub-Saharan Africa [Simooya et al., 1991; Abouya et al., 1995] that the chest X-ray can appear normal in HIV-positive PT patients.

Studies in sub-Saharan Africa revealed that tuberculous patients with HIV infection are more likely to have atypical chest radiographic appearances (pulmonary infiltrates with no cavities, lower-lobe involvement, intrathoracic lymphadenopathy, and even normal appearance) than tuberculous patients without HIV infection [Harries et al., 1998b; Banda et al., 2000]. In areas of high HIV and tuberculosis prevalence, 75% of patients with smear-negative tuberculosis are likely to have atypical chest radiographic findings [Tessema et al., 2001]. Patients with smear-negative tuberculosis are less likely to have cavities on the chest radiograph (odds ratio 2·56) than patients with smear positive tuberculosis [Samb et al., 1999]. In addition, smear-negative patients can also present with normal or only slightly abnormal chest radiographs [Harries et al., 1998a]. A study confirmed pulmonary tuberculosis by sputum culture in 21% of patients with suspected tuberculosis and negative smears and normal or slightly abnormal chest radiographs. 47% of such patients were found to have typical radiographic features after 3 months. A third of the culture-negative patients also developed typical radiographic signs of tuberculosis during follow-up. Authors from that study suggested that close monitoring of smear-negative patients with suspected tuberculosis and normal or slightly abnormal chest radiographs is useful in areas with high prevalence of HIV infection and tuberculosis.

5.1.3 Sputum smear microscopy

Microscopy for the detection of AFB is rapid, low cost, and detects the most infectious cases of tuberculosis, but needs maintenance of equipment, consistent supply of reagents, and proper training in interpretation of the slides [Foulds and O'Brien, 1998]. International guidelines recommend the microscopic examination of three serial sputum specimens for acid-fast bacilli (AFB) in the investigation of pulmonary TB suspects, and define a positive case as a case with at least two smear-positive results [WHO 2003]. Recent studies have shown that under routine conditions, evaluating TB suspects with two sputum smears is as effective as with three sputum smears and is accompanied with less laboratory work and thus reductions in the cost related to the TB workup [Ipuge et al., 1996; Gopi et al., 2004]. This strategy could leave more time for the examination of each slide, should the workload dictate a reduction in the number of examinations. For a smear to be positive, there must be at least 5000-10 000 acid-fast bacilli per mL sputum, but these bacilli could be released only intermittently from cavities [WHO 2004]. If the sensitivity of smear microscopy could be improved, it would be a valuable instrument for TB control [Angeby et al., 2004] and would improve the diagnosis of tuberculosis in both adults. Many investigators have suggested sputum liquefaction and concentration through centrifugation to improve detection of AFB in negative smears through direct microscopy. Liquefaction of sputum with sodium hypochlorite and concentration by either centrifugation or sedimentation is the most widely studied procedure [Angeby et al., 2004]. Studies carried out in developing countries have shown an increase of almost two fold in the sensitivity of AFB detection compared with direct microscopy [Gebre et al., 1995; Habeenzu et al., 1998]. A systematic review also showed that studies that used sputum processing with chemicals including bleach and centrifugation yielded a mean 18% increase in sensitivity and an incremental yield (positives with bleach minus positives with Ziehl-Neelsen stain only) of 9% [Steingart et al., 2006]. Specificity ranged from 96% to 100% with the bleach method alone and from 95% to 100% with the Ziehl-Neelsen method alone [Angeby et al., 2004]. In HIV-positive patients, sensitivity increased from 38·5% to 50·0% after concentration [Bruchfeld et al., 2000]. This improvement was less remarkable when compared with the sensitivity of direct microscopy supported by clinicians' judgment in diagnosing pulmonary tuberculosis. The main disadvantages of the bleach method are the additional processing time, the technique lacks standardisation, and its advantages over other sputum concentration methods are not clear [Colebunders and Bastian, 2000].

Fluorescence microscopy increases the probability of detecting AFB, especially if the sputum contains few bacteria, and hence improves the sensitivity of microscopy in HIV-positive patients. A systematic review of studies that used fluorescence microscopy showed that on average, in comparison with Ziehl-Neelsen microscopy, fluorescence microscopy showed a 10% increase in sensitivity and 9% incremental yield, and this improvement was not affected by HIV status [Kivihya-Ndugga et al., 2003; Steingart et al., 2006]. The methods had similar specificity, but fluorescence microscopy done on one or two specimens was more cost effective than the Ziehl-Neelsen method used on three sputum specimens [Kivihya-Ndugga et al., 2003].

6. Differential diagnosis of smear-negative TB

There have been a number of research studies in sub-Saharan Africa, using either induced sputum or fibre-optic bronchoscopy with bronchoalveolar lavage and transbronchial biopsy, to determine the range of pulmonary diseases found in patients with respiratory illness and negative AFB sputum smears. AFB microscopy lacks sensitivity compared with culture. In patients with culture-confirmed pulmonary TB, the sensitivity of AFB microscopy ranges from 22 to 80% [Kim et al., 1984]. In the setting of low income countries as elsewhere, there are a number of factors that influence the diagnosis of smear negative tuberculosis. These factors include the prevalence of tuberculosis in the population, the prevalence of HIV infection, and finally, the prevalence of other infections that may mimic tuberculosis. In under-resourced, over-worked TB control programmes, laboratories cannot cope with the influx of diagnostic and follow-up smear examinations, and smears may not be done at all. For example, in Botswana in 1992, 48% of patients reported with pulmonary tuberculosis had no smear examinations performed [De Cock and Wilkinson, 1995]. Alternatively, the sputum specimens collected may be inadequate in quality or number. Ipuge et al. [Ipuge et al., 1996] found that 83.4% of smear-positive cases were detected on the first specimen, 12.2% on the second, and 4.4% on the third, by Ziehl-Neelsen staining under routine programme conditions in Tanzania. Finally, the performance of the smears may be technically inadequate. Declining quality of smear examination is a particular problem in overburdened laboratories in HIV-endemic countries. When, as part of an epidemiological study of TB and HIV in Tanzania, Chum et al. [Chum et al., 1996] compared the sputum microscopy results obtained in local and reference laboratories, 29% of new smear-negative cases (on the basis of local microscopy) were found to be smear-positive by the reference laboratory. False-negative results can be due to inadequate staining, under- or over-decolourisation, or inspection of too few fields (i.e., a minimum of 100 fields of a Ziehl-Neelsen smear must be examined before reporting a negative result and this examination takes about 5–10 minutes) [WHO 1998].

Other diseases identified in patients suspected of having TB include bacterial pneumonia due to a wide range of pathogens, Pneumocystis carinii pneumonia (PCP), Kaposi's sarcoma, nocardiosis and fungal infections with Cryptococcus neoformans and Aspergillus fumigatus. Bacterial pneumonia is the main differential diagnosis in HIV-positive and HIV-negative individuals, while PCP, cryptococcosis, and nocardiosis are of increased importance in HIV-positive subjects. The reported rates of PCP in African HIV-positive patients with respiratory symptoms vary between 0 and 33%. [Abouya et al., 1992; Kamanfu et al., 1993; Batungwanayo et al., 1994; Greenberg et al., 1995; Malin et al., 1995; Daley et al., 1996; Grant et al., 1998].

This variation has not been fully explained, but has been attributed to differences in patient selection, the level of immunodeficiency of HIV-positive patients in Africa, the limited availability of specialized laboratory diagnostics, the failure to diagnose PCP in the presence of multiple other infections, and geographic differences in the prevalence of PCP [Batungwanayo et al., 1994; Malin et al., 1995]. HIV-associated nocardiosis may also be under diagnosed. Lucas et al. [Lucas et al., 1994] conducted an autopsy study of 247 HIV-positive cases in Abidjan, Ivory Coast, and found one case of nocardiosis for every nine TB cases. These medical conditions account for significant morbidity and mortality in patients presenting with 'smear-negative pulmonary disease' in HIV- and TB endemic developing countries. However, the pre-eminent position of TB as the major pathogen in these circumstances must be emphasised. Moreover, it is necessary to emphase the importance of appropriate diagnosis of smear negative tuberculosis, both in terms of public health to identify early infectious sources more rapidly, and in terms of individual health, to identify specific diseases that can be treated. "In areas of high prevalence of tuberculosis, the most common disease that occurs in someone with the clinical signs of tuberculosis but has a negative sputum smear is still tuberculosis

7. Conclusion and future perspective

Smear-negative pulmonary TB is an increasing clinical problem in developing countries affected by the dual HIV/TB epidemic. It is clear that in sub-Saharan Africa more information is required to help solve some of the problems surrounding the diagnosis of smear negative TB. Clear diagnostic criteria need to be developed and agreed upon, and these may vary from country to country according to the availability of diagnostic facilities. Management algorithms that have been validated by local studies should improve case detection. Where current WHO guidelines have been implemented, clinical audits have the potential to improve the quality of diagnosis of smear-negative tuberculosis. Wider use of sputum induction and evaluation of novel sputum processing techniques may also improve the investigation of these patients. Some authors have argued for the wider availability of

TB culture facilities in developing countries; however, these Utopian interventions will require increased financial and technical support from the international community. The contribution of false negative sputum smears to the overall burden of smear-negative TB and the deficiencies in the system that lead to false-negative results need to be addressed. Rates of misdiagnosis of smear-negative tuberculosis can be reduced by development of diagnostic tools, which incorporate the diagnosis of other non-tuberculosis pulmonary disorders. Extensive basic research to develop rapid, simple, and accurate tuberculosis diagnostic tools that can be used in laboratories and remote locations is essential. Increased political commitment, greater scientific interest, and massive investment are needed. At the same time, innovative means need to be sought to address the human resources issues in the diagnosis problem, such as strategic efforts to train adequate and efficient laboratory staff at all levels. New diagnostic techniques are required in addition to AFB microscopy for the identification of smear-negative tuberculosis. These need to be appropriate for use in low income countries. Research into development of more cost-effective microbiological and serological diagnostic solutions is under way. However, until such tests are widely available, diagnostic scoring systems and algorithms must be developed and validated to assist clinicians working in resource-poor settings. Research collaboration is required between countries with similar HIV prevalence to address these research needs and to develop joint management guidelines, which can be applied and evaluated in different situations.

8. References

Aber VR, Allen BW, Mitchison DA, Ayuma P, Edwards EA, Keyes AB: Quality control in tuberculosis bacteriology. 1. Laboratory studies on isolated positive cultures and the efficiency of direct smear examination. Tubercle 1980;61:123-133.

Abouya L, Coulibaly IM, Coulibaly D, Kassim S, Ackah A, Greenberg AE, Wiktor SZ, De Cock KM: Radiologic manifestations of pulmonary tuberculosis in hiv-1 and hiv-2-infected patients in abidjan, cote d'ivoire. Tuber Lung Dis 1995;76:436-440.

Abouya YL, Beaumel A, Lucas S, Dago-Akribi A, Coulibaly G, N'Dhatz M, Konan JB, Yapi A, De Cock KM: Pneumocystis carinii pneumonia. An uncommon cause of death in african patients with acquired immunodeficiency syndrome. Am Rev Respir Dis 1992;145:617-620.

Affolabi D, Akpona R, Odoun M, Alidjinou K, Wachinou P, Anagonou S, Gninafon M, Trebucq A: Smear-negative, culture-positive pulmonary tuberculosis among patients with chronic cough in cotonou, benin. Int J Tuberc Lung Dis;15:67-70.

Angeby KA, Hoffner SE, Diwan VK: Should the 'bleach microscopy method' be recommended for improved case detection of tuberculosis? Literature review and key person analysis. Int J Tuberc Lung Dis 2004;8:806-815.

Antonucci G, Girardi E, Raviglione MC, Ippolito G: Risk factors for tuberculosis in hiv-infected persons. A prospective cohort study. The gruppo italiano di studio tubercolosi e aids (gista). JAMA 1995;274:143-148.

Apers L, Wijarajah C, Mutsvangwa J, Chigara N, Mason P, van der Stuyft P: Accuracy of routine diagnosis of pulmonary tuberculosis in an area of high hiv prevalence. Int J Tuberc Lung Dis 2004;8:945-951.

Banda H, Kang'ombe C, Harries AD, Nyangulu DS, Whitty CJ, Wirima JJ, Salaniponi FM, Maher D, Nunn P: Mortality rates and recurrent rates of tuberculosis in patients with smear-negative pulmonary tuberculosis and tuberculous pleural effusion who have completed treatment. Int J Tuberc Lung Dis 2000;4:968-974.

Banda HT, Harries AD, Welby S, Boeree MJ, Wirima JJ, Subramanyam VR, Maher D, Nunn PA: Prevalence of tuberculosis in tb suspects with short duration of cough. Trans R Soc Trop Med Hyg 1998;92:161-163.

Bassett I, Chetty S, Wang B, et al. Intensive TB screening for HIV infected patients ready to start ART in Durban, South Africa: limitations of WHO guidelines. In: Program and abstracts of the 16th Conference on Retroviruses and Opportunistic Infections (Montreal). 2009. Abstract 779.

Batungwanayo J, Taelman H, Dhote R, Bogaerts J, Allen S, Van de Perre P: Pulmonary tuberculosis in kigali, rwanda. Impact of human immunodeficiency virus infection on clinical and radiographic presentation. Am Rev Respir Dis 1992;146:53-56.

Batungwanayo J, Taelman H, Lucas S, Bogaerts J, Alard D, Kagame A, Blanche P, Clerinx J, van de Perre P, Allen S: Pulmonary disease associated with the human immunodeficiency virus in kigali, rwanda. A fiberoptic bronchoscopic study of 111 cases of undetermined etiology. Am J Respir Crit Care Med 1994;149:1591-1596.

Behr MA, Warren SA, Salamon H, Hopewell PC, Ponce de Leon A, Daley CL, Small PM: Transmission of mycobacterium tuberculosis from patients smear-negative for acid-fast bacilli. Lancet 1999;353:444-449.

Brenchley JM, Knox KS, Asher AI, Price DA, Kohli LM, Gostick E, Hill BJ, Hage CA, Brahmi Z, Khoruts A, Twigg HL, 3rd, Schacker TW, Douek DC: High frequencies of polyfunctional hiv-specific t cells are associated with preservation of mucosal cd4 t cells in bronchoalveolar lavage. Mucosal Immunol 2008;1:49-58.

Brenchley JM, Price DA, Douek DC: Hiv disease: Fallout from a mucosal catastrophe? Nat Immunol 2006a;7:235-239.

Brenchley JM, Price DA, Schacker TW, Asher TE, Silvestri G, Rao S, Kazzaz Z, Bornstein E, Lambotte O, Altmann D, Blazar BR, Rodriguez B, Teixeira-Johnson L, Landay A, Martin JN, Hecht FM, Picker LJ, Lederman MM, Deeks SG, Douek DC: Microbial translocation is a cause of systemic immune activation in chronic hiv infection. Nat Med 2006b;12:1365-1371.

Brown CA, Draper P, Hart PD: Mycobacteria and lysosomes: A paradox. Nature 1969;221:658-660.

Bruchfeld J, Aderaye G, Palme IB, Bjorvatn B, Britton S, Feleke Y, Kallenius G, Lindquist L: Evaluation of outpatients with suspected pulmonary tuberculosis in a high hiv prevalence setting in ethiopia: Clinical, diagnostic and epidemiological characteristics. Scand J Infect Dis 2002;34:331-337.

Bruchfeld J, Aderaye G, Palme IB, Bjorvatn B, Kallenius G, Lindquist L: Sputum concentration improves diagnosis of tuberculosis in a setting with a high prevalence of hiv. Trans R Soc Trop Med Hyg 2000;94:677-680.

Chintu C, Mwaba P: Tuberculosis in children with human immunodeficiency virus infection. Int J Tuberc Lung Dis 2005;9:477-484.

Chum HJ, O'Brien RJ, Chonde TM, Graf P, Rieder HL: An epidemiological study of tuberculosis and hiv infection in tanzania, 1991-1993. AIDS 1996;10:299-309.

Colebunders R, Bastian I: A review of the diagnosis and treatment of smear-negative pulmonary tuberculosis. Int J Tuberc Lung Dis 2000;4:97-107.

Connolly C, Reid A, Davies G, Sturm W, McAdam KP, Wilkinson D: Relapse and mortality among hiv-infected and uninfected patients with tuberculosis successfully treated with twice weekly directly observed therapy in rural south africa. AIDS 1999;13:1543-1547.

Daley CL, Mugusi F, Chen LL, Schmidt DM, Small PM, Bearer E, Aris E, Mtoni IM, Cegielski JP, Lallinger G, Mbaga I, Murray JF: Pulmonary complications of hiv infection in dar es salaam, tanzania. Role of bronchoscopy and bronchoalveolar lavage. Am J Respir Crit Care Med 1996;154:105-110.

Day RB, Wang Y, Knox KS, Pasula R, Martin WJ, 2nd, Twigg HL, 3rd: Alveolar macrophages from hiv-infected subjects are resistant to mycobacterium tuberculosis in vitro. Am J Respir Cell Mol Biol 2004;30:403-410.

De Cock KM, Soro B, Coulibaly IM, Lucas SB: Tuberculosis and hiv infection in sub-saharan africa. JAMA 1992;268:1581-1587.

De Cock KM, Wilkinson D: Tuberculosis control in resource-poor countries: Alternative approaches in the era of hiv. Lancet 1995;346:675-677.

Desta K, Asrat D, Lemma E, Gebeyehu M, Feleke B: Prevalence of smear negative pulmonary tuberculosis among patients visiting st. Peter's tuberculosis specialized hospital, addis ababa, ethiopia. Ethiop Med J 2009;47:17-24.

Dheda K, Chang JS, Breen RA, Haddock JA, Lipman MC, Kim LU, Huggett JF, Johnson MA, Rook GA, Zumla A: Expression of a novel cytokine, il-4delta2, in hiv and hiv-tuberculosis co-infection. AIDS 2005;19:1601-1606.

Dheda K, van Zyl-Smit RN, Meldau R, Meldau S, Symons G, Khalfey H, Govender N, Rosu V, Sechi LA, Maredza A, Semple P, Whitelaw A, Wainwright H, Badri M, Dawson R, Bateman ED, Zumla A: Quantitative lung t cell responses aid the rapid diagnosis of pulmonary tuberculosis. Thorax 2009;64:847-853.

Edwards D, Vogt M, Bangani N, et al. Baseline screening for TB among patients enrolling in an ART service in South Africa. In: Program and abstracts of the 16th Conference on Retroviruses and Opportunistic Infections (Montreal). 2009. Abstract 780.

Elliott AM, Luo N, Tembo G, Halwiindi B, Steenbergen G, Machiels L, Pobee J, Nunn P, Hayes RJ, McAdam KP: Impact of hiv on tuberculosis in zambia: A cross sectional study. BMJ 1990;301:412-415.

Elliott AM, Namaambo K, Allen BW, Luo N, Hayes RJ, Pobee JO, McAdam KP: Negative sputum smear results in hiv-positive patients with pulmonary tuberculosis in lusaka, zambia. Tuber Lung Dis 1993;74:191-194.

Foulds J, O'Brien R: New tools for the diagnosis of tuberculosis: The perspective of developing countries. Int J Tuberc Lung Dis 1998;2:778-783.

Gebre N, Karlsson U, Jonsson G, Macaden R, Wolde A, Assefa A, Miorner H: Improved microscopical diagnosis of pulmonary tuberculosis in developing countries. Trans R Soc Trop Med Hyg 1995;89:191-193.

Geldmacher C, Schuetz A, Ngwenyama N, Casazza JP, Sanga E, Saathoff E, Boehme C, Geis S, Maboko L, Singh M, Minja F, Meyerhans A, Koup RA, Hoelscher M: Early depletion of mycobacterium tuberculosis-specific t helper 1 cell responses after hiv-1 infection. J Infect Dis 2008;198:1590-1598.

Gopi PG, Subramani R, Selvakumar N, Santha T, Eusuff SI, Narayanan PR: Smear examination of two specimens for diagnosis of pulmonary tuberculosis in tiruvallur district, south india. Int J Tuberc Lung Dis 2004;8:824-828.

Graf P. Tuberculosis control in high-prevalence countries. In: Davies PDO, ed. Clinical tuberculosis 1994. London, Chapman & Hall, 1994: 325-339.

Grant AD, Sidibe K, Domoua K, Bonard D, Sylla-Koko F, Dosso M, Yapi A, Maurice C, Whitaker JP, Lucas SB, Hayes RJ, Wiktor SZ, De Cock KM, Greenberg AE:

Spectrum of disease among hiv-infected adults hospitalised in a respiratory medicine unit in abidjan, cote d'ivoire. Int J Tuberc Lung Dis 1998;2:926-934.

Greenberg AE, Lucas S, Tossou O, Coulibaly IM, Coulibaly D, Kassim S, Ackah A, De Cock KM: Autopsy-proven causes of death in hiv-infected patients treated for tuberculosis in abidjan, cote d'ivoire. AIDS 1995;9:1251-1254.

Greenberg SD, Frager D, Suster B, Walker S, Stavropoulos C, Rothpearl A: Active pulmonary tuberculosis in patients with aids: Spectrum of radiographic findings (including a normal appearance). Radiology 1994;193:115-119.

Gutierrez MG, Master SS, Singh SB, Taylor GA, Colombo MI, Deretic V: Autophagy is a defense mechanism inhibiting bcg and mycobacterium tuberculosis survival in infected macrophages. Cell 2004;119:753-766.

Habeenzu C, Lubasi D, Fleming AF: 'improved sensitivity of direct microscopy for detection of acid-fast bacilli in sputum in developing countries. Trans R Soc Trop Med Hyg 1998;92:415-416.

Hargreaves NJ, Kadzakumanja O, Phiri S, Nyangulu DS, Salaniponi FM, Harries AD, Squire SB: What causes smear-negative pulmonary tuberculosis in malawi, an area of high hiv seroprevalence? Int J Tuberc Lung Dis 2001;5:113-122.

Hargreaves NJ, Phiri S, Kwanjana J, Nyangulu DS, Squire SB: Unrecognised mycobacterium tuberculosis. Lancet 2000;355:141; author reply 142-143.

Harries AD: Tuberculosis and human immunodeficiency virus infection in developing countries. Lancet 1990;335:387-390.

Harries AD, Banda HT, Boeree MJ, Welby S, Wirima JJ, Subramanyam VR, Maher D, Nunn P: Management of pulmonary tuberculosis suspects with negative sputum smears and normal or minimally abnormal chest radiographs in resource-poor settings. Int J Tuberc Lung Dis 1998a;2:999-1004.

Harries AD, Maher D, Nunn P: An approach to the problems of diagnosing and treating adult smear-negative pulmonary tuberculosis in high-hiv-prevalence settings in sub-saharan africa. Bull World Health Organ 1998b;76:651-662.

Harries AD, Nyangulu DS, Kangombe C, Ndalama D, Wirima JJ, Salaniponi FM, Liomba G, Maher D, Nunn P: The scourge of hiv-related tuberculosis: A cohort study in a district general hospital in malawi. Ann Trop Med Parasitol 1997;91:771-776.

Hernandez-Garduno E, Cook V, Kunimoto D, Elwood RK, Black WA, FitzGerald JM: Transmission of tuberculosis from smear negative patients: A molecular epidemiology study. Thorax 2004;59:286-290.

Hopewell PC: Impact of human immunodeficiency virus infection on the epidemiology, clinical features, management, and control of tuberculosis. Clin Infect Dis 1992;15:540-547.

Ipuge YA, Rieder HL, Enarson DA: The yield of acid-fast bacilli from serial smears in routine microscopy laboratories in rural tanzania. Trans R Soc Trop Med Hyg 1996;90:258-261.

Jones BE, Young SM, Antoniskis D, Davidson PT, Kramer F, Barnes PF: Relationship of the manifestations of tuberculosis to cd4 cell counts in patients with human immunodeficiency virus infection. Am Rev Respir Dis 1993;148:1292-1297.

Kalsdorf B, Scriba TJ, Wood K, Day CL, Dheda K, Dawson R, Hanekom WA, Lange C, Wilkinson RJ: Hiv-1 infection impairs the bronchoalveolar t-cell response to mycobacteria. Am J Respir Crit Care Med 2009;180:1262-1270.

Kamanfu G, Mlika-Cabanne N, Girard PM, Nimubona S, Mpfizi B, Cishako A, Roux P, Coulaud JP, Larouze B, Aubry P, et al.: Pulmonary complications of human immunodeficiency virus infection in bujumbura, burundi. Am Rev Respir Dis 1993;147:658-663.

Kanaya AM, Glidden DV, Chambers HF: Identifying pulmonary tuberculosis in patients with negative sputum smear results. Chest 2001;120:349-355.

Kang'ombe CT, Harries AD, Ito K, Clark T, Nyirenda TE, Aldis W, Nunn PP, Semba RD, Salaniponi FM: Long-term outcome in patients registered with tuberculosis in zomba, malawi: Mortality at 7 years according to initial hiv status and type of tb. Int J Tuberc Lung Dis 2004;8:829-836.

Kassu A, Mengistu G, Ayele B, Diro E, Mekonnen F, Ketema D, Moges F, Mesfin T, Getachew A, Ergicho B, Elias D, Aseffa A, Wondmikun Y, Ota F: Coinfection and clinical manifestations of tuberculosis in human immunodeficiency virus-infected and -uninfected adults at a teaching hospital, northwest ethiopia. J Microbiol Immunol Infect 2007;40:116-122.

Keane J, Remold HG, Kornfeld H: Virulent mycobacterium tuberculosis strains evade apoptosis of infected alveolar macrophages. J Immunol 2000;164:2016-2020.

Kim TC, Blackman RS, Heatwole KM, Kim T, Rochester DF: Acid-fast bacilli in sputum smears of patients with pulmonary tuberculosis. Prevalence and significance of negative smears pretreatment and positive smears post-treatment. Am Rev Respir Dis 1984;129:264-268.

Kivihya-Ndugga LE, van Cleeff MR, Githui WA, Nganga LW, Kibuga DK, Odhiambo JA, Klatser PR: A comprehensive comparison of ziehl-neelsen and fluorescence microscopy for the diagnosis of tuberculosis in a resource-poor urban setting. Int J Tuberc Lung Dis 2003;7:1163-1171.

Klausner JD, Ryder RW, Baende E, Lelo U, Williame JC, Ngamboli K, Perriens JH, Kaboto M, Prignot J: Mycobacterium tuberculosis in household contacts of human immunodeficiency virus type 1-seropositive patients with active pulmonary tuberculosis in kinshasa, zaire. J Infect Dis 1993;168:106-111.

Kyei GB, Dinkins C, Davis AS, Roberts E, Singh SB, Dong C, Wu L, Kominami E, Ueno T, Yamamoto A, Federico M, Panganiban A, Vergne I, Deretic V: Autophagy pathway intersects with hiv-1 biosynthesis and regulates viral yields in macrophages. J Cell Biol 2009;186:255-268.

Lawn SD, Bekker LG, Middelkoop K, Myer L, Wood R: Impact of hiv infection on the epidemiology of tuberculosis in a peri-urban community in south africa: The need for age-specific interventions. Clin Infect Dis 2006;42:1040-1047.

Long R, Scalcini M, Manfreda J, Jean-Baptiste M, Hershfield E: The impact of hiv on the usefulness of sputum smears for the diagnosis of tuberculosis. Am J Public Health 1991;81:1326-1328.

Lucas SB, Hounnou A, Peacock C, Beaumel A, Kadio A, De Cock KM: Nocardiosis in hiv-positive patients: An autopsy study in west africa. Tuber Lung Dis 1994;75:301-307.

Malin AS, Gwanzura LK, Klein S, Robertson VJ, Musvaire P, Mason PR: Pneumocystis carinii pneumonia in zimbabwe. Lancet 1995;346:1258-1261.

Markowitz N, Hansen NI, Wilcosky TC, Hopewell PC, Glassroth J, Kvale PA, Mangura BT, Osmond D, Wallace JM, Rosen MJ, Reichman LB: Tuberculin and anergy testing in hiv-seropositive and hiv-seronegative persons. Pulmonary complications of hiv infection study group. Ann Intern Med 1993;119:185-193.

Mukadi Y, Perriens JH, St Louis ME, Brown C, Prignot J, Willame JC, Pouthier F, Kaboto M, Ryder RW, Portaels F, et al.: Spectrum of immunodeficiency in hiv-1-infected patients with pulmonary tuberculosis in zaire. Lancet 1993;342:143-146.

Munyati SS, Dhoba T, Makanza ED, Mungofa S, Wellington M, Mutsvangwa J, Gwanzura L, Hakim J, Nyakabau M, Mason PR, Robertson V, Rusakaniko S, Butterworth AE, Corbett EL: Chronic cough in primary health care attendees, harare, zimbabwe: Diagnosis and impact of hiv infection. Clin Infect Dis 2005;40:1818-1827.

Mwandumba HC, Russell DG, Nyirenda MH, Anderson J, White SA, Molyneux ME, Squire SB: Mycobacterium tuberculosis resides in nonacidified vacuoles in endocytically competent alveolar macrophages from patients with tuberculosis and hiv infection. J Immunol 2004;172:4592-4598.

Nunn P, Gicheha C, Hayes R, Gathua S, Brindle R, Kibuga D, Mutie T, Kamunyi R, Omwega M, Were J, et al.: Cross-sectional survey of hiv infection among patients with tuberculosis in nairobi, kenya. Tuber Lung Dis 1992;73:45-51.

Nyirenda TE, Harries AD, Banerjee A, Salaniponi FM: Accuracy of chest radiograph diagnosis for smear-negative pulmonary tuberculosis suspects by hospital clinical staff in malawi. Trop Doct 1999;29:219-220.

Oddo M, Renno T, Attinger A, Bakker T, MacDonald HR, Meylan PR: Fas ligand-induced apoptosis of infected human macrophages reduces the viability of intracellular mycobacterium tuberculosis. J Immunol 1998;160:5448-5454.

Palomino JC, Cardoso S, Ritacco V (2007) Tuberculosis 2007: from basic science to patient care. Available: http://www.tuberculosistextbook.com/ tuberculosis2007.pdf. Accessed 2011 Jul 5.

Parry CM: Sputum smear negative pulmonary tuberculosis. Trop Doct 1993;23:145-146.

Patel NR, Koziel H. Lung defenses in the immunosuppressed patient. In: Agusti C, Torres A, editors. Pulmonary infection in the immunocompromised patient. Oxford: Wiley-Blackwell; 2009

Patel NR, Swan K, Li X, Tachado SD, Koziel H: Impaired m. Tuberculosis-mediated apoptosis in alveolar macrophages from hiv+ persons: Potential role of il-10 and bcl-3. J Leukoc Biol 2009;86:53-60.

Patel NR, Zhu J, Tachado SD, Zhang J, Wan Z, Saukkonen J, Koziel H: Hiv impairs tnf-alpha mediated macrophage apoptotic response to mycobacterium tuberculosis. J Immunol 2007;179:6973-6980.

Pedro-Botet J, Gutierrez J, Miralles R, Coll J, Rubies-Prat J: Pulmonary tuberculosis in hiv-infected patients with normal chest radiographs. AIDS 1992;6:91-93.

Perkins MD, Cunningham J: Facing the crisis: Improving the diagnosis of tuberculosis in the hiv era. J Infect Dis 2007;196 Suppl 1:S15-27.

Raviglione MC, Harries AD, Msiska R, Wilkinson D, Nunn P: Tuberculosis and hiv: Current status in africa. AIDS 1997;11 Suppl B:S115-123.

Russell DG: Mycobacterium tuberculosis: Here today, and here tomorrow. Nat Rev Mol Cell Biol 2001;2:569-577.

Samb B, Henzel D, Daley CL, Mugusi F, Niyongabo T, Mlika-Cabanne N, Kamanfu G, Aubry P, Mbaga I, Larouze B, Murray JF: Methods for diagnosing tuberculosis among in-patients in eastern africa whose sputum smears are negative. Int J Tuberc Lung Dis 1997;1:25-30.

Samb B, Sow PS, Kony S, Maynart-Badiane M, Diouf G, Cissokho S, Ba D, Sane M, Klotz F, Faye-Niang MA, Mboup S, Ndoye I, Delaporte E, Hane AA, Samb A, Coulaud JP, Coll-Seck AM, Larouze B, Murray JF: Risk factors for negative sputum acid-fast bacilli smears in pulmonary tuberculosis: Results from dakar, senegal, a city with low hiv seroprevalence. Int J Tuberc Lung Dis 1999;3:330-336.

Saukkonen JJ, Bazydlo B, Thomas M, Strieter RM, Keane J, Kornfeld H: Beta-chemokines are induced by mycobacterium tuberculosis and inhibit its growth. Infect Immun 2002;70:1684-1693.

Schaible UE, Winau F, Sieling PA, Fischer K, Collins HL, Hagens K, Modlin RL, Brinkmann V, Kaufmann SH: Apoptosis facilitates antigen presentation to t lymphocytes through mhc-i and cd1 in tuberculosis. Nat Med 2003;9:1039-1046.

Selwyn PA, Pumerantz AS, Durante A, Alcabes PG, Gourevitch MN, Boiselle PM, Elmore JG: Clinical predictors of pneumocystis carinii pneumonia, bacterial pneumonia and tuberculosis in hiv-infected patients. AIDS 1998;12:885-893.

Siddiqi K, Lambert ML, Walley J: Clinical diagnosis of smear-negative pulmonary tuberculosis in low-income countries: The current evidence. Lancet Infect Dis 2003;3:288-296.

Simooya OO, Maboshe MN, Kaoma RB, Chimfwembe EC, Thurairajah A, Mukunyandela M: Hiv infection in newly diagnosed tuberculosis patients in ndola, zambia. Cent Afr J Med 1991;37:4-7.

Sonnenberg P, Glynn JR, Fielding K, Murray J, Godfrey-Faussett P, Shearer S: How soon after infection with hiv does the risk of tuberculosis start to increase? A retrospective cohort study in south african gold miners. J Infect Dis 2005;191:150-158.

Sonnenberg P, Murray J, Glynn JR, Shearer S, Kambashi B, Godfrey-Faussett P: Hiv-1 and recurrence, relapse, and reinfection of tuberculosis after cure: A cohort study in south african mineworkers. Lancet 2001;358:1687-1693.

Steingart KR, Ng V, Henry M, Hopewell PC, Ramsay A, Cunningham J, Urbanczik R, Perkins MD, Aziz MA, Pai M: Sputum processing methods to improve the sensitivity of smear microscopy for tuberculosis: A systematic review. Lancet Infect Dis 2006;6:664-674.

Sudre P, ten Dam G, Kochi A: Tuberculosis: A global overview of the situation today. Bull World Health Organ 1992;70:149-159.

Sutherland R, Yang H, Scriba TJ, Ondondo B, Robinson N, Conlon C, Suttill A, McShane H, Fidler S, McMichael A, Dorrell L: Impaired ifn-gamma-secreting capacity in mycobacterial antigen-specific cd4 t cells during chronic hiv-1 infection despite long-term haart. AIDS 2006;20:821-829.

Tessema TA, Bjune G, Assefa G, Bjorvat B: An evaluation of the diagnostic value of clinical and radiological manifestations in patients attending the addis ababa tuberculosis centre. Scand J Infect Dis 2001;33:355-361.

Toman K. Tuberculosis case-finding and chemotherapy. Questions and answers. Geneva, World Health Organization, 1979.

Tostmann A, Kik SV, Kalisvaart NA, Sebek MM, Verver S, Boeree MJ, van Soolingen D: Tuberculosis transmission by patients with smear-negative pulmonary tuberculosis in a large cohort in the netherlands. Clin Infect Dis 2008;47:1135-1142.

van Cleeff MR, Kivihya-Ndugga L, Githui W, Nganga L, Odhiambo J, Klatser PR: A comprehensive study of the efficiency of the routine pulmonary tuberculosis diagnostic process in nairobi. Int J Tuberc Lung Dis 2003;7:186-189.

Whalen C, Horsburgh CR, Hom D, Lahart C, Simberkoff M, Ellner J: Accelerated course of human immunodeficiency virus infection after tuberculosis. Am J Respir Crit Care Med 1995;151:129-135.

Whalen C, Horsburgh CR, Jr., Hom D, Lahart C, Simberkoff M, Ellner J: Site of disease and opportunistic infection predict survival in hiv-associated tuberculosis. AIDS 1997;11:455-460.

Laboratory Services in Tuberculosis Control. Technical Series: Microscopy. WHO/TB/98.258. Geneva: World Health Organization, 1998.

Worl Health Organization (WHO): Global tuberculosis control, WHO report 2002 [http://www.who.int/gtb/publications] accessed 2011 Jul 13

World Health Organization. Treatment of tuberculosis. Guidelines for national programs. WHO/CDS/TB/2003.313. Geneva, Switzerland: WHO, 2003.

World Health Orgainization. Toman's Tuberculosis: Case detection, treatment and monitoring-questions and answers. WHO/HTM/TB/2004.334. Geneva: World Health Organization, 2004.

Worl Health Organization (WHO): Improving the diagnosis and treatment of smear-negative pulmonary and extra-pulmonary tuberculosis among adults and adolescents: recommendations for HIV-prevalent and resource-constrained settings. Geneva, World Health Organization, 2007. WHO/HTM/TB/2007.379 WHO/HIV/2007.01

World Health Organization. Global tuberculosis control: a short update to the 2009 report. December 2009. Geneva: World Health Organization, 2009.

World Health Organization. Global tuberculosis control: epidemiology, strategy, financing. WHO report 2009. Geneva, Switzerland: WHO; 2009

Wilkinson D, Davies GR: The increasing burden of tuberculosis in rural south africa--impact of the hiv epidemic. S Afr Med J 1997;87:447-450.

Williams BG, Dye C: Antiretroviral drugs for tuberculosis control in the era of hiv/aids. Science 2003;301:1535-1537.

Winau F, Weber S, Sad S, de Diego J, Hoops SL, Breiden B, Sandhoff K, Brinkmann V, Kaufmann SH, Schaible UE: Apoptotic vesicles crossprime cd8 t cells and protect against tuberculosis. Immunity 2006;24:105-117.

Yassin MA, Takele L, Gebresenbet S, Girma E, Lera M, Lendebo E, Cuevas LE: Hiv and tuberculosis coinfection in the southern region of ethiopia: A prospective epidemiological study. Scand J Infect Dis 2004;36:670-673.

Zachariah R, Spielmann MP, Harries AD, Salaniponi FL: Voluntary counselling, hiv testing and sexual behaviour among patients with tuberculosis in a rural district of malawi. Int J Tuberc Lung Dis 2003;7:65-71.

Zhang M, Gong J, Iyer DV, Jones BE, Modlin RL, Barnes PF: T cell cytokine responses in persons with tuberculosis and human immunodeficiency virus infection. J Clin Invest 1994;94:2435-2442.

7

Diagnostic Methods for *Mycobacterium tuberculosis* and Challenges in Its Detection in India

Shamsher S. Kanwar
Department of Biotechnology
Himachal Pradesh University, Summer Hill, Shimla
India

1. Introduction

Tuberculosis (TB) is one of the world's oldest and most important disseminating infectious diseases that still accounts for a high morbidity and mortality among adults. Despite high prevalence, case detection rates are low, posing major hurdles for TB control in developed and developing countries. Traditional diagnosis of TB bacilli depends upon smear positivity in sputum samples, culture and chest radiography. All these tests have known limitations. Conventional tests for detection of drug resistance are slow, tedious and difficult to perform in field conditions. For rapid diagnosis, new methods include newer versions of nucleic acid amplification tests, immune-based assays, skin patch test and rapid culture systems. For drug resistance analysis line-probe assays, bacteriophage-based assays, molecular beacons and microscopic observation drug susceptibility assay are available. An ideal test for TB is still not available and fast emergence of drug resistant tubercle strains aided by the ever-increasing HIV AIDS-epidemic in third-world countries has stressed the need of rapid diagnostic test(s) to show the presence of mycobateria in the clinical samples. Microscopy and culture are still the major backbone for laboratory diagnosis of tuberculosis; new methods including molecular diagnostic tests have evolved over a period of time. The majority of molecular tests have been focused on: (i) detection of nucleic acids both DNA and RNA, which are specific to *Mycobacterium tuberculosis*, by amplification techniques such as polymerase chain reaction (PCR) focusing on detection and molecular epidemiology of *M. tuberculosis*; and (ii) detection of mutations in the genes which are associated with resistance to anti-tuberculosis drugs by sequencing or nucleic acid hybridization. The development and use of rapid diagnostic tools become increasingly important in addressing the emergence and treatment of multi-drug resistant (MDR) and extreme-drug (XDR) resistant *M. tuberculosis* strains.

Tuberculosis remains one of the most challenging bacterial diseases in spite of development of a realm of antibiotics and diagnostic molecular biology techniques. The tubercle bacillus was discovered more than two hundred years ago and substantial advancements have been made in our knowledge about the development of tuberculosis in human. The organism seems to evolve over a period of time in terms of its ability to survive the action of front line anti mycobacterial antibiotics by developing appropriate antibiotic resistant mechanisms. The estimated mortality by World Health Organization reports over 1.7 million deaths in 2006 and 9 million new cases of tuberculosis [WHO 2008]. The economic burden of management of disease in patients in the prime of their age is enormous because of prolonged antibiotic treatment. In spite of availability of anti mycobacterial drugs, tuberculosis remains one of the major health problems facing mankind particularly in developing countries. Presently, about one third of word's population is infected with *Mycobacterium tuberculosis*. Currently, the number of people dying of tuberculosis is more than any other infectious diseases. Death from tuberculosis comprises 25% of all avoidable deaths in developing countries [Ramachandran and Parmasivan 2003]. Nearly 95% of all tuberculosis cases and 98% of deaths due to tuberculosis are in developing countries and 75% of tuberculosis cases are in the economically productive age group. Currently, more people die of tuberculosis than from any other infectious disease. In India, out of a total population of more than 1 billion, approximately 2 million develop active disease and up to half a million die of tuberculosis. It also imparts a financial burden on the economy in terms of out-put losses because of premature deaths and ill health. To add to the existing cost burden, the cumulative effect is seen because of ever increasing number of new TB cases associated with HIV patients and about 1.8 million of these are co-infected with TB [Ramachandran and Paramasivan 2003].

2. Traditional methods of tuberculosis detection, management and limitations

Robert Koch discovered the tubercle bacillus in 1882, and there after methods of staining these microorganisms were developed to assist the diagnosis of the disease. Early diagnosis of the tuberculosis in the patients is a challenging task especially in the pauci-bacillary and extra-pulmonary forms. The conventional methods that are still the mainstay of the diagnosis of TB like Tuberculin test/ Montoux test, radiological examination and other imaging methods and sputum smear microscopy have their own limitations. Sputum smear microscopy requires 10,000 to 1,00,000 organisms/ ml and acid fast bacilli could be any pathogenic or saprophytic mycobacteria. Although smear microscopy may be made more convenient by using various fluorochromes (auramine, rhodamine, FITC etc.) but the scarce presence of tuber bacilli in the sputum has its own disadvantage. The smear positivity has to be supplemented with the culture positivity that has its own limitations because of failure of bacilli to grow or often become contaminated with other microbes. The slow growth of the tubercle bacilli on medium lingers on the confirmation of the causative organism. Histopathology is characteristic but there could be problems to get representative specimen, and non-specific features. Immunoassay based approaches are doubtful as the antibodies and the antigens may persist for some time after control of the clinical or sub-clinical disease. Thus Acid Fast Bacilli (AFB) staining of clinical material followed by smear microscopy remains the most cost effective, frequently used microbiological test for detection of TB. The major drawback of sputum smear microscopy is its poor sensitivity, especially to be ~70% in a recent review [Steingart et al., 2006]. Although the AFB staining is easy to perform in the field settings especially in the poor third world countries as well in the developing countries but the sensitivity of sputum smear microscopy is clearly less in many settings and may be sometimes as low as ~35% in some situations with high rates of TB and HIV co-infection [Khatri and Frieden 2002]. Compounding the poor test sensitivity is in adequate or absent test quality assurance in some recourse-constrained settings, further cut down the over all yield of the microscopy, driving up the laboratory workload as more sputum tests per patient are performed in an effort to reach a diagnosis, and increasing delay in diagnosis and patient's compliance to repeated follow-up [Dorman 2010]. Moreover drug-susceptibility status cannot be determined from the smear microscopy.

Unfortunately, the world's largest democracy India has over 1.2 billion people and this overpopulated country also has the highest burden of tuberculosis in the world. India accounts for about 20% incidence of tuberculosis besides a high incidence of global occurrence of multi drug resistant (MDR) tuberculosis. The poor sanitation conditions, thickly populated urban and rural area, scanty medical services in villages and rural area, malnourishment, insensitivity of private sector towards quick diagnosis, treatment and management of TB positive patients and higher cost of non-standard methods of diagnosis of TB are some of the important reasons of concern. It is obvious that any global effort towards control and eradication of TB and fast emerging MDR-TB is invariably dependent upon success of concerted efforts to contain the spread of this contagious disease. In India, the National TB Programme (NTP) was initiated in 1962. However, the poor infrastructure, inadequate funding, administrative lack-luster approach, irregular drug supply, non-standard and multiple anti-tuberculosis drug therapy, irregularity or non-compliance of patients to the clinician and a long treatment period had little effect on containing the spread of TB and controlling the emerging MRD-TB strains. The management and control of TB was further compounded and complicated with low rates of TB case detection, compliance of treatment regimen (30%), high rate of default (40-60%) and continuing high mortality (1: 2000) the NTP programme had little success rate. To overcome the deficiencies of NTP a Revised National Tuberculosis Control Programme (RNTCP) was launched by the Government of India in 1997, based on the global DOTS (Directly Observed Treatment, Short Course) approach that was used to exert an epidemiological impact by achieving 70% case detection and 85% cure rate. It was an encouraging sign that by 2002, 100% of the Indian population was covered by the India's own drug-delivery model - the DOTS programme, making this extended coverage as India's most significant public health accomplishment. The RNTCP thus achieved a pronounced success in cure rates (>80% in new infectious cases), substantial decline in mortality with low rate (<10%) of default [Khatri and Frieden 2002; TB India 2009; Bhargava et al., 2011].

3. Tuberculosis and HIV epidemic

In spite of improvement in public health system, participation of private sector in TB detection and management still the sputum smear microscopy test is most commonly used in public health settings to detect pulmonary TB. This method has roughly 50% chance of detection. Unfortunately, a significant number of people outside the public health sector, where the most common test is the serological (various types of ELISA for detection of *M. tuberculosis* antigens; or anti-*M. tuberculosis* IgG or IgM antibodies) that are expensive and means nothing. The global impact of converging dual epidemics of tuberculosis and human immunodeficiency virus (HIV) is one of the major challenges of the present time. In India, there are 2.5 million people living with HIV and AIDS at the end of 2007 while the incidence of TB was `1.8 million cases per year [WHO 2008, WHO Global Tuberculosis Program 1992].

In a survey carried out among new TB patients by RNTCP in 2007, HIV sero-prevalence varied widely and ranged from 1-13.8% across the 15 districts [Swaminathan and Narendran 2008]. Pulmonary involvement occurs in about 75% of all HIV-infected patients with TB [Devivanayagam et al., 2001; Ahmad and Shameen 2005]. Moreover, the interaction between HIV and TB in persons co-infected with HIV and TB is bi-directional and synergistic. As HIV progresses, there is cutaneous anergy as well as impaired tissue containment of mycobacteria leading to widespread dissemination of mycobacteria. While TB can develop at any CD4 count, extra-pulmonary and disseminated forms of the diseases are more common as immunodeficiency increases. Thus HIV infection is associated not only with an increased incidence of TB but also with altered clinical manifestations especially in the advanced stages of the disease. The cost management of anti-HIV and anti-TB therapy in the patients becomes a daunting task that compromises the success rate of containment and spread of TB from HIV infected patients. Current guidelines recommend that irrespective of HIV status, TB management require a minimum of 6 months of treatment with four drugs (including rifampin) in the intensive phase and two drugs in the continuation phase. In India, under the RNTCP, patients with newly diagnosed TB receive a 6-month thrice-weekly regimen 9cat I – 2EHRZ$_3$/4RH$_3$) while those with relapse, default or failure receive an 8-months regimen (cat II – 2SEHRZ$_3$/1SEHRZ$_3$/5EHR$_3$). The lifetime risk of TB in immuno-competent persons is 5% to 10%, but HIV positive individuals; there is a 5% to 15% annual risk of developing active TB diseases [Swaminathan et al., 2000]. WHO estimated 9.2 million new cases of TB globally in 2006 (139 per 100,000); of whom 7,09,000 (7.7%) were HIV positive (WHO 2008). India, China, Indonesia, South Africa and Nigeria rank 1st to 5th in terms of incident TB cases.

The first and foremost step in the diagnosis of TB is its accurate and early detection. To achieve this objective a number of methods have been developed and reported (Table 1) that achieve early growth of *M. tuberculosis* [Katoch and Sharma 1997; Katoch 2004].

4. Anti-TB drug resistance

The overall pattern of drug resistance to first line anti TB therapy is similar in HIV positive and negative patients; however, MDR-TB is marginally higher (3-4%) in HIV positive patients with newly diagnosed tuberculosis status [Swaminathan 2005]. Rifampicin mono-resistance is more common in HIV infected patients and arises independently from mutations in drug susceptible strains. Treatment of MDR-TB should employ at least 3-4 new drugs. The regimen should include an aminoglycoside and be given under direct observation. Extensively drug resistant (XDR) TB strains have emerged and have been reported from India [Singh et al., 2007; Thomas et al., 2007]. Such strains appeared to be as an outcome of the mismanagement of TB. It seems that XDR-TB is practically untreatable and thus an attempt may be made to limit its spread by strengthening the TB control programme. Presently, there is no national policy regarding TB preventive therapy for HIV positive patients in India [Swaminathan and Narendran 2008]. A clinical trial conducted at the Tuberculosis Research Center, Chennai investigated two different regimens; a 6-month regimen of ethambutol and isoniazid vs. a 3-year regimen of isoniazid alone, in order to establish ideal duration of therapy. In a TB-endemic country like India, consideration shall be given to provide preventive therapy to HIV-infected persons. Line probe assays, a family

S. No.	Method	Concept	Reference(s)
1	BACTEC system	Generation and detection of radioactive CO_2 from substrate palmitic acid. Used world-over, detection of growth in 5-7 d. Inclusion of (NAP: beta nitro alpha acetylamine beta hydroxy propiophenone) distinguishes *M. tuberculosis* [inhibition] from other mycobacteria.	Venkataram et al., 1998; Bemer et al., 2002
2	Mycobacteria growth indicator tube (MGIT)	Developed by Becton Dickinson, growth detection by non-radioactive fluorochrome detection; useful in drug screening, early detection of mycobacterium growth in 7-12 d.	Bemer et al., 2002; Tortoli et al., 1999
3	MB/BacT system	Developed by Organon Technika; colorimetric detection of bacterial growth in, cultures; also useful for drug susceptibility testing	Brunello and Fontana 2000
4	TK Medium	Developed by Salubris, Inc., MA, USA is a novel colorimetric system that indicates growth of mycobacteria by changing its color, also discriminates between mycobacteria and contamination, and enables drug susceptibility testing. Test is low cost and simple. Sensitivity of TK medium is comparable to the LJ-medium.	Kocagoz et al., 2004; Salubris, Inc.
5	Septi-Check	Bi-phase system developed by Roche. Consists of enriched selective broth and a slide having non-selective Middlebrook agar on one side and two sections on other side: one with NAP + egg-containing agar, and second with chocolate agar for detection of contaminating microbes.	Isenberg et al., 1991

S. No.	Method	Concept	Reference(s)
6	Reporter phages/ Bronx box	Use of mycobacterium-specific phage(s) and a reporter gene (luciferase) for detection of growth and drug-susceptibility to anti-TB drugs. Viability detection by either emission of light from microbe due to activation of luciferase gene or production of plaque on an indicator strain of mycobacteria; results availability in 2 d.	Riska et al., 1999; Wilson et al., 1997; Krishnamurthy et al., 2002
7	E-test	Use of gradient of drug on a paper-strip; useful for drug susceptibility testing of *M. tuberculosis*.	Kirk et al., 1998
8	Flow cytometry	Use of FACS for drug susceptibility testing, high cost of equipment and trained operator are the drawbacks.	Kakkar et al., 2000
9	Line-probe assay	A novel DNA strip-based test that uses PCR and reverse hybridization methods for rapid detection of mutations associated with drug resistance. Designed to identify *M. tuberculosis* complex and simultaneous detection of mutations associated with drug resistance.	Morgan et al., 2005

Table 1. Methods of early detection of *M. tuberculosis*.

of novel DNA strip-based tests use PCR and reverse hybridization methods for the rapid detection of mutations associated with drug resistance. These kits [INNO-LiPA Rif TB kit, Innogenetics NV, Gent, Belgium; GenoType MTBDR assay; Hain Life-science GmbH, Nehren, Germany] are not currently FDA approved for use in USA. Line-probe assays are designed to identify *M. tuberculosis* complex and simultaneously detect mutations associated with drug resistance. In June 2008, WHO announced a new policy statement endorsing the use of line probe assays for rapid screening of patients at risk of MRD-TB (http://www.who.int/tb/en/). However, the line probe assays are not recommended as a complete replacement for conventional culture and drug susceptibility testing. Culture is still required for smear-negative specimens and conventional drug susceptibility testing is still necessary to confirm XDR-TB.

5. Ineffective TB diagnostics in India

Ineffective TB diagnostics are a lucrative market in India. Patients seeking TB care in the private medical institutes are commonly subjected to diagnostic tests i.e. the anti-body-based blood tests, including ELISA that are completely ineffective at detecting TB. This is because a large number of the world's population has anti-TB antibodies, though only 10% of them do develop the active form of the disease. Obviously if patients who do not have TB are misdiagnosed, they could undergo 6-months of nasty toxic anti-TB chemotherapy. If patients have active TB and the test missies it, the disease may worsen and they may continue to spread the disease in their community. According to a preliminary analysis of over 80 labs in India, it is estimated that patients undergo more than 1.5 million useless TB antibody tests each year (WHO recommends against inaccurate tuberculosis tests by Kelly Morris; www.thelancet.com vol 377 Jan 8, 2011). The absence of any regulatory mechanisms results in the import of these dubious diagnostics from France, UK, USA and other countries, where these tests are not approved for TB diagnosis. These tests generate at least US $ 15 million. In a country that has ~100,000 labs this is probably a fraction of the enormous total market. Accurate diagnose is critical to the control of tuberculosis in India, particularly in view of the fact that India has set new targets as a part of RNTCP, which includes early detection of 90% of all TB cases by year 2015.

6. Molecular diagnosis of TB in Indian context

In India various institutes working on TB have sufficient technical expertise and financial affordability to use molecular diagnostic methods for detection of tubercle bacilli in the samples. For a laboratory with good sample load and which is using rapid methods for early growth detection the additional cost of sample analysis shall not be significant. If 10-25 isolates/ growths are assessed for identity simultaneously, additional cost for each isolate using a non-radioactive detection system like digoxigenin (DIG) should not be more than 200-250 rupees (~US $ 4-5). Similarly for a PCR system using primers, which are not patented, cost should be in similar range as prices of primers and reagents have considerably been reduced during the last couple of years [Katoch 2004]. The nucleic acid amplification tests (NAATs) are designed to amplify nucleic acid regions specific to the *Mycobacterium tuberculosis* complex. Such tests may be used directly on clinical samples/ sputum samples. Nucleic acid amplification test (NAAT) commercial kits are available under various brands like Amplified *M. tuberculosis* Direct Test (MTD; Gen-Probe Inc., CA, USA), the Amplicor *M. tuberculosis* (MTB) tests (Roche Molecular Diagnostics, CA, USA and the BD ProbeTec ET assay (BD Biosciences, MD, USA. Besides in-house lab developed PCR assays vary widely in their protocols and vary from lab to lab. In-house NAAT are cheap and are often used in research in developing countries where commercial NAATs are quite expensive to test large number of samples and thus in-house PCR technique/ protocol(s) provide a cheap option (Pai 2004). However, all the detection methods including the conventional AFB-staining, skin tuberculin test and new generation NAAT tests have some advantages as well as limitations (Table 2).

Method	Use	Intended use	Advantages	Limitations
AFB smear microscopy	Rapid tubercle bacilli detection	Community	Needs moderate training, microscope and low investment	Low sensitivity
Culture on solid media	Mycobacterial growth and drug susceptibility assay	Referral lab	Good sensitivity; gold standard	Long time to detect growth of bacteria
Chest radiography	Pulmonary TB detection	Referral by clinician	Indications and use not restricted to TB	Low specificity & sensitivity, trained clinician needed
Tuberculin skin test	Detection of *M. tuberculosis*	Community	Extensive clinical and published experience	Sensitivity decreases in immuno-comprised persons, positive reaction in BCG vaccinees
γ-Interferon release assay	Detection of *M. tuberculosis* infection	Referral to reference lab	Highly specific for *M. tuberculosis*	Trained manpower, poor sensitivity especially in immunocompro mised hosts
Automated, non-integrated NAAT	Pulmonary TB detection	Reference lab	High sensitivity, rapidity and detection of mutations in MDR-TB strains.	Moderately trained personnel and equipment, laborious and possible cross-contamination among specimens
Culture in liquid media [MGIT; BacT/ Alert and others]	TB detection and as a prerequisite to drug-susceptibility testing	Referral lab	High sensitivity (more sensitivity than liquid media)	Long time for detection; less than solid medium but high contamination rate in some settings

Method	Use	Intended use	Advantages	Limitations
Line probe assay	TB detection and drug susceptibility testing	Reference lab	Poor sensitivity in smear-negative samples, short analysis time	Labor intensive, potential for cross-contamination, requires extensive training
Strip-based Mycobacterium species identification	Species identification i.e. TB versus non-TB in cultures positive for mycobacterial growth	Referral lab	Accurate, requires minimal-training/ equipment/ consumables	Moderate training in handling of pathogenic microbes

Adapted from references: Pai et al., 2006; Perkins and Cunningham 2007; Nyendak et al., 2009; WHO and Stop TB Partnership 2009; Dorman 2010.

Table 2. Tuberculosis diagnostic methods in use, recently endorsed by WHO and under development.

7. Challenges in the TB care and control

At present a vigorous approach is needed to proactively detect the TB cases under RNTCP. The DOT service providers may be actively involved in identifying fresh potential TB patients in their community and getting them diagnosed for TB. Another possibility is contact tracing of both adults and children diagnosed to have TB. Such approach is currently being followed in HIV programs and could be considered to improve upon the case detection rate. Further prevalence studies in different parts of India may be conducted systematically to determine the existing burden of TB. The district level data will be quite helpful in achieving a realistic figure of TB cases.

Lab strengthening: In most cases among the poorest strata of people living in slums or rural areas the sputum transportation is difficult to reach populations is a major consideration and TB is quite commonly said to be poor man's disease. Thus inadequate number of microscopic centers/ labs put the burden on existing microscopic centers that causes a delay in the reporting of the results of the sputum samples. Most labs conduct AFB testing and are ill equipped to perform culture of tubercle bacilli.

Migrant populations: Presently, there is no national level strategy and guidelines for tuberculosis care and control for the migrant population in India who move from one state or place to another one as a part of their jobs or in search of jobs. Millions of migrants are currently working in unorganized job sectors with no health facilities, insurance facilities and work place policy for disease care and control like TB, HIV etc. Such workers are solely dependent on the relatively expensive private health sector for their healthcare. Accessing those migrants at their residences and working places with the key messages of TB, DOTS and RNTCP is extremely challenging because of the geographically scattered areas and huge number of migrants. Also women engaged in unorganized job sectors are particularly prone to tuberculosis due to continuous exploitation by the employers. The migrant workers should be mapped in the urban and peri-urban areas (construction sites, street dwellers, illegal residents along the railway tracts, brick kilns etc.) and should be provided RNTCP services (like sensitization on TB, identification of suspected TB cases, referral and tracking) through community-based programs as part of the extended TB monitoring and care program and activities. Moreover, the TB component may be introduced into the existing HIV programs for migrant workers after collaboration with National AIDS Control Programs (NACO).

New TB testing tools: For 100% detection of the TB cases new technologies and techniques shall be establishes that are reasonably cheap, rapid and easily available. Recently a new PCR based diagnostic kit has been developed through a partnership between Cepheid and Foundation for Innovative New diagnostics, the University of Medicine and Density of New Jersey, the Bill and Melinda Gates Foundation and national Institute of Health (U.S.). The study demonstrated high sensitivity and specificity, identifying 98% of patients with TB and correctly identified 98% of bacteria resistant to rifampin.

Besides PCR, some novel tests involving use of beacons for the rapid detection of mutations associated with drug resistance have been reported [Varma-Basil et al., 2004]. Employing Xpert/RIF kit 1,700 patients were screened at five sites across the world including Mumbai, and using this PCR 98% of patients with TB and resistant to rifampin were correctly identified. This PCR needed about 100 minutes compared to current tests that may take up to 3 months to have results. Unfortunately, the PCR NAATs are performed in a few national labs and specialized private hospitals only. Facilities for culture and drug susceptibility testing of TB cultures in India are grossly inadequate [Bhargava 2011]. As of 2008, only 17 accredited facilities were doing culture and drug-susceptibility testing (~0.1 facility/ 10 million residents against 1/ 10 million). Efforts are underway to enhance the number of labs/ facilities to 43 to perform drug-susceptibility testing. The RNTCP has started to include rapid diagnostic methods to perform culture and drug-susceptibility testing so as to prevent delay in management of MDR-TB patients.

8. Conclusion

TB one of the most communicable diseases is still evading accurate diagnosis because of lack and development of cheap, less labor/ equipment intensive, highly specific and sensitive methods. Culture positivity in sputum positive samples is still considered to be a gold standard as this method provides a further lead in accessing the drug susceptibility of the grown mycobacterial cultures. Currently, most of the tools/ techniques in demonstration or late-stage validation are sputum based and thus are likely to result in incremental gains in rate of TB detection. Still there is an urgent need to develop and validate a mycobacterial culture based or NAAT-based technique that is close to 100% specificity and sensitivity. The need to fast develop such techniques is urgent because of development of MDR mycobacterial strains in third-world countries as these countries are also experiencing an increased burden of HIV-positive patients. The previous decade has shown how despite '100% coverage' and impressive case detection and cure rates, TB continues to be an epidemic of magnanimous magnitude in India. Thus in India a staunch collaboration between RNTCP, NACO and private partners is the need of the hour to contain the fast spread of MRD *M. tuberculosis* strains.

9. References

Ahmad Z and Shameem M (2005). Manifestations of tuberculosis in HIV infected patients. JIACM 6: 302-305.

Bemer P, Palicova F, Rusch-Gerdes S, Dugeon HB and Pfyffer GE (2002). Multicentre evaluation of fully automatic BACTEC mycobacteria growth indicator tube 960 system for susceptibility testing of *Mycobacterium tuberculosis*. J Clin Microbiol 40: 150-154.

Bhargava A, Pinto l and Pai M (2011). Mismanagement of tuberculosis in India: causes, consequences and the way forward. Hypothesis 9: 1-13.

Brunello F and Fontana R (2000). Reliability of the MB-BactT system for testing susceptibility of *Mycobacterium tuberculosis* complex strains to anti-tuberculous drugs. J Clin Microbiol 38: 872-873.

Deivanayagam CN, Rajasekaran S, Senthilnathan V, Krishnarajasekhar R, Raja K, Chandrasekar C, Palanisamy S, Samuel DA, Jothivel G and Elango SV (2001). Clinico-radiological spectrum of tuberculosia among HIV-sero-positives – a Tambaram study. Indian J Tuberc 49: 123-127.

Dorman SE (2010). New diagnostic tests for tuberculosis: Bench, bedside and beyond. Clin Infect Dis 50: S173-S177.

Isenberg HD, D'Amate RF, Heifets L, Murray PR, Scardamaglia M, Jacob MC et al., (1991). Collaborative feasibility study of a biphasic system (Roche Septi-Chek AFB) for rapid detection and isolation of mycobacteria. J Clin Microbiol 29: 1713-1722.

Kakkar N, Sharma M, Ray P, Seth S and Kumar S (2000). Evaluation of E-test for susceptibility testing of mycobacteria to primary antitubercular drugs. Indian J Med Res 111: 168-171.

Katoch VM (2004). Newer diagnostic techniques for tuberculosis. Indian J Med Res 120: 418-428.

Katoch VM and Sharma VD (1997).Advances in the diagnosis of mycobacterial diseases. Indian J Med Microbiol 15: 49-55.

Khatri GR and Frieden T (2002). Controlling tuberculosis in India. N Engl J Med 347: 1420-1425.

Kirk SM, Schell RF, Moore AV, Callister SM and Mazurek GH (1998). Flow cytometric testing of susceptibilities of *Mycobacterium tuberculosis* isolates to ethambutol, isoniazid and rifampicin in 24 hours. J Clin Microbiol 36: 1568-1571.

Kocagoz T, O'Brien R and Perkins M (2004). A new colorimetric culture system for the diagnosis of tuberculosis. Int J Tuberc Lung Dis 8: 1512-1513.

Krishnamurthy A, Rodrigues C and Mehta AP (2002). Rapid detection of rifampicin resistance in *Mycobacterium tuberculosis* by phage assay. Indian J Med Microbiol 20: 211-214.

Morgan M, Kalantri S, Flores L and Pai M (2005). A commercial line probe assay for the rapid detection of rifampicin resistance in Mycobacterium tuberculosis. A systemic review and meta-analysis. BMC Infect Dis 5: 62.

Nyendak MR, Lewinsohn DA and Lewinsohn DM (2009). New diagnostic methods for tuberculosis. Curr Opin Infect Dis 22: 174-182.

Pai M (2004). The accuracy and reliability of nucleic acid amplification tests in the diagnosis of tuberculosis. Natl Med J India 17: 233-236.

Pai M, Kalantri S and Dheda K (2006). New tools and emerging technologies for the diagnosis of tuberculosis: Part II. Active tuberculosis and drug resistance. Expert Rev Mol Diagn 6: 423-432.

Perkin MD and Cunningham J (2007). Facing the crisis: Improving the diagnosis of tuberculosis in the HIV era. J Infect Dis 196(Suppl 1): S15-S27.

Ramachandran R and Parmasivan CN (2003). What is new in the diagnosis of tuberculosis? Part I: Techniques for diagnosis of tuberculosis. Indian J Tuberculosis 50: 133-141.

Riska PF, Su Y, Bardarov S, Freundlish L, Sarkis G, Hatfull G et al., (1999). Rapid film-based determination of antibiotic susceptibility of *Mycobacterium tuberculosis* strains by using a luciferase reporter phage and the Bronx box. J Clin Microbiol 37: 1144-1149.

Singh S, Sankar MM and Gopinath K (2007). High rate of extensively drug-resistant tuberculosis in Indian AIDS patients. AIDS 21: 2345-2347.

Steingart KR, Henry M, Ng V et al., (2006). Fluorescence versus conventional smear microscopy for tuberculosis: A systemic review. Lancet Infect Dis 6: 570-581.

Swaminathan S and Narendran G (2008). HIV and tuberculosis in India. J Biosci 33: 527-537.

Swaminathan S, Paramasivan CN, Ponnuraja C, Iliayas S, Rajasekaran S and naryanan PR (2005). Anti-tuberculosis drug resistance tuberculosis in South India. Int J Tuberc Lung Dis 9: 896-900.

Swaminathan S, Ramachandran R, Baskaran G and Paramsivan CN (2000). Risk of development of tuberculosis in HIV infectd patients. Int J Tuberc Lung Dis 4: 839-844.

TB India (2009). RNTCP status report.

Thomas BE, Ramachandran R, Anitha S and Swaminathan S (2007). Feasibility of routine HIV testing among TB patients through a voluntary, counseling and testing center VCTC). Int J Tuberc Lung Dis 11: 1296-1301.

Tortoli E, Cichero P, Piersimoni C, Simonetii T, Gesu G and Nistta D (1999). Use of BACTEC MGIT for recovery of mycobacteria from clinical specimens: multicentric study. J Clin Microbiol 37: 3578-3582.

Varma-Basil M, El-Hajj H, Colangeli R et al., (2004). Rapid detection of rifampin resistance in *Mycobacterium tuberculosis* isolates from India and Mexico by a molecular beacon assay. J Clin Microbiol 42: 5512-5516.

Venkataraman P, Herbert D and Paramasivan CN (1998). Evaluation of BACTEC radiometric method in the early diagnosis of tuberculosis. Indian J Med Res 108: 120127.

WHO (2008). Global tuberculosis control: surveillance, planning, financing. WHO report 2008. WHO/HTM/TB/2008.393. Geneva.

WHO Global Tuberculosis Program (1992). Tuberculosis programme review, India, September 1992.

Wilson S, Al-Suwaidi A, McNerny R, porter J and Drobniewski F (1997). Evaluation of a new rapid bacteriophage based method for the drug susceptibility testing of *Mycobacterium tuberculosis*. Nature Med 3: 415-418.

World Health Organization (1997). Prevalence and incidence of tuberculosis in India. A comprehensive review. WHO/TB/97, 231.

World Health Organization Stop TB partnership (2009). New laboratory diagnosis tools for tuberculosis control. http://www.apps.who.int/tdr.

8

Immunologic Diagnosis of Neurotuberculosis

Iacob Simona Alexandra[1], Banica Dorina[1], Iacob Diana Gabriela[2],
Panaitescu Eugenia[2], Radu Irina[3] and Cojocaru Manole[4]
[1]*National Institute of Infectious Diseases "Matei Bals", Bucharest,*
[2]*The University of Medicine and Pharmacy "Carol Davila" Bucharest,*
[3]*The University of Bucharest,*
[4]*The "Titu Maiorescu" University*
Romania

1. Introduction

Tuberculosis (TB) is one of the most prevalent infectious diseases in the world, particularly in developing countries. The high incidence and mortality of TB in these countries mainly resides in the limited financial resources, the emergence of multiresistant strains and the spread of HIV infections. The key element for controlling TB is a rapid and early diagnosis which ensures the correct treatment and eradication of the infection source in the community. Current strategies for the development of a rapid and accurate diagnosis address 3 major objectives: improving the present diagnostic tools through better knowledge, developing new tests and increasing the accessibility to such diagnostic possibilities (Who Strategic Directions, 2006). The gold standard of diagnosis in TB is the identification of mycobacteria in the pathologic product using acid-fast smear microscopy and mycobacterial culture. Nevertheless the bacteriologic diagnosis is presently inefficient due to increasing number of smear-negative TB forms. This has led to the development of various complementary diagnostic methods such immunologic assays. The aim of the present chapter is to outline the literature data on the importance of the immunologic diagnosis in neurotuberculosis, a lethal localization of TB. It presents the current immunological assays and their practical value in the diagnosis of neurotuberculosis as complementary methods.

2. General data

Neurotuberculosis is represented by various central nervous system (CNS) tuberculous manifestations including : tuberculoma, tuberculous abscess, meningoencephalitis , spinal arachnoiditis and cerebral miliary tuberculosis. This diverse neurological frame mostly emerges as a result of the invasive potential as well as of the immune pathogeny of neurotuberculosis. The difficulty in the diagnosis of neurotuberculosis lies in the atypical clinical presentation and non-specific changes recorded by various diagnostic assays. The bacteriological exams of the cerebrospinal fluid (CSF) are still regarded as the sole diagnostic tools in the confirmation of neurotuberculosis. Nevertheless the bacteriological assay in neurological forms of TB has a low sensitivity and a considerable delay. As a rule, owing to the rapid evolution and increased mortality, the suspected neurotuberculosis patients frequently receive antituberculous treatment before bacteriological confirmation (Donald & Schoeman, 2004). A complete antituberculous treatment requires 6-12 months, during which serious adverse reactions could occur. On the other hand nontuberculous CNS infections with different treatment and high mortality could be overlooked. Therefore multiple research studies based on new diagnostic methods have been developed over the last 30 years aiming to improve the diagnostic efficiency in neurotuberculosis.

3. Diagnostic methods in neurotuberculosis

CSF analysis represents the basic element in the diagnosis of neurotuberculosis. The isolation and identification of mycobacteria in CSF are crucial for the diagnosis of neurotuberculosis. However as the CSF is a paucibacillar product, these methods often fail. All the same the CSF could present characteristic cytological and chemical changes which could be suggestive for the neurotuberculosis diagnosis in a specific clinical context. In several cases, especially in children and immunosupressed patients, the cytochemical changes of the CSF lack even these particular findings and the neurotuberculosis diagnosis is then ommited. During the past decades various complementary methods have been implemented to assist these difficulties. These currently include : nucleic acid amplification tests (NAATs), CSF adenosindeaminase (ADA) detection and immunologic assays.

3.1 Advantages and disadvantages of current diagnostic techniques in neurotuberculosis

Below are the main findings, advantages and disadvantages of each current diagnostic method in neurotuberculosis (Desai et al, 2006; Sonmeza et al, 2008; Nyendak et al, 2009; Davies & Pai 2008)

a. **CSF cytology.** *Main findings*: at the onset mixed pleocytosis with mainly lymphocytes(80-90%) and the presence of neutrophils (10-20%); in the later stages, only lymphocytes.

Advantages: rapid, inexpensive, sensitive method. *Disadvantages*: 1) Variable CSF cytology in the evolution of the disease, 2) Many atypical CSF aspects at the onset or throughout the evolution in immunodepressed hosts and children 3)Low specificity; 4)Normal CSF cytology cannot rule out localized forms of neurotuberculosis

b. **Biochemical CSF exam.** *Main findings*: high CSF protein level and low glucose.

Advantages: rapid, inexpensive. *Disadvantages*: 1) Very low specificity: many infections of the CNS share similar changes ; 2) CSF biochemical analysis is normal in localized forms of neurotuberculosis.

c. Bacteriologic CSF exam.

CSF smear. *Main findings*: the CSF smear detects mycobacteria using acid-fast bacilli stains (Ziehl-Neelsen or the Kinyoun method) as well as fluorescence staining.

Advantages: rapid, inexpensive, simple, specific, low technical demand. *Disadvantages*: 1) Very low sensitivity of 13-53%; nevertheless, fluorescence microscopy and certain processing methods have been developed to improve the sensitivity; 2) The CSF smear cannot distinguish between different species of mycobacteria ; moreover, it is difficult to detect nontuberculous mycobacteria; 3) The procesessing is prone to contamination with environmental or water-borne saprophitic mycobacteria; 4) Results depend on the CSF volume (a positive result requires >6ml of CSF) and on the number of samples (repeated analysis of lumbar punctures increases diagnostic yield); 5) False negative smear results in localized forms of cerebral TB.

CSF culture. *Main findings*: isolation and identification of mycobacteria on selective media (solid or liquid media).

Advantages: 1) Represents the definitive proof of active TB (gold standard). 2) Enables the performance of an antibiogram; 3) better sensitivity, than the CSF smear. *Disadvantages*: 1) Sensitivity depends on the number of samples, CSF volume and mycobacteria loading (CSF enrichment techniques could be used); 2) Large differences between media on efficiency and price; 3) Adequate laboratory infrastructure and trained personnel are necessary; 4) Detection requires minimum 14 days even on selective media; 5) Negative CSF culture in localized neurotuberculosis.

d.   **Nucleic acid amplification tests (NAATs).** *Main findings*: detect mycobacteria nucleic acid in serum and CSF using the *PCR* assay.

Advantages: NAATs exhibits a high specificity (88%-100%), good positive predictive value and rapid processing. Due to its specificity it could be used for treatment monitoring. *Disadvantages*: 1) NAATs have a highly variable sensitivity and low negative predictive value, especially in smear-negative and extrapulmonary TB; the sensitivity of the *PCR* method (33% to 90%) is highly dependent on the mycobacteria loading and variable for each *PCR* technique; 2) *PCR* becomes rapidly negative after treatment; 3) In-house *NAATs* produces highly variable results compared to commercial, standardized *NAATs*. Nevertheless, commercial *NAATs* show a potential role in confirming the diagnosis of TB meningitis, although their overall low sensitivity precludes the use of these tests to rule out the diagnosis with certainty; 4) The high price makes them prohibitive in poor countries with the highest prevalence of TB.

e.   **The adenosine deaminase (ADA) detection**

Advantages: rapid; inexpensive; high diagnostic accuracy. *Disadvantages:* 1) Low specificity: it cannot rule out bacterial meningitis. 2) Not standardized.

f.   **Histologic exam.** *Main findings*: reveals tissue mycobacteria and characteristic granulomatous aspects.

Advantages: 1) Very high specificity. 2) The main diagnosis method for localised cerebral TB. *Disadvantages:* 1) Invasive method; 2) Histology does not distinguish between mycobacteria or different granulomatous diseases; 4)Belated result (requires one or two days)

g.   **Imaging methods.** *Main findings:* indicates complications of neurotuberculosis (hydrocephalus, vasculitis) and localized forms of neurotuberculosis. *Advantages*: improves the differential diagnosis and treatment evaluation. *Disadvantages*: 1) Images are not pathognomonic for TB; 2) High exposure to radiation; 3) Very expensive.

Conclusion: None of the current methods meets the criteria required by an efficient diagnostic test: rapid, accurate and readily applicable. Treatment in neurotuberculosis is therefore implemented according to the association of epidemiological, clinical criteria, bacteriologic CSF examination and different complementary laboratory methods dependent on the technical level of each laboratory. The decision on which tests to use should consider country-level technical facilities and other relevant factors, such as cost and availability. The lack of standardisation in the use of these methods renders their comparison more difficult.

3.2 Reason for the development of immunologic assays in neurotuberculosis

Unlike latent TB, neurotuberculosis is characterized by active CNS lesions accompanied by an intense cellular and humoral immune response. Both T cells and B cells are active during mycobacteria replication suggesting the potential use of immune markers in cerebral TB. Immune diagnostic tools also assessed antigens released by *M.tbc* in the CSF or specific antibodies. Beginning with 1990, numerous antigens and antibodies were screened for the diagnosis of neurotuberculosis in endemic areas. Studies on these methods proved a good specificity and simple, inexpensive and rapid results. Nevertheless the low sensitivity and the development of molecular techniques decreased the importance of these methods in neurotuberculosis diagnosis. The immunological diagnosis continues to be considered in TB endemic areas due to the increasing number of immunological biomarkers detection (Walzl et al, 2011). Over the past years, T cell-based IFNg release assays (IGRAs) performed on T cell isolated from the CSF, were found senzitive and specific for TB meningitis. IGRAs restored the interest in the immunological methods for TB diagnosis even in countries with high financial support. (Thomas et al, 2008).

3.3 The advantages and disadvantages of immunologic diagnostic methods in the diagnosis of neurotuberculosis

a.   Determination of mycobacterial antigens or antimycobacterial antibodies in serum and CSF fluid. (Thomas et al, 2008; Patel et al, 2010)

Advantages: 1) Rapid , inexpensive, simple technique, minimal training requirements compared to molecular methods. 2) Specific detection of the intrathecal synthesis of antimycobacterial antibodies and of mycobacterial antigens in the CSF.

Disadvantages: 1) Highly inconsistent estimates of sensitivity and specificity correlated with the method used, detected type of antigen or antibody and mycobacteria load; however combinations of select antigens provide higher sensitivity compared to single antigens. 2) False negative results particularly in immunodepressed hosts; 3) Specificity can be affected by cross reactions between different mycobacteria or other bacterial species (*Nocardia, Leishmania*); 4) Some methods (*ELISA*) require specific equipment, skilled technicians and refrigerated reagents.

b.   **IFN-γ release assays (IGRAs)** The two methods presently used are *QuantiFERON-Gold (QFT-G)* method and *T-SPOT.TB* method. Both can substitute the tuberculin skin test (*TST*) in routine clinical practice, especially where *BCG* vaccination is prevalent.

Avantages: rapid and specific. 2) Applied in few studies of neurotuberculosis with a sensitivity of 90% and specificity of 100% in cases of negative bacteriological TB meningitis.

Disadvantages: 1) Requires appropiate lab-facility; 2) Expensive; 3) T cell lymphopenia and anergy resulting from disseminated TB or advanced HIV infection, lead to the lack of *ELISPOT* responses. 4) False negative results in patients with atypical CSF (few lymphocytes). 5) False positive results in the case of blood contamination during puncture.

Conclusion. The immunological diagnosis in neurotuberculosis reflects the present knowledge related to the immune pathogenesis of TB. Addition of new immunologic data and a more complex interpretation of the results could improve the diagnostic value of these methods.

4. Imunologic response in NTB

TB is primarily a pulmonary disease. The protective immunity in infections with *M.tbc* is ensured by the macrophageal activity, CD4T cell response and Th1 cytokines. Consequently, the immune response frequently leads to the formation of granuloma, an organized and efficient form of defence. The granulomas include mycobacteria with a modified metabolism and potential of active replication which increases in case of immunodepression. The granulomas adjacent to the meninges or cerebral vessels increase the risk of CSF mycobacteria invasion. Mycobacteria reaching the subarachnoidial space release antigens and induce an intense inflammatory response. Since 1990, these antigens have been acknowledged as potential markers for the diagnosis of TB meningitis.

4.1 Mycobacterial antigens (general data, classification, role)

M.tbc encodes about 4000 proteins. As mycobacteria are extremely dynamic they release a variable number of antigens according to the clinical form of TB, the duration of the infection and the host immune response. The recognition of relevant mycobacterial antigens by T cell subsets is an essential step in triggering the protective immunity in TB. A functional classification of these antigens is presently unavailable, nor is the selection of antigens for the development of efficient serological diagnostic tools. Sequencing of the M.tbc genome in 1998 and the knowledge in proteogenomics led to the identification of numerous immunogenic antigens specific for *M. tbc* and *M .bovis*. These specific antigens differ from environmental mycobacterias or BCG vaccine strains and could be used in the immunologic TB diagnosis. However no specific antigen or set of antigens has been yet recognized in TB and no set of antigens has been established for diagnosis with confidence. The release of a certain antigen is induced by a large number of factors such as the type of infection (active or inactive), the host immune status (imunocompetent or immunodeppressed), local immune metabolism or ph conditions, mycobacteria viability (viable mycobacteria release other antigens than dormant bacilli), mycobacteria virulence and the infection site. The immunogenicity of these antigens also differs: only a small number of the antigens released in the culture media (25%) induced the synthesis of specific antibodies. (Samanich et al, 2000). The variability of released antigens under different conditions and their immunogenicity hinders an accurate selection and represents a serious obstacle in the immunodiagnostic development of TB. A cocktail combining a large number of antigens (10 to 12 recombinant antigens or poly-proteins) appears to be a reasonable choice for increasing both the sensitivity and the specificity of immunologic diagnostic methods (Raja et al, 2008). The classification and nomenclature of mycobacteria antigens is not unitary. There are more names and classifications for one antigen depending on localization (cellular wall, cellular membrane and cytoplasm antigens) and structure (lipids, proteins, polysaccharides and their complexes). Proteic antigens are secreted in active lesions and have proved a great potential in the serological diagnosis, either alone or in poly-protein complexes (Houghton et al, 2002) , while glycolipidic antigens are released in immunodepressed hosts especially. A detailed presentation of mycobacteria antigens belongs to Young (Yang et al, 1992). Several of these proteic antigens have already been included in diagnostic tests for neurotuberculosis: antigens of 38 kDa, 16 kDa, 88 kDa, MPT51, CFP-10, antigen 85B (associated to the protein 30-31 kDa), lipoarabinomannan (LAM), antigen A60, antigen 5, cord factor. The roles assigned to mycobacteria antigens are often contradictory and not fully understood. The documented activity of mycobacteria antigens is diverse: enhancing the immune response (antigen 85, P320, A60) , triggering the delayed-type hypersensitivity (proteic antigens), interfering with the adhesion of mycobacteria on host cells, promoting phagosome-lysososme fusion. Certain antigens (LAM, 30kDa antigen, antigen 6) also induce cellular immunodepression by inhibiting various functions of the macrophages, or T Lymphocytes and assisting in the formation of granulomas.

4.2 Antimycobacterial antibodies (general data, relevance, dynamics)

M. tbc is resistant to antimycobacterial antibodies. Stimulation of the humoral immunity using polysaccharide conjugated vaccines has not been efficient and antimycobacterial antibodies are not considered protective (Glatman-Freedman et al, 2000). Nevertheless their presence could influence the immune response. Thus the presence of B lymphocytes surrounding granulomas suggests the involvement of humoral immunity in latent forms of TB .The appearance of plasmocytes in the CSF also suggests a potential role of specific antibodies in TB meningitis. Numerous studies have attempted to identify specific antibodies in active TB but the present data is incomplete. The antigenic variability of mycobacteria is mirrored by the heterogenity of the released antibiodies. The repertoir of released antibodies appears to be diverse and correlated to many factors (the lesion's evolution and localization, the immune status etc) (Davidow et al, 2005). As in the case of antigens, the type of the released antibodies in different hosts and different forms of TB is unpredictable. Thus anti 38kDa are elevated in pulmonary TB while LAM antibodies and anti 16 kda increase in the CSF of patients with TB meningitis; anti 38 kDa have been associated with a poor outcome, while anti 19kda suggested a good prognosis. Anti38kDa are released in the presence of cavitary lesions and have not been found in patients who do not present such lesions such as immunodeppresed hosts. Anti 85 complex are present in large quantities in disease forms confirmed by positive smear as well as in severe forms. By comparison, lower amounts were found in forms with negative smears or minimal lesions. (Wiker & Harboe, 1992). Antibody responses are correlated with the bacillary load. Under these circumstances the level of IgG was regarded by some authors as an index for the antigenic load with possible implications in treatment follow-up (Fadda et al, 1992). The present knowledge on the role of antimycobacterial antibodies is the result of numerous immunologic diagnostic studies but their implication in the TB pathogenesis is still little known. IgM antibodies were found in different groups of patients with TB including vaccinated patients and are frequently found in HIV patients. Their presence marks the colonization with mycobacteria or the risk of TB relapse. IgA antibodies are rarely found.

They are detected in the CSF, pericardial and pleural liquid. They could appear in a state of anergy or in the absence of IgG antibodies, sometimes indicating an aberrant immune response Th2 like. Immune complexes are frequently correlated with IgA antibodies and severe disease. A protective effect of IgA of short duration has been observed in the early stages of TB. IgG antibodies appear during chronic disease; high titres are maintained even during treatment. These are the main type of antibodies observed in neurotuberculosis (Maes, 1991).

The dynamic synthesis of antimycobacterial antibodies

Different stimuli were documented to trigger the antimycobacterial antibodies in the primary versus post primary infection or active versus inactive TB. The hummoral immune response following BCG vaccination indicates that IgM anti PPD increase progressively until the third month, followed by an increase of IgG. The antibody dynamics in TB infection could be similar (Maes et al, 1989), but it also depends on the clinical form and treatment starting. IgA serum antibodies appear immediately after IgM and precede IgG, but the CSF dynamics could vary. IgG antibodies are prevalent in both active and inactive cases (Kaplan & Chase, 1980). During treatment for primary tuberculosis antimycobacteria antibodies are present in low titres, exhibit a slow increase and are directed against a low number of antigens. (Kaplan & Chase, 1980). Only 11-46% of patients display an initial titre of antibodies, but the number of cases subsequently increases to 60%. In relapse forms of TB the serum reacts with a larger number of antigens, the IgG titre is higher and rapidly increases under treatment. A detectable IgG titre is initially recorded in 66% of patients but reaches 75-100% of patients in the later stages. Similar conclusions were published in other studies in which TB relapse forms produced a positive serology in 100% of patients compared to 11% in primary TB (Julian et al, 1997). Seroconversion under treatment in patients with TB exceeds 3-8 weeks in patients with a negative titre at the onset, while in those with positive onset titres the antibody increase is rapid and immediate. The titre of antimycobacterial antibodies in the serum and CSF is higher in treated compared to untreated patients (Kaplan & Chase 1980). Some authors consider that in primary TB the maximum titre could emerge after 3 months of treatment. The presence of antimycobacterial antibodies in large quantities in relapse as well as in the treated forms is a significant advantage in the serodiagnosis of neurotuberculosis (as the latter frequently occurs as a relapse). The main disadvantage is related to the slow antibody dynamics in primary infections.

4.3 The intrathecal synthesis of antimycobacterial antibodies in NTB

CNS dissemination of mycobacteria is assisted by alveolar macrophages and their interaction with epithelial cells. Although the hematomeningeal barrier ensures the CNS protection from systemic immune reactions, the nevrax is still the site of intense inflammatory reactions. The intracerebral immune reactions are supported by the phagocytic cells of CNS, such as astrocytes and endothelial cells. (de Micco & Toga, 1988) The complex of astrocytes and endothelial cells is also connected to microglial cells, oligodendrocytes and hematopoetic stem cells. All these cells could activate lymphocytes and release inflammatory cytokines. Moreover, the lymphocytes crossing the hematomeningeal barrier synthesize intrathecal immunoglobulins (Ig). The intrathecal synthesis of specific antibodies was first observed in neurotuberculosis by Kinman. He showed that the stimulation of CSF lymphocytes by PPD leads to their intense proliferation

(Kinnman et al, 1981). Subsequent studies revealed a local production of antimycobacterial antibodies anti PPD in the CSF (Kalish et al, 1983). In 1990, Sindic proved the presence of IgG in the CSF against the antigen of M. *tbc* H37Ra and A60 (Sindic et al, 1990) In this study antimycobacterial antibodies appeared in the subarachnoid space as early as 15 days after clinical onset and persisted up to 69 months. The delayed immune response after the disappearance of the antigenic stimulus could persist as a result of immune disorders of active B cells clones. A similar response was also observed in other nontuberculous meningoencephalitis even 8 years later. IgG generally dominate the CNS humoral immune response, but in some cases IgA are also present (Felgenhauer & Schädlich, 1987). The antimycobacterial antibodies synthesis could be detected and quantified in the CSF, resulting in titres that could be higher in the CSF compared to the serum. Furthermore the increase of the Ig index in the CSF is a proof of the local synthesis of antimycobacterial antibodies (Kinman et al, 1981). The intrathecal synthesis of antimycobacterial antibodies released in the CSF is specific for cerebral TB and thus represents a solid argument in favor of the neurotuberculosis diagnosis.

5. Immunologic methods used in the diagnosis of neurotuberculosis

Immunological assays are rapid and easy to process but their use in TB is disputed due to contradictory results on sensitivity. Nevertheless, immunologic methods could be considered as complementary diagnostic tools especially in poor areas and smear-negative CSF neurotuberculosis. The most commonly used serological assay in neurotuberculosis is enzyme-linked immunosorbent assay (ELISA). Rapid methods (such as immunodot) are only seldom used. ELISA is automated and able to simultaneously analyse a high number of samples and different antibodies (Ig G, IgM or IgA). The evaluation of serological assays requires the accuracy of the following parameters: the sensitivity (probability of a positive test in people with neurotuberculosis), the specificity (probability of a negative test in uninfected people), the positive predictive value (probability that the person is infected when the test is positive) and the negative predictive value (probability that the person is uninfected when the test is negative).

5.1 The enzyme-immuno-assay (ELISA) technique

ELISA technique was first introduced in the serological diagnosis of TB in 1976. It detects the antigen/antibody-enzyme linked complexes, with the antigen affixed to a solid adsorbent surface. Despite its highly variable sensitivity and specificity, studies on pulmonary TB proved that it is rapid and simple to process, suggesting its use in the extrapulmonary TB diagnosis. There are several comercial ELISA kits (Anda Biological using antigen A60, Omerga Pathozyme TB using antigen 38 kDa, Pathozyme TB complex with antigen 38 kDa and antigen 16 kDa, Pathozyme Myco with antigen 38 kDa and lypopolissaharidic antigen), and various in-house antibody-ELISA detection tests. Numerous ELISA studies were performed for the detection of different antigens and antibodies released in the pulmonary and extrapulmonary TB. Daniel and Debanne published a reference study in 1987 (Daniel & Debanne, 1987) analysing ELISA results in different forms of TB. They concluded that ELISA sensitivity of 25-100% and specificity of 76-100% were highly variable depending on the used antigen. A subsequent systematic revue on ELISA studies also revealed an extremely variable sensitivity of 0-100% and specificity of 59-100% in pulmonary TB and modest results in TB meningitis (sensitivity of 48% and specificity of 82%) (Steingart et al, 2007).

5.2 Interferon-γ-release assays (IGRAs)

There are currently 2 methods measuring the IFN-γ released by sensitized T cells: QuantiFERON-Gold *In Tube* (Cellestis Ltd) which measures IFN-γ-released in whole blood following *ex vivo* stimulation with ESAT-6, CFP-10 and TB 7.7 antigens and the T-SPOT.TB method (Oxford Immunotec Ltd) which measures IFN-γ-released by peripheral blood mononuclear cells following *ex vivo* stimulation with ESAT-6 and CFP-10. These 2 methods were initially approved for the diagnosis of latent TB, displaying a higher efficiency compared to tuberculin skin tests (TST). Their use was later extended for the diagnosis of active TB including HIV-infected patients. Recent studies on TB meningitis using both methods revealed only modest results. (Thomas et al, 2008, Patel et al, 2010). Thus the specificity in the diagnosis of active TB was generally low (59-79%) while the sensitivity was between 79% (non HIV patients) and 64% (HIV patients) (Sester et al, 2011). Nevertheless more optimistic results in TB meningitis were also reported (Murakami et al, 2008).

5.3 Other techniques used in the immune diagnosis of neurotuberculosis

The immunoblot technique is based on the electrophoretic separation of proteins (antigens or antibodies from serum or CSF), blotting for separate fractions on nitrocelulosis and identification of each proteic fraction with a specific anti-serum conjugated with a complex of streptavidin-biotin preoxidase (calitative reaction). The immunoblot technique was previously used by several authors in the diagnosis of mycobacterial infections. Most antigens recorded in these studies weighted between 30-45 kDa. However, only a part of the serum antigens identified in pulmonary TB were also recorded in the CSF in TB meningitis. In a study by Mathai the patients with TB meningitis presented 27 kDa, 30kDa, 45 kDa and 5kDa *M.tbc* antigens (Mathai et al, 1994). The latter was found in another study in 70% of patients with TB meningitis (Mathai et al, 1991). Patil also identified 30-40kDa antigens in the CSF but lower amounts of 14kDa and 18-25kDa antigens (Patil et al, 1996). Katti identified mostly 30-32kDa and 71kDa antigens in the CSF of patients with TB meningitis (Katti, 2001). Literature data also reveals the predominance of 30kDa antigen in the CSF. Research proved that 30 kDa protein is also a member of the Ag 85 complex (Ag 85 A and Ag 85 B), an antigen frequently detected in TB meningitis. This emphasizes the importance of 30 kDa antigen as a CSF marker in various forms of TB meningitis. **ImmunoDOT** is an rapid-test format, dipstick ELISA that allows patients to be tested for multiple parameters simultaneously. Up to five or six different tests may be completed simultaneously on a single sample, making it ideal for users who require fast, and reliable diagnostic tests in a single patient format. ImmunoDot or other rapid techniques are suitable for low CSF volumes and limited resources laboratories. **Haemagglutination assays** such as reverse passive haemagglutination (RPHA) using polyclonal or monoclonal antibodies, could be used in the serum and CSF, with a variable sensitivity in the diagnosis of TB meningitis. (Venkatesh et al, 2007). The use of a polyclonal serum generally proved more efficient. The main limitation of this method was connected to the variable sensitivity (50-94%) and to the short shelf-life of red-cell labelled antibodies; both listed drawbacks could be amended (Katti, 2001). The method is interesting from the perspective of using a single sample for the detection of both antibodies and antigens in biologic products and for measuring antigens and antibody dilutions needed in treatment monitoring. **Radioimmunoassay (RIA)** has been used for the TB diagnosis since 1987, with variable results. The method could follow the antigens level in the CSF during treatment which enables its use in treatment monitoring (Kadival et al, 1987). In conclusion, neurotuberculosis presently employs a wide range ofimmunologic diagnostic techniques. Their results however are not influenced by the method as much as by the detected antigens or antibodies. Presented below is the diagnostic value of the main antigens and antibodies detected in the serum and CSF in patients with neurotuberculosis.

6. Diagnostic value of immunological assays in studies of adults with neurotuberculosis

6.1 Mycobacterial antigens detection in neurotuberculosis

The mycobacterial antigens detection in CSF samples evidence active meningeal infection and could hold a diagnostic value. Hence, several *M.tbc* antigens have been analyzed as potential markers for the TB menigitis diagnosis. Moreover, quantitative determination of antigens could be useful for treatment monitoring. Attempts to detect mycobacterial antigens in neurotuberculosis have been made since 1984 employing mostly agglutination tests, *ELISA* with different variants or other methods (Venkatesh et al, 2007; Sumi et al, 2002; Radhacrishnan et al, 1990; Katti, 2001; Kashyap et al, 2009). Numerous antigens were evaluated: 55-kDa antigen, 14 kDa, PPD, 62 kDa, ag 85 complex , 30-32 kDa protein, LAM, Ag Mtbc, *M. tbc* H37Rv. The main conclusions of these studies are listed below.

a. **Method efficiency.** The specificity of methods: 69-100%. The sensitivity variation depended on the diagnosis criteria: in bacteriologically confirmed TB meningitis 79-100%; 67-92% in unconfirmed cases and 50-100% in both confirmed and unconfirmed cases.

b. **Comments**. The evaluated antigens were extremely different for each study. The sensitivity of methods was highly variable too. No method or specific antigen rendered a higher efficiency, although more studies have confirmed the presence of 30Kda antigen (ag 85 complex) in the CSF and simultaneous use of more antigens improved the methods sensitivity. The highly variable results could derive from the reduced level of antigen in the CSF, as well as from the lack of complete information connected with the precise type of antigens released in the CSF in TB meningitis.

6.2 Antimycobacterial antibodies detection in neurotuberculosis

Irrespective of localisation, antigentic stimulation in mycobacteria infections induces the synthesis of specific antibodies in the serum. In neurological localizations however, antibodies also appear in the CSF as a result of intratechal synthesis (Sindic et al, 1990; Kinmann et al, 1981; Kalish et al, 1983) and active secretion by choroidal plexuses. False positive antibodies in the CSF are possible in areas endemic for TB, where healthy persons or patients with pulmonary TB present high serum levels of antimycobacterial antibodies able to difusse from the serum to the CSF. The assesment of the intratechal synthesis of antimycobacterial antibodies could help ascertain such false positive reactions. Most studies analyzing the presence of the antimycobacterial antibodies in CSF were performed in imunocompetent adults with TB meningitis. The detected antibodies involved more antigens either isolated or simultaneous (LAM, PPD, A60, M.tbc, Ag 5, 14kDa, 19 kDa, 27 kDa, 30 kDa, 35 kDa, 40 kDa, Ag H37Ra, LAM, 30 kDa, 65 kDa heat shock protein, ESAT-6 antigen). In addition, most authors focused on the detection of IgG type antibodies using ELISA. Below are the main findings of these studies (Thakur & Mandal, 1996; Maheshwari et al, 2000; Patil1et al, 1996; Kashyap et al 2009; Mudaliar et al, 2006).

a. **Method's efficiency.** The specificity of antimycobacterial antibodies detection ranged between 92-100% but the positive predictive value was high. False positive results were recorded in patients who also presented pulmonary TB or as a result of cross-reactivity; 65 antigen kDa belonging to stress proteins was most frequently involved in cross reactions with other bacteria. The sensitivity of methods was highly variable: 30-100% in the studies with a single tested antigen and 61-100% when testing multiple antigens Chandramuki et al, 1989; Mathai et al, 1990a). The sensitivity was correlated with diagnosis criteria as follows: 80-90% sensitivity in bacteriologically confirmed tuberculous meningitis, 30-62% sensitivity in unconfirmed cases, 58% sensitivity in histologically confirmed tuberculomas and 70-87% sensitivity in clinically TB meningitis Large differences between studies were also noticed depending on antibodies detection (for LAM, the sensitivity varied between 58-85% and for A60, the sensitivity ranged from 38 to 100%).

b. **Comments.** Almost all studies were perfomed in patients with TB meningitis. Nevertheless, a study on tuberculoma revealed A60 antibodies in these patients too. This indicates the potential use of the serodiagnosis in localized forms of neurotuberculosis, in which noninvasive diagnostic tools are presently unavailable. The variability of the recorded results was connected with more factors: 1) the use of different antigens (several studies indicate LAM antigen as immunodominant in the CSF; 2) the use of different dilutions: higher dilutions of the CSF decreased the sensitivity; 3) the immune status of different patients: low antibody detection in immunodepressed patients (only 10%) compared to immunocompetent hosts (50%); 4) almost all studies analyzed IgG antibodies, while only few also considered IgM or IgA. The antigens which induced IgM antimycobacterial antibodies were different from those responsible for IgG. IgG antibodies were mostly directed against LAM or 14 kDa antigen (74% of the total patients), suggesting that using these antigens could raise the efficiency. 5) some studies disclosed that simultaneous detection of serum and CSF antimycobacterial antibodies improved the CSF results compared to serum detection only. (Srivastava et al, 1994); however other studies reported inferior CSF sensitivity compared to the serum sensitivity.(Ghoshal et al, 2003). 6) the sensitivity of antibodies detection increased during treatment with 18% for both IgG and IgA detection.

Conclusion. There is a large number of serological studies dedicated to neurotuberculosis, with extremely different results. They are hard to compare as a result of using different study protocols and different antibodies detection. Despite the unconfindence which these studies arose, serologic diagnosis is widely used in poor countries. The standardisation of the methods in what regards the recommended antigens (type, concentration) and the immunological assay, could help improve the immunological diagnosis. One advantage of this method is the CSF specificity of antigens and intrathecal antimycobacterial antibodies synthesis and also the increased antibody level during antituberculous treatment, which renders this method useful for a retrospective diagnosis.

6.3 Intrathecal synthesis of antimycobacterial antibodies in neurotuberculosis

TB meningitis prompts a vigorous humoral local response proved by CSF intrathecal synthesis of antimycobacterial antibodies. Sindic proved that most antibodies synthesized intrathecally are directed against antigen A60 (Sindic et al, 1990). He also revealed the presence of Ig in the subarahnoidian space after 14-27 days of disease and their persistence after several years. A higher Ig G index is presently regarded as a strong argument in favor of the humoral local response induced by mycobacteria. All the same not all Ig detected in the CSF belong to antimycobacterial antibodies. Unspecific IgG were also found in other diseases affecting the CNS as a results of an immunosuppresive abberation. This immune impairment allows B cell multiplication and antibody persistence accounting for false positive results. Fals positive CSF results could also be found after passive transfer of antimycobacterial antibodies from the serum in the subarachnoid space. The mathematical evaluation of the intrathecal synthesis takes into account the presence of antibodies and IgG level in serum and CSF could highlight these false positive results.

6.4 Personal contribution. The intrathecal synthesis of antimycobacterial antibodies in patients with TB meningitis

The sole presence of antimycobacterial antibodies in the CSF cannot define the local inflammatory response since any form of TB accompanied by high titres of antibodies could promote their passive transfer in the CSF. The intrathecal synthesis was instead acknowledged as a typical finding in neurotuberculosis and an alternative for improving the specificity and positive predictive value of diagnosis in TB meningitis.The aim of our study was to evaluate the presence of antimycobacterial antibodies released as a result of the intrathecal synthesis in TB meningitis and to differentiate them from unspecific Ig.

Subjects. The study was performed on 21 adult patients with TB meningitis. A total of 34 CSF samples were collected, all having proved positive for antimycobacterial antibodies. The samples were collected after starting the antituberculous treatment, between 3 and 140 days after the clinical onset of the disease. Diagnosis criteria of TB meningitis were based on clinical characteristic features, CSF characteristic features (CSF lymphocytosis, increased protein and decreased sugar), evidence of pulmonary or extrapulmonary TB and positivity of CSF Lowenstein culture (for 3 patients only). Antimycobacterial antibodies were detected through ELISA using glycolipidic (GL) antigens and A60antigen.

Methods. Two types of comparative antigens were used for ELISA: GL antigen (0,1 ml sol of 10micrograms/ml of purified glycolipid in hexan obtained from Cantacuzino laboratories, Romania) and A60 (Andaelisa mycobacteria IgG, IgM, IgA kits, from Anda Biologicals, Strasbourg, France).

a. Elisa anti GL antigen detection method steps: 0,1 ml of ½ diluted CSF and 0,1 ml of conjugate (protein A–peroxidase) were distributed in microplates at 37^0 C for 1 hour; 0,1 ml *OPD* (peroxide and ortophenylendiamine) substrate in citric acid-sodium citrate buffer, 0,1 M, pH =5, was used. The reaction was prolonged for 30 minutes, at 37^0C, at dark. The optical densities (OD) were read with a Multiscan MCC Reader, at 450 nm. Serum Ig isolated from immunised rabbits with *Mtbc* suspension were used as positive controls. Cut off was established at two standard deviations above the level considered normal. The level of antibodies was expressed in international units (UI). The baseline serounit for the CSF fluid was 0 UI.

b. Elisa antiA60 detection steps: the CSF fluid was diluted 1/10 according to the kit instructions; anti-human IgG, IgA, IgM were conjugated to peroxidase (one hour at 37⁰C). The baseline serounits were: 125 for IgG, 200 for IgA serounits and 0.8 for IgM antibodies. Supplementary analysis in all subjects included: serum and CSF albumin expressed in mg/ml) (Ortodiagnosis) and serum and CSF Ig (radial passive immunodifussion). Albumin index, IgG index and IgG intratechal synthesis were calculated using the following mathematical formula (Tibbling 1977):

1. **Albumin index** (mg/ml)= CSF albumin/ serum albumin ratio. The normal value of CSF albumin was considered < 35mg% and between 3500-5000 mg% for serum albumin. The normal value of the *albumin index* is < 7×10^{-3} (0.007). Higher values suggest the permeability of the hematomeningeal barrier and the possibility of a passive transfer of antimycobacterial antibodies from the blood to the CSF.

2. **IgG index** (mg/ml)= (CSF IgG/serum IgG) / (CSF albumin /serum albumin) ratio.The normal value of the IgG index is ≤0.7. Higher values indicate increased IgG synthesis.

3. **IgG intratechal synthesis** of antimycobacterial antibodies was acquired using the formula: (CSF antimycobacterial antibodies of IgG type/CSF IgG) / (serum antimycobacterial antibodies of IgG type/serum IgG) ratio. Antimycobacterial antibodies of IgG type were measured in *ELISA* units. Serum and CSF IgG were quantified in mg/ml. The normal value of the intratechal synthesis calculated using this formula is < 1.

Results. The intrathecal synthesis was present 3 days after clinical onset and persisted up to 140 days after onset. The intrathecal synthesis against GL antigen was assessed in 31 samples while anti A60 antibodies were assessed only in 19 samples, out of the total of 34 CSF samples. 19 CSF samples were studied comparatively for the intrathecal synthesis of anti GL antibodies and antiA60: anti GL antibodies were detected in 7 samples only (22,58%) and anti A60 in 15 patients (78,94%).Eighteen from the 19 CSF samples (94,73%) presented the intrathecal synthesis of either anti GL antibodies or anti A60.Results are displayed in table 1.

Antimycobacterial antibodies of IgG type	Total CSF samples	CSF samples positive for the intrathecal antibody synthesis	CSF samples positive for a high albumin index	CSF samples positive for a high IgG index
GL-IgG antibodies	31	7 from 31 samples (22,58%)	33 from 34 samples (97,05%)	24 from 34 samples (70,58%)
A60-IgG antibodies	19	15 from 19 (78,94%)		
GL and A60 IgG antibodies	19	18 from 19 (94,73%)		

Table 1. Results of the albumin index, IgG index and the intrathecal synthesis of antimycobacterial anti GL and A60 in patients with TB meningitis

Observations. High values of the IgG index were recorded in 70, 58% cases and high values of the albumin index suggesting an increased permeability of the hematomeningeal barrier were noticed in 97,05% of patients. Only a part of the patients positive for CSF anti GL or A60 antibodies also exhibited an intrathecal synthesis. This finding confirms the transfer of antibodies from the serum into the CSF, through the hematomenigeal barrier. We also observed a significantly lower anti GL intrathecal synthesis compared to anti A60. In our study the simultaneous detection of intrathecal synthesis increased the CSF detection of antimycobacterial antibodies.

Conclusions. This study recorded the intrathecal synthesis of at least one type of antimycobacterial antibodies (GL or A60) in 94,73% of the TB meningitis patients even after specific treatment starting. The current study is also one of the few confirming the intrathecal synthesis of antimycobacterial antibodies in TB meningitis. Our findings support the value of the immunologic diagnosis, be it retrospective, after specific treatment starting.

7. Diagnostic value of immunological assays in children with neurotuberculosis

TB meningitis in children develops after hematogenic dissemination from the pulmonary infection site. Thus it manifests as a progressive primary disease, while in adults it commonly arises as a relapsing form of TB. The neurologic signs and symptoms become obvious 2 weeks after the onset. CSF changes are frequently unspecific and cases with a normal CSF examination have also been described in TB encephalopathy. The first obstacle in the diagnosis lies in obtaining adequate CSF and sputum samples. Moreover the bacteriological diagnosis in TB meningitis is disappointing: acid fast bacilli stain is positive in only 15% of cases and culture in only 30% of cases. The prognosis is poor and a rapid diagnosis is imperious. Most treatment regimens in children TB meningitis are initiated based on clinical, epidemiological data and pulmonary radiological features, without a bacteriological confirmation. The most adequate methods in the neurotuberculosis diagnosis in children are the molecular techniques (Lawn & Zumla, 2011). These are rapid and specific, but the high cost prevents their use on a wider scale in poor countries. At the same time, some countries are reluctant to employ molecular techniques in the TB diagnosis in children (Consensus Statement on Childhood Tuberculosis, 2010). Therefore the serological methods could be an alternative, but there are few studies on children and their efficiency is variable. The lack of knowledge related to the type of antigen released in this age group causes highly unspecific results. The serologic diagnosis is based on antigens randomly chosen, considered as immunodominant in adult TB (Raja et al, 2001). However certain results yielded by serologic techniques deserve credit for having revealed additional information on the immune pathogenesis of TB in children. According to these the titre of antimycobacterial antibodies and TST in children under 2 years are influenced by BCG vaccination which prompts persistent titres of antimycobacterial antibodies. Children between 0-4 years display a decreased humoral immune response despite a strong cellular immune response. (Seth et al, 1993). Subsequently the titre of antimycobacterial antibodies increases with age (Delacourt et al, 1993). Children with primary lesions of TB or calcified lesions also present increased titres of serum antibodies. As a result there is a high risk of false positive reactions in TB endemic areas. Thus the serologic diagnosis of active TB is not regarded as a plausible alternative for diagnosis in children. In addition, the serologic results in children with pulmonary and extrapulmonary TB exhibit an extremely varied sensitivity (20.7%-85%) (Rosen, 1990, Alde et al, 1989). Results with a better sensitivity were retrieved for A60, antigen 85 complex, 30 kDa or combinations of multiple antigens (Delacourt et al, 1993, Dayal et al, 2008, Raja et al, 2001). The specificity depends on the antigen used or the type of detected antibodies (Raja, 2001, Delacourt et al, 1993). There are also studies suggesting a correlation between the titre of antibodies and the antituberculous treatment. This implies the monitoring of antibodies titre in the pediatric management of TB. (Sireci et al, 2007). However the above mentioned results are considered of little practical value and irrelevant for the current diagnostic methods in TB. Other immunologic assays such as IGRAs although unrelated to the BCG vaccination and with a high specificity appear not to be advantageous in all cases of active TB in children. (Kampmann et al, 2009). There are few serologic studies in children with TB meningitis which displayed a high variable sensitivity. A comparative analysis on these studies is hindered by the diverse antigens used and discordant results (Dole et al, 1989; Srivastava et al, 1998) (table 9). Serious errors of interpretation are important for the above mentioned reasons.

The efficiency of serologic techniques in children with neurotuberculosis is low: sensitivity of 30%-100% and specificity of 62-96%. The sensitivity was influenced by the CSF dilution, the type of detected antibody and the chosen antigen. The sensitivity was similar for the serum and CSF.

Comments. ELISA was the technique most commonly used. Best results involved antimycobacterial antibodies A60, 30 Kda and *M. bovis* BCG towards Ag 5 and LAM. Some studies considered the detection of IgM more relevant than IgG. The detection of antigens in the CSF proved more useful compared to the finding of antibodies in TB meningitis.

8. Diagnostic value of immunological assays in studies of HIV patients with neurotuberculosis

The neurotuberculosis diagnosis in HIV infected patients is probably overevaluated. The TB patients with HIV often present miliaria forms, extrapulmonary localisations of TB and extensive vasculisis, accompanied by specific HIV manifestations. The difficulty to recognize the neurologic forms of TB increases with the advancing immunodepression. The low inflammatory response in HIV patients generates an atypical CSF aspect and repeated confusions with meningitis of other aetiology. At the same time, the TB aetiology should always be included in the differential diagnosis due to its frequency in the evolution of the HIV infection. TB meningitis usually appears as a relapse and only rarely during primary infection. Bacteriological confirmation is delayed and its sensitivity is under dispute: some authors recorded a higher number of false negative smear sample results while others maintained that the sensitivity is similar in both HIV and non-HIV infected patients. Therefore in order to raise the cases diagnosed one should consider the addition of invasive investigations and high cost molecular techniques. The immunologic methods of diagnosis in immunodepressed hosts have been little evaluated. HIV patients display a decreasing Th1 count, sustaining the Th2 stimulation of B cells and the synthesis of antimycobacterial antibodies. Specific tests of cell immunity (IGRAs, TST) are disappointing (Pai & Lewinsohn, 2005) but the humoral immune response appears to persist for a long time. An advantage of the serologic diagnosis is that of the high titres of antimycobacterial antibodies in relapse forms which comprise the majority of TB forms in HIV patients. Certain authors observed an increased IgG in the serum of HIV patients with pulmonary TB compared to controls (Van Vooren et al,1994). No difference has been observed between pulmonary TB and extrapulmonary TB in what regards humoral immunity (Daleine et al, 1995). The essential difference resides in the released antigens. A serologic study in HIV patients with TB infection concluded that only 14 antigens induced the antibody synthesis in these patients. Interestingly, most antigens between 32-45KDa (except for 38 Kda) failed to elicit a humoral reponse (Zhou et al, 1996). The best results involved glycolipidic antigens , especially LOS, LAM, DAT, PGL (Patel et al, 2009) and high molecular weight proteic antigens (ag 85Kda, 88Kda) (Laal et al, 1997). LAM positivity has been associated with HIV co-infection and low CD4 T cell count. Below are the conclusions of ten studies performed in patients with HIV and TB infection using Elisa and numerous antigens (LOS, LAM , 88kDa , PPD , 38 kDa, 88 kDa, A60 or antigen combinations such as PPD and DAT, PPD and SLIV or PPD and LAM.

Main findings. Various studies revealed an extremely variable sensitivity (0-95%), not only for different antigens included in the same study, but also for the same antigen in different studies (such as the high variable sensitivity for LAM in different studies: 35-95%). Only the selection of LOS antigen has led to concordant results between studies. Despite the dysfunctional cellular immune responses in HIV patients, several investigators have reported the presence of antibodies against *M. tbc*, TB16.3, TB9.7, MPT 51, MTB 81 and 88 kDa antigens (Laal et al, 1997). Comparative studies also revealed that the sensitivity for certain antigens (PPD, *M.tbc*) doubles in patients who are HIV negative compared to HIV positive. Moreover the sensitivity is higher in HIV patients compared to AIDS patients. However the level of anti A60 IgG remains elevated in patients with AIDS or with a negative TST result. Despite the low sensitivity the specificity of the Mycodot test was high.

Comments. Secondary TB elicits a stronger serologic response than primary TB and could account for the differences between the different groups of patients (Maes, 1991). However none of the mentioned studies classified the patients as primary or secondary TB. On the other hand an attempt to classify according to the bacteriological confirmation revealed a higher detection sensitivity for antimycobacterial antibodies in patients with confirmed TB (57%) than in patients with unconfirmed TB (30%) (Kameswaran et al, 2002). Antimycobacterial antibodies could predict tuberculosis in HIV patients in some studies. A study by Amicosante proved the appearance of antimycobacterial antibodies one year before the clinical onset of tuberculosis in 67% of HIV infected patients. (Amicosante et al, 1994). The early prediction and diagnosis of neurotuberculosis rendered by antibodies are extremely important for an early starting of antituberculous chemotherapy. Unfortunately only few HIV patients with neurotuberculosis are recorded in the evaluation of extrapulmonary TB and it is difficult to estimate the real value of serologic methods.

9. Diagnostic value of immunological assays in patients with neurologic nonmycobacterial infections

Nontuberculous mycobacteria infections with neurologic or systemic localizations exhibit a low titre of IgG (Oliver et al, 2001). In addition the presence of corresponding antibodies in HIV patients suggests colonization (usually involving the digestive tract) rather than infection (Maes 1991). Thus studies on patients with AIDS and disseminated infection with

M.avium failed to detect any IgG antimycobacterial antibodies in the serum, unlike patients with AIDS and pulmonary infection with *M.avium* (Daniel et al, 1990). A study on the IgG, IgM, IgA released against antigen LAM has triggered no immune response in mycobacteria infections other than TB (Demkow et al, 2006). There are also studies upholding the possibility of a serologic diagnosis in HIV patients with nontuberculous mycobacteria infection using antigens extracted from PPD-B /M. intracellulare, PPD-Y/M. kansasii, PPD-F/M. fortuitum) Nevertheless the serologic diagnosis is presently impractical in the case of nontuberculous mycobacteria infections and there are no available studies regarding HIV patients with neurotuberculosis.

10. The interpretation of serologic results in the diagnosis of neurotuberculosis. Reasons for false positive and negative results

Immunoenzymatic techniques are the most frequently used techniques for the detection of antimycobacterial antibodies in the CSF. The detection of CSF and serum antimycobacterial antibodies through such methods is specific, inexpensive, rapid, but displays a moderate sensitivity and requires a correct interpretation of the data.

Reasons for false negative results. Most false negative results are related to the low level of antimycobacterial antibodies in the serum or CSF, along with inadequate technical parameters. The low titre of antibodies could be the consequence of: a) decreased antigenic stimulation induced by reduced metabolism of mycobacteria; b) reduced antibodies synthesis as a result of a congenital or acquired immunodeficiency; c) antigen fixation in the immune complexes; d) early detection. The use of inadequate technical parameters correlates with: a) a cut off too highly set; b) too high dilutions (the current CSF dilutions of 1/10 appear to exceed the titre of antibodies); c) belated CSF processing; d) improper storing conditions.

Reasons for false positive results in the CSF: a) excessive amount of serum antibodies able to cross the blood barier (a finding usually related to pulmonary TB); b) cross reaction with other infections (Nocardia, Corynebacterium) , the rheumatoid factor, or other diseases (sarcoidosis, pulmonary neoplasm, autoimmune diseases); c) immune hiperreactivity unable to suppress the antibody synthesis after the disappearance of the stimulus; f) insufficient purification of the antigens; g) high prevalence of TB and a low cut-off.

11. Improvement possibilities of serologic techniques in neurotuberculosis

The improvement of immunologic results in neurotuberculosis diagnosis is first related to the knowledge advance of TB immunopathology. The current improvement strategies focus on the following: a) The discovery of highly specific antigens; b) Polyproteins or multiple antigens concurrent detection; c) Cut-off value adapted to the geographic area TB endemicity and to the CSF sample (the predicted cut off value for the CSF is of 40 serounits of IgG instead of 200 serounits required by pulmonary TB); d) The removal of immune complexes; e) Repeated serologic detection after onset and during treatment; f) Simultaneous screening for antibodies IgM, IgG, IgA; g) Simultaneous detection of antibodies and antigenes using rapid techniques; h)The use of low dilutions for the immunosuppressed patients); i) Intrathecal synthesis detection; j) Correlation with immunologic markers (the CD4 level, immunogram) for a correct interpretation of the immune status.

12. Conclusions

a.   The value and limits of the immunologic diagnosis in NTB

The detection of mycobacteria antigens and antimycobacterial antibodies in the CSF, as well as in the serum of patients with neurotuberculosis could augment the diagnosis suspicion and ensure a rapid treatment. Increasing the efficiency of the immunologic diagnosis in neurotuberculosis requires antigens that are specific for neurological localizations as well as standardized and sensitive methods. Immunoserological studies on neurotuberculosis generally involve methods with a good specificity and acceptable senzitivity. The rapidity and increased specificity are the main advantages of these methods. Still, these diagnostic methods cannot replace the bacteriological exam and are presently unstandardised, which hinders the results comparison. In addition, the correct interpretation requires complex data (not always available) related to the onset, treatment, medical history, other localizations of tuberculosis and the immunologic status. In the absence of these data, the results obtained through serological methods cannot be relevant.

b.   The possibilities of performing the immunologic diagnosis in NTB

Despite the numerous diagnostic tools presently available, the neurologic forms of TB often remain undetected and lead to an increased mortality. Neurologic localizations are mostly smear negative and require a rapid diagnosis. The only rapid diagnosis method employs molecular techniques which are too expensive for developing countries. Moreover, starting antituberculous treatment before the collection of specific pathological products decreases the sensitivity of both bacteriological and molecular methods. The immunologic methods are inexpensive and could also be used after treatment starting. The rapid methods (Dot) do not even require trained personnel, the results are available without delay and the reagents are easy to store. As long as the interpretation of the results is correct, the serological methods deliver significant information and a rapid orientation in the diagnosis at a low cost.

c.   The practical value of the immunologic diagnosis as a complementary method in developing countries with a high prevalence of TB

The immunologic methods studied in neurotuberculosis hold a practical value once their results are included in an internationally accepted algorithm for diagnosis. However, the use of these diagnostic methods and reports on cost-efficiency are regarded with reluctance. Literature data published between 2004-2008 on TB case definitions includes only 1 study which considers ELISA IgM detection useful in TB meningitis (Kalita et al, 2007).Three other studies consider that a positive TST test could exhibit only a potential utility in the diagnosis of TB. (Marais et al, 2010) There is also insufficient experience in order to appreciate the efficiency of IGRAs assays in the diagnosis of neurotuberculosis. Therefore the immunologic diagnosis in neurotuberculosis is not currently accepted in the international guidelines as a complementary diagnosis for the confirmation of the diagnosis of neurotuberculosis. Nevertheless serologic diagnostic methods are in use in developing countries and provide rapid orientative data in TB meningitis. However each assay should be validated using controls from that specific area and a part of the technical criteria are also to be adapted to that area in terms of cut off value and used antigens. Standardised diagnostic criteria for TB meningitis as well as standardised immunologic methods could render correct forthcoming comparisons between immunologic studies. It could also establish the real value of these methods especially in poor countries with a high prevalence for tuberculosis and reduced possibilities of diagnosis.

13. Acnowledgments

This work was supported by CNCSIS-Grant project 1165/2508/2008

14. References

Alde, S., Piñasco, H., Pelosi F., Budani H., Palma-Beltran O. & Gonzalez-Montaner LJ. (1989). Evaluation of an enzyme-linked immunosorbent assay (ELISA) using an IgG antibody to Mycobacterium tuberculosis antigen 5 in the diagnosis of active tuberculosis in children. *Am Rev Respir Dis.*, Vol.139, No.3, (Mar 1989), pp. 748-751.

Amicosante, M., Richeldi, L., Monno, L., Cuboni, A., Tartoni, P., Angarano, G., Orefici, G. & Saltini C. (1997). Serological markers predicting tuberculosis in human immunodeficiency virus-infected patients. *Int J Tuberc Lung Dis.* No 5 (Oct 1997), pp 435-440.

Chandramuki, A., Bothamley, G., Brennan, P.& Ivanyi J. (1989). Levels of antibody to defined antigens of Mycobacterium tuberculosis in tuberculous meningitis. *J Clin Microbiol.* Vol. 27, No. 5, (May 1989), pp. 821-825.

Cho, T., Park, S., Cho, S., Lee, H., Kim, S., Kim, S.& Lee, B.(1995). Intrathecal synthesis of immunoglobulin G and Mycobacterium tuberculosis-specific humoral immune response in tuberculous meningitis. *Clin Diagn Lab Immunol.* Vol.2, No.3, (May 1995), pp. 361-364.

Consensus Statement on Childhood Tuberculosis Working group on Tuberculosis, Indian Academy of Pediatrics (IAP), (2010). *Indian Pediatrics,* Vol. 47 (Jan 17, 2010), pp. 41-55.

Daleine, G.& Lagrange, P. (1995). Preliminary evaluation of a Mycobacterium tuberculosis lipooligosaccharide (LOS) antigen in the serological diagnosis of tuberculosis in HIV seropositive and seronegative patients. *Tuber Lung Dis.*, Vol.76, No.3, (Jun 1995), pp. 234-239.

Daniel, P., Kataaha, P.& Eriki, P.(1990). AIDS patiens with coexisting tuberculosis can be diagnosic serologicaly while thouse wih M. avium disease cannot, *ARRD* 141, Vol.141, No.4 (Feb 1990), A264.

Daniel, T.& Debanne, S. (1987). The serodiagnosis of tuberculosis and other mycobacterial diseases by enzyme-linked immunosorbent assay. *Am Rev Respir Dis.* Vol.135, No.5, (1987 May), pp.1137-1151.

Davidow, A., Kanaujia, G., Shi, L., Kaviar, J., Guo, X., Sung, N.& Kaplan, G.(2005). Menzies D, Gennaro ML. Antibody profiles characteristic of Mycobacterium tuberculosis infection state. *Infect Immun.* , Vol.73, No.10 (Oct 2005), pp. 6846-6851.

Davies, P., Pai, M.,(2008). The diagnosis and misdiagnosis of tuberculosis. *Int J Tuberc Lung Dis.*Vol 12, No 11, (Nov 2008), pp. 1226-1234Dayal, R., Singh, A., Katoch, V., Joshi,

B., Chauhan, D., Singh, P., Kumar, G.& Sharma V. (2008).Serological diagnosis of tuberculosis. *Indian J Pediatr.* Vol.75, No.12, (Dec 2008), pp. 1219-21.

Dayal, R., Singh, A., Katoch, V., Joshi, B., Chauhan, D., Singh, P., Kumar, G.& Sharma V. (2008).Serological diagnosis of tuberculosis. *Indian J Pediatr.* Vol.75, No.12, (Dec 2008), pp. 1219-21.

de Micco C.& Toga, M. (1988). The immune status of the central nervous system. *Rev Neurol (Paris), Vol.* 144, No.12, (1988) pp.776-788.

Delacourt C, Gobin J, Gaillard JL, de Blic J, Veron M, Scheinmann P.Value of ELISA using antigen 60 for the diagnosis of tuberculosis in children. *Chest.*,Vol. 104, No.2, (Aug 1993) ,pp. 393-398.

Demkow, U., Białas-Chromiec, B., Filewska, M., Zielonka, T., Michałowska-Mitczuk, D., Kuś, J., Broniarek-Samson, B., Augustynowicz-Kopeć, E., Zwolska, Z.& Rowińska-Zakrzewska, E. (2006). Humoral immune response against mycobacterial antigens in patients with tuberculosis and mycobacterial infections other than tuberculosis. *Pneumonol Alergol Pol.* Vol.74, No. 2, (2006), pp. 203-208

Desai, D., Nataraj, G., Kulkarni, S., Bichile, L., Mehta, P., Baveja, S., Rajan, R., Raut, A.& Shenoy, A. (2006). Utility of the polymerase chain reaction in the diagnosis of tuberculous meningitis. *Res Microbiol.* Vol. 157, No.10, (Dec 2006), pp. 967-70.

Dole, M., Maniar, P., Lahiri, K.& Shah, M. (1989). Enzyme-linked immuno-assay for the detection of mycobacterium tuberculosis specific IgG antibody in the cerebrospinal fluid in cases of tuberculous meningitis. *J Trop Pediatr.* Vol. 35, No.5, (Oct 1989), pp. 218-220.

Donald, P. & Schoeman, J. (2004). Tuberculous meningitis. *N Engl J Med* Vol. 351 (Oct 21, 2004), pp. 1719-1720

Fadda, G., Grillo, R., Ginesu, F., Santoru, L., Zanetti, S.& Dettori, G. (1992). Serodiagnosis and follow up of patients with pulmonary tuberculosis by enzyme-linked immunosorbent assay. *Eur J Epidemiol.* Vol.8, No.1, (Jan 1992), pp. 81-87.

Felgenhauer, K. & Schädlich, H. (1987). The compartmental IgM and IgA response within the central nervous system. *J Neurol Sci.* Vol.77, No 2-3, (Feb 1987), pp.125-135.

Ghoshal, U., Kishore, J., Kumar, B.& Ayyagari, A. (2003). Serodiagnosis of smear and culture-negative neurotuberculosis with enzyme linked immunosorbent assay for anti A-60 immunoglobulins. *Indian J Pathol Microbiol.* Vol.46, No.3, (Jul 2003), pp. 530-534.

Glatman-Freedman, A., Casadevall, A., Dai, Z., Jacobs, WR Jr., Li, A., Morris, S., Navoa, J, Piperdi, S., Robbins, J., Schneerson, R., Schwebach, .&J Shapiro, M. (2004). Antigenic Evidence of Prevalence and Diversity of Mycobacterium tuberculosis Arabinomannan , *J Clin Microbiol.* Vol. 42, No 7, (Jul 2004), pp. 3225-3231.

Houghton, R., Lodes, M., Dillon, D., Reynolds, L., Day, C., McNeill, P., Hendrickson, R., Skeiky, Y., Sampaio, D., Badaro, R, Lyashchenko, K.& Reed, S.(2002). Use of multiepitope polyproteins in serodiagnosis of active tuberculosis. *Clin Diagn Lab Immunol.*Vol.9, No. 4, (Jul 2002), pp. 883-891

Julián, E., Matas, L., Ausina, V.& Luquin, M. (1997). Detection of lipoarabinomannan antibodies in patients with newly acquired tuberculosis and patients with relapse tuberculosis. *J Clin Microbiol.*, Vol.35, No.10, (Oct 1997), pp. 2663-2664.

Kadival, G., Samuel, A., Mazarelo, T. & Chaparas, S. (1987). Radioimmunoassay for detecting Mycobacterium tuberculosis antigen in cerebrospinal fluids of patients with tuberculous meningitis. *J Infect Dis.*, Vol.155, No. 4, (Apr 1987), pp. 608-611Kalish, S., Radin, R., Levitz, D., Zeiss, C.& Phair, J. (1983). The enzyme-linked immunosorbent assay method for IgG antibody to purified protein derivative in cerebrospinal fluid of patients with tuberculous meningitis. *Ann Intern Med.*, Vol.99, No.5, (Nov 1983), pp. 630-633.

Kalita, J., Misra, U.& Ranjan, P. (2007). Predictors of long-term neurological sequelae of tuberculous meningitis: a multivariate analysis. *Eur J Neurol.*Vol.14, No.1, (Jan 2007), pp 33-37.

Kameswaran, M., Shetty, K., Ray, M., Jaleel, M.& Kadival, G.. (2002). Evaluation of an in-house-developed radioassay kit for antibody detection in cases of pulmonary tuberculosis and tuberculous meningitis. *Clin Diagn Lab Immunol.*, Vol.9, No. 5, (Sep 2002), pp. 987-993.

Kaplan, M.& Chase, M. (1980). Antibodies to mycobacteria in human tuberculosis. I. Development of antibodies before and after antimicrobial therapy. *J Infect Dis.*, Vol.142, No.6, (Dec 1980), pp. 825-834.

Kashyap, R., Ramteke, S., Morey, S., Purohit, H., & Daginawala, H.(2009). Diagnostic value of early secreted antigenic target-6 for the diagnosis of tuberculous meningitis patients. *Infection.* Vol.37, No.6, (Dec 2009), pp. 508-513.

Kampmann, B., Whittaker, E., Williams, A., Walters, S., Gordon, A., Martínez-Alier N, et al.(2009). Interferon-gamma release assays do not identify more children with active TB than TST. *Eur Respir J.*, Vol.33, (2009), pp. 1374-1378

Katti, M. (2001). Immunodiagnosis of tuberculous meningitis: rapid detection of mycobacterial antigens in cerebrospinal fluid by reverse passive hemagglutination assay and their characterization by Western blotting. *FEMS Immunol Med Microbiol.*,Vol.31, No.1, (Jul 2001), pp. 59-64.

Kinnman, J., Link, H. & Frydén, A. (1981). Characterization of antibody activity in oligoclonal immunoglobulin G synthesized within the central nervous system in a patient with tuberculous meningitis. *J Clin Microbiol.* , Vol.13, No 1, (Jan 1981), pp. 30-35.

Laal, S.,Samanich, K., Sonnenberg,M., Zolla-Pazner, S., Phadtare J.& Belisle J. (1997). Human humoral responses to antigens of Mycobacterium tuberculosis: immunodominance of high-molecular-mass antigens. *Clin Diagn Lab Immunol.*, Vol.4, No.1, (Jan 1997), pp. 49–56.

Lawn, S.& Zumla, A. (2011). Tuberculosis. *Lancet.* Vol 2, No 378(9785), (Jul 2011), pp. 57-72.

Maes, R., Homasson, J., Kubin, M.& Bayer M.(1989). Development of an enzyme immunoassay for the serodiagnostic of tuberculosis and mycobacterioses. *Med Microbiol Immunol.*, Vol.178, No.6, (1989), pp. 323-335.

Maes, R. (1991). Clinical usefulness of serological measurements obtained by antigen 60 in mycobacterial infections: development of a new concept. *Klin Wochenschr.*, Vol. 69, No.15, (Oct 1991), pp. 696-709.

Maheshwari, A., Gupta, H., Gupta, S., Bhatia, R.& Datta, K.(2000). Diagnostic utility of estimation of mycobacterial antigen A60 specific immunoglobulins in serum and CSF in adult neurotuberculosis. *J Commun Dis.*,Vol.32, No. 1, (Mar 2000), pp. 54-60.

Marais, S., Thwaites, G., Schoeman, J., Török, M., Misra, U., Prasad, K., Donald, P., Wilkinson, R.& Marais, B. (2010). Tuberculous meningitis: a uniform case definition for use in clinical research. *Lancet Infect Dis.*, Vol.10, No.11, (Nov 2010), pp. 803-12.

Mathai, A., Radhakrishnan, V.& Shobha S.Diagnosis of tuberculous meningitis confirmed by means of an immunoblot method. *J Infect.*, Vol.29, No.1, (Jul 1994), pp. 33-39.

Mathai, A., Radhakrishnan, V.& Thomas, M. (1991). Rapid diagnosis of tuberculous meningitis with a dot enzyme immunoassay to detect antibody in cerebrospinal fluid. *Eur J Clin Microbiol Infect Dis.*, Vol.10, No.5, (May 1991), pp. 440-443.

Mudaliar, A., Kashyap, R., Purohit, H., Taori, G.& Daginawala, H. (2006).Detection of 65 kD heat shock protein in cerebrospinal fluid of tuberculous meningitis patients. *BMC Neurol.*, Vol. 15, No.6, (Sep 2006), pp.34-36.

Murakami, S., Takeno, M., Oka, H., Ueda, A., Kurokawa, T., Kuroiwa, Y.& Ishigatsubo Y. (2008). Diagnosis of tuberculous meningitis due to detection of ESAT-6-specific gamma interferon production in cerebrospinal fluid enzyme-linked immunospot assay. *Clin Vaccine Immunol.*, Vol.15, No. 5, (May 2008), pp. 897-899.

Nyendak, M., Lewinsohn, D.& Lewinsohn, D. (2009). New diagnostic methods for tuberculosis. *Current Opinion in Infectious Diseases*, Vol.22, No 2, (April 2009), pp. 174-182

Oliver, A., Maiz, L., Cantón, R., Escobar, H., Baquero, F.& Gómez-Mampaso, E. (2001). Nontuberculous mycobacteria in patients with cystic fibrosis. *Clin Infect Dis.*, Vol.1, No 32(9), (May 2001), pp. 1298-303.

Park, S., Lee, B., Cho, S., Kim, W., Lee, B. & Kim, J. (1993). Diagnosis of tuberculous meningitis by detection of immunoglobulin G antibodies to purified protein derivative and lipoarabinomannan antigen in cerebrospinal fluid. *Tuber Lung Dis.*,Vol.74, No.5, (Oct 1993), pp. 317-322.

Patel, V., Bhigjee, A., Paruk, H., Singh, R., Meldau, R., Connolly, C.& Dheda, K. (2009). Utility of a novel lipoarabinomannan assay for the diagnosis of tuberculous meningitis in a resource-poor high-HIV prevalence setting. *Cerebrospinal Fluid Res.*, Vol.6, (Nov 2, 2009), pp.13-18.

Patel, V., Singh, R., Connolly, C., Kasprowicz, V., Zumla, A. & Dheda K. (2010). Comparison of a clinical prediction rule and a LAM antigen-detection assay for the rapid diagnosis of TBM in a high HIV prevalence setting. *PLoS One*, Vol.5, No. 12, (Dec 22, 2010) : e15664.Patil, S., Gourie-Devi, M., Chaudhuri, J.& Chandramuki, A. (1996). Identification of antibody responses to Mycobacterium tuberculosis antigens in the CSF of tuberculous meningitis patients by Western blotting. *Clin Immunol Immunopathol.*, Vol.81, No.1, (Oct 1996), pp. 35-40.

Radhakrishnan, V., Annamma, M.& Shobha S. (1990). Correlation between culture of Mycobacterium tuberculosis and IgG antibody to Mycobacterium tuberculosis antigen-5 in the cerebrospinal fluid of patients with tuberculous meningitis. *J Infect.*, Vol.21, No.3, (Nov 1990), pp. 271-277.

Raja, A., Ranganathan, U.& Bethunaickan, R. (2008). Improved diagnosis of pulmonary tuberculosis by detection of antibodies against multiple Mycobacterium tuberculosis antigens., *Diagn Microbiol Infect Dis.* ,Vol.60, No.4, (Apr 2008), pp. 361-368.

Rosen E. (1990). The diagnostic value of an enzyme-linked immune sorbent assay using adsorbed mycobacterial sonicates in children. *Tubercle*, Vol.71, No.2, (Jun 1990), pp. 127-130.

Samanich, K., Keen, M., Vissa, V., Harder, J., Spencer, J., Belisle, J., Zolla-Pazner, S.& Laal S. (2000). Serodiagnostic potential of culture filtrate antigens of Mycobacterium tuberculosis. *Clin Diagn Lab Immunol.* ,Vol.7, No.4, (Jul 2000), pp. 662-668.

Sester, M., Sotgiu, G., Lange, C., Giehl, C., Girardi, E., Migliori, G., Bossink, A., Dheda, K., Diel, R., Dominguez, J., & Manissero D. (2010). Interferon-γ release assays for the diagnosis of active tuberculosis: a systematic review and meta-analysis. *Eur Respir J.*,Vol.37, No.1, (Jan 2011), pp 100-111.

Seth, V., Kabra, S., Beotra, A. & Semwal OP. (1993).Tuberculous meningitis in children: manifestation of an immune compromised state. *Indian Pediatr.* Vol.30, No.10, (Oct 1993), pp. 1181-1186.

Sindic, C., Boucquey, D., Van Antwerpen, M., Baelden, M., Laterre, C.& Cocito C. (1990). Intrathecal synthesis of anti-mycobacterial antibodies in patients with tuberculous meningitis. An immunoblotting study. *J Neurol Neurosurg Psychiatry.*, Vol.53, No.8, (Aug 1990), pp. 662-666.

Sireci, G., Dieli, F., Di Liberto, D., Buccheri, S., La Manna, M., Scarpa, F., Macaluso, P., Romano, A., Titone, L., Di Carlo, P., Singh, M., Ivanyi, J.& Salerno A. (2007). Anti-16-kilodalton mycobacterial protein immunoglobulin m levels in healthy but purified protein derivative-reactive children decrease after chemoprophylaxis. *Clin Vaccine Immunol.*, Vol.14, No.9, (Sep 2007), pp. 1231-1234.

Sonmeza, G., Ersin Ozturka, E., Sildiroglua, O., Mutlua, H., Cucea, F.,M. Senolb, G., Kutluc, A., Basekima, C.& Kizilkaya E. (2008). MRI findings of intracranial tuberculomas, *Clinical Imaging,* Vol. 32, No. 2, (March 2008), pp. 88-92

Srivastava, K., Bansal, M., Gupta, S., Srivastava, R., Kapoor, R., Wakhlu, I.& Srivastava BS. (1998). Diagnosis of tuberculous meningitis by detection of antigen and antibodies in CSF and sera. *Indian Pediatr.*, Vol.35, No.9, (Sep1998), pp. 841-850.

Srivastava, L., Prasanna, S.& Srivastava, V.(1994). Diagnosis of tuberculous meningitis by ELISA test. *Indian J Med Res.*, Vol.99, (Jan 1994), pp. 8-12.

Steingart, K., Ramsay, A.& Pai, M. (2007). Commercial serological tests for the diagnosis of tuberculosis: do they work? *Future Microbiol.*, Vol.2, No.4, (Aug 2007), pp. 355-359.

Sumi, M., Mathai, A., Reuben, S,. Sarada, C., Radhakrishnan, V., Indulakshmi, R., Sathish, M., Ajaykumar, R.& Manju, Y. (2002). A comparative evaluation of dot immunobinding assay (Dot-Iba) and polymerase chain reaction (PCR) for the laboratory diagnosis of tuberculous meningitis. *Diagn Microbiol Infect Dis.*, Vol. 42, No.1, (Jan 2002), pp. 35-38.

Thakur, A.& Mandal, A. (19960. Usefulness of ELISA using antigen A60 in serodiagnosis of neurotuberculosis. *J Commun Dis.*,Vol.28, No.1, (Mar 1996), pp. 8-14.

Thomas, M., Hinks, T., Raghuraman, S., Ramalingam, N., Ernst, M., Nau R., Lange C., Kösters K., John, G., Marshall, B.& Lalvani A. (20087). Rapid diagnosis of Mycobacterium tuberculosis meningitis by enumeration of cerebrospinal fluid antigen-specific T-cells. *Int J Tuberc Lung Dis.* Vol.12, No.6, (Jun 2008), pp. 651-657

Tibbling, I. (1977). Establishment of reference values. Scand. J. Clin.G., H. Link, and S. Ohman. Principles of albumin and IgG analyses in neurological disorders. *Lab. Invest.*, No. 37, (1977), pp. 385-390.

Van Vooren, J., Launois, P., Huygen, K., Leguenno, B.& Drowart A. (1994). Detection of anti-85A and anti-85B IgG antibodies in HIV-infected patients with active pulmonary tuberculosis. *Eur J Clin Microbiol Infect Dis.*, Vol.13, No.5, (May 1994), pp. 444-446.

Venkatesh, K., Parija, S., Mahadevan, S.& Negi, V. (2007). Reverse passive haemagglutination (RPHA) test for detection of mycobacterial antigen in the cerebrospinal fluid for diagnosis of tubercular meningitis. *Indian J Tuberc.*, Vol.54, No.1, (Jan 2007),pp. 41-48.

Young, D., Kaufmann, S., Hermans, P. & Thole, J. (1992). Mycobacterial protein antigens: a compilation. *Mol Microbiol.*, Vol.6, No.2, (Jan 1992), pp. 133-145.

Walzl, G., Ronacher, K., Hanekom, W., Scriba, T.& Zumla,A. (2011). Immunological biomarkers of tuberculosis, *Nature Reviews Immunology*, Vol.11, No.5, (May 2011), pp.343-354.

Wiker & Harboe M, (1992). The antigen 85 complex: a major secretion product of Mycobacterium tuberculosis. *Microbiol Rev.*, Vol.56, No.4,(Dec 1992), pp. 648-661.

9

Mycobacterium tuberculosis:
Biorisk, Biosafety and Biocontainment

Wellman Ribón

Universidad Industrial de Santander, Bucaramanga
Colombia

1. Introduction

1.1 Biorisk, biosafety and biocontainment: A life or death process

Safety at workplaces, occupational diseases, pandemics, international travel, public transportation, day care centers, nursing homes, and jails, among others, are situations we are frequently involved in and whose impact and risks we are not aware of but could change the course of our lives. When we travel abroad on business or vacation usually our expectations are high, but we have no information on the process undertaken to secure passengers health, as well as community and environmental safety. When we share a closed space such as an airplane, we should be aware of some diseases, especially air borne diseases, to be able to assess exposure risk and minimize it by adopting biosafety measures (individual, collective or both), and have the proper infrastructure to contain or isolate such risk.

Based on this multifactor approach, scientists and experts on *Mycobacterium tuberculosis* biology, on chemical agents, personal protective equipment (PPE), industrial air purifiers, building design, laboratory equipment and different transportation means join their efforts to harmonize the life of communities around the planet.

Every community should make an effort to acquire a culture aimed at preserving their physical integrity and environmental quality because this process is not restricted to expert laboratories. Anti-pandemic plans presently emphasize that communities are the main pillar to contain these devastating events and such a perspective must transcend the usual scenarios such as hospitals, laboratories, universities, public transportation, supermarkets, movie theaters, etc.

The debate today is heated, and there is an extensive and sometimes emphatic documentation. Many of the aspects involved are described separately, but we must remember that they should be integrated so as to avoid implementing isolated components that may have been successful elsewhere but are not reproducible in our own settings. The present chapter is no exception: we collected the minimum information required to develop the safety data sheet and start the risk assessment; we describe the basic, most general biosafety measures adopted internationally, and we offer a guide on essential biocontainment measures (some of which are described in the section dedicated to biosafety). Such a structure responds solely to academic purposes, but we have to remember that in reality they are inclusive, inseparable processes aimed at the same results. They are the starting point to strengthen the process in any institution, and, therefore, risk assessment should be done together with experts from different disciplines and based on updated knowledge, as well as on the identification of protection elements that may be included in the process and adapted to specific infrastructures and resources. This is the only way to develop a practical and reliable process. Besides, contingency plans should be designed to respond to unexpected catastrophic events such as bioterrorist attacks (Wheelis 2002) and natural disasters.

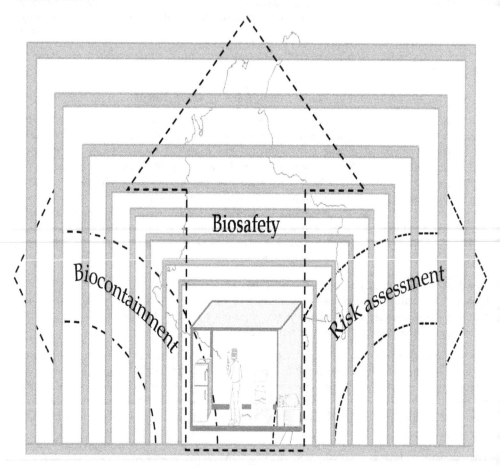

Fig. 1. Calculating risk levels and negative and positive impact according to the safety procedures.

Finally, as this is a complex and dynamic process, you should determine a specific, known and daily situation and then identify exposure risks, the PPE presently in use and consider and assess if you can contain the risk and prevent it from having greater magnitude. Figure 1 will help you in calculating risk levels and negative and positive impact according to your present procedures. Remember human fragility and the fact that probably many of the elements mentioned are no at your disposal, but you can resort to those available in your day-to-day scenario. Human beings are not disposable or reusable, but they are biodegradable or incinerable depending on the circumstances, and that is why the process described in this chapter must be seen as conducive to a better quality of life or to death.

2. Biorisk

The following is a description of various characteristics of the microorganism which are useful in understanding biorisk, biosafety, and biocontainment. *M. tuberculosis* is a pathogen that has been extensively studied; the majority of information required for risk-evaluation of each procedure or work situation can be easily consulted in publications of such renowned international organizations as: The World Health Organization (WHO); The Centers for Disease Control and Prevention (CDC); the National Institutes of Health (NIH); Sandia National Laboratories; American Biological Safety Association (ABSA); Asociación Mexica de Bioseguridad (AMEXBIO), and in the domestic regulations of each country. The updated versions of this information can be accessed through the systematic review of professional scientific publications. Each institutional biosafety committee is responsible for implementing, and ensuring compliance with, the relevant guidelines and regulations. The *M. tuberculosis* safety data sheet should be prepared in each laboratory, posted in a conspicuous location, and accessible to all personnel who work in the area. Staff should be diligent in the risk assessment of their tasks and procedures, request the required PPE, and comply with containment measures in order to guarantee their safety and that of their colleagues and the environment.

2.1 Safety date sheet

2.1.1 Identification of the microorganism, (Riley 1961, Kunz 1982, Wayne 1984 and Grange 1990)

Agent name: *Mycobacterium tuberculosis*

Taxonomy

Domain: Bacteria

Phylum: Actinobacteria

Class: Actinomycetes

Order: Actinomycetales

Family: Mycobacteriaceae

Genus: *Mycobacterium*

Specie: *tuberculosis*

2.1.2 Biological characteristics

Condition: bacteria aerobic

Grow: slow-growing

Motility: non-motile

Spore: non-endospore forming* (aspect in discussion by Ghosh 2009 and Traag 2010)

Acid-Fast Bacillus (AFB)

Allergenic: no

Cancerous: no

Abortive: no

Toxins forming: no

Immunosupressor: no

Capable of mutating in the host: yes

Recommended pictogram:

2.1.3 Mode of transmission

Usually airborne human to human (inhalation of infectious aerosols or infected droplets) or dermal inoculation and possible ingestion, it is not transmitted through sexual contact, and there has been no documentation of vertical transmission. (Wells 1955 and Verhagen 2011)

Disease:

Tuberculosis (TB) (second leading cause of death worldwide)

Latent TB infection

Multidrug resistant TB (MDR TB)

Extensively drug resistant TB (XDR TB)

Host:

Humans, nonhuman primates, and commonly used laboratory animals: pigs, cats, dogs, sheep, cattle, rodents and seals. Some domestic animals, in contact with people suffering from TB, are able to develop TB and become themselves a source of infection. (Grange 1990, National Research Council. 1997 and 2003, Hankenson 2003, Krauss 2003, and Cousins 2003)

Infectious dose for humans: is very low (ID_{50} 1-10 bacilli by inhalation route), a sputum of an infected patient can contain several millions of bacilli per milliliter.(Riley, 1957 and 1961 and CDC 1999)

Communicability: high, human to human with symptoms.

Incubation period: long (years), may progress to pulmonary or disseminated disease.

Vectors: none

Zoonosis: by inhalation or direct contact with infected animal or tissues from infected animal.

Survival on inanimate surfaces at different relative humidities: *M. tuberculosis* can survive for several days on inanimate surfaces; 70 days on carpet, 45 days on clothing, 105 days on paper, 90 to 120 days on dust, 6 to 8 months in sputum in a cool and dark room, 45 days in manure, and 49 days in guinea pig tissue.(Kunz 1982, and Rubin 1991)

Geographical localization: worldwide

2.1.4 Detection

Latent TB infection has been traditionally identified by the tuberculin skin test (TST, Mantoux or PPD); currently the new generation of test entails interferon gamma (IFN-γ) release assays (IGRAs: Quantiferon and T-SPOT.TB).

Diagnosis of TB: acid fast stain of sputum samples, culture, phenotypic and genotypic identification of *M. tuberculosis*, DNA fingerprinting (Rozo 2010) and drug susceptibility testing and tissue exams.

Possibility of viewing the bacillus in clinical specimens: yes, through examination of clinical sample for acid-fast bacilli (AFB), fluorescence microscopy and light-emitting diode (LED)

Growth in culture media: yes, frequently in Lowenstein-Jensen (LJ), Ogawa Kudoh (OK) or liquid culture as modified Middlebrook 7H9 broth, the *M. tuberculosis* is of slow growth, between 4 to 8 weeks, from clinical samples. (Welch 1993)

Rapid identification of *M. tuberculosis*: through the employment of methods such as nucleic acid hybridization methods, lateral flow assays, line probe assays, and DNA sequencing.

2.1.5 Epidemiology

Risk population: it is relatively more prevalent in immigrants, minorities, the elderly, persons with acquired immunodeficiency syndrome (AIDS) and among healthcare workers, and laboratory personnel who are occupationally exposed.

Mortality and morbidity: mortality for TB, depending on the country, MDR TB 50% to 70% of the patients not treated within a period of two years. Mortality is higher in patients with TB/AIDS. The morbidity in TB is high.

Perception of malicious use: low

2.1.6 Surveys of laboratory-acquired infection and prophylaxis

Laboratory personnel should undergo an annual PPD or IGRAs, and workers with a positive test should be evaluated for active TB; in accidental exposure the laboratory personnel should be tested 3 to 6 months after the event and should be offered prophylaxis if is required in TB, but the referenced isoniazid (INH) prophylaxis is not applicable in MDR TB.

Vaccine: Bacille Calmette Guerin (BCG), attenuate live vaccine, with limited protection. (Lietman 1999)

Treatment: therapy with multiple drugs

First line: INH, rifampin (RIF), pyrazinamide (PZA), ethambutol (EMB), streptomycin (SM).

Second line: Amikacin, capreomycin, ciprofloxacin, ethionamide, kanamycin, levofloxicin. Ofloxacin and *para*-aminosalicylic acid for MDR TB and XDR TB.

2.1.7 Prevention and control

Exposure control-personal protection: PPE such as respiratory protection (fit-tested respirators with N-95 rating) (Occupational Safety and Health Administration –OSHA- 2003 and 2004), hand protection, eye protection, skin and body protection, and hygiene measures.

Containment:

Objective: to prevent aerosol exposure or dermal inoculation.

Biosafety level (BSL) 2 can be used for low-risk procedures, such as making smear and diagnosis activities including primary culture of clinical specimens potentially infected by bacilli of *M. tuberculosis* s with PPE. (Welch 1993)(American Thoracic Society 1993)

BSL-3 can be used for high-risk procedures, such as handling solid and liquid positive culture, secondary cultures for diagnostic or research activities, DNA or RNA extraction (only in the initial stages of the procedure)(Castro 2009, Warren 2006, and NIH 2002), biochemical test, centrifugations, pipetting, mechanical homogenizing, sonication, heating or boiling, work with bacteriological loops, preparation and manipulation of frozen sections, animal studies, infected clinical specimens and others with PPE. (CDC. 1999 and 2006, and Hankenson 2003)

2.1.8 Disinfection, inactivation and sterilization of *M. tuberculosis*

Efficient disinfectants are:

0.4-5 phenol during 10 minutes

5% formaldehyde during at least 10 minutes

1-2% Glutaraldehyde during 30 minutes

0.2-5% Sodium hypochlorite for one minute

70-96% Ethyl alcohol during 2 minutes

3-10% Hydrogen peroxide during 5 minutes

2-10%, 75ppm Iodophore

Mix of iodine + iodophores or ethyl alcohol

Mix of paraformaldehyde + glutaraldehyde or formalin

Susceptible to moist heat sterilization at 121°C for 15 minutes at 121 pounds of pressure in autoclave.

Note: quaternary ammoniums inhibit tubercle bacilli but do not kill them. Please check the efficacy of each disinfectant in your own laboratory conditions.

Ultraviolet dosage required: 10.000 µW-s/cm² at 254 nanometer for 99.9% destruction of bacillus.

2.1.9 Transport information

WHO classification of infective microorganisms by risk groups (RG):

RG 3 (high individual risk, low community risk): a pathogen that usually causes serious human or animal disease but does not ordinarily spread from one infected individual to another. Effective treatment and preventive measures are available (WHO 2004).

Cultures positives for *M. tuberculosis* require packing measures, and labeled as "Infectious substance". The triple packaging should be utilized according to the International Air Transport Association (IATA) and Dangerous Goods regulation and WHO recommendations. *M. tuberculosis* (cultures only) is included in Category A, UN 2814 (Infectious Substances, affecting humans) see table 1. (IATA 2006)

Infections substance	Class	Division	Category	Proper shipping name	UN Number	Packing instruction (PI)
M. tuberculosis cultures only	6	6.2	A	Infections substance	2814	602

Table 1. General information of *M. tuberculosis* for international shipping.

2.1.10 Biosafety functions officer

Mistakes and accidents, which result in over-exposure to infectious materials, should be immediately reported and corrective measures should be taken to avoid a repetition of the event.

Mandatory: personnel concerned with mycobacteria activity should be experienced and under the supervision of the head of the laboratory.

2.2 Epidemiology of hospital and laboratory acquired TB

The epidemiology is defined as the study of the distribution and determinants of diseases and injuries in human populations. Inherent in the definition of epidemiology is the necessity of measuring the amount of disease in a population by relating the number of cases to a population base. One of the unfortunate consequences of working with infectious materials is the potential for acquiring an infection. The laboratory acquired infections (LAI) due to a wide variety of viruses, bacteria, parasites and fungi have been described. In the absence of precise data on LAIs, epidemiological methods provide the necessary tools to evaluate the extent and nature of personnel exposures. Although the precise risk of infection after an exposure remains poorly defined, surveys of LAIs suggested that *Brucella* species, *Shigella* species, *Salmonella* species, *M. tuberculosis* and *Neisseria meningitidis* are the most common causes. Early surveys of laboratory acquired TB found an incidence of TB among laboratory personnel 3-9 times greater than that in the general population (Harrintong 1976 and Reid 1957). The *M. tuberculosis*, the causative organism of TB, has distinction of repeatedly being ranked within the top five most commonly LAI (Pike 1976, 1978, and 1979). The OSHA in 1996, 1997, 2003 and 2004, promulgated withdrawal of the 1997 proposed standard on occupational exposure to TB. Along with the withdrawal of the 1997 standard, the respirator-specific standard, 29 CFR 1910.139, was also withdraw. The effect of withdrawing these standards is the application of the general industry respiratory protection standard, 29 CFR 1910.134, for all occupations, to those workplaces that provide respiratory protection from TB.

According to WHO, TB remains the second leading cause of death worldwide, killing 2 million people each year. In many developed countries, TB is considered a disease of the past. However, the impact of this disease can be devastating even today specially in poor countries. An estimated 9.4 million new cases of TB globally, with most cases occurring in resource limited or resource poor countries. In addition to that, much of deadliness of TB epidemic has to do with the virulent synergy between Human Immunodeficiency Virus (HIV) and TB. Recently, MDR-TB and XDR TB have had devastating effects on populations of HIV infected individuals in developing countries.

2.3 Risk assessment

Risk assessment was defined by Boa (Boa 2000), as "the use of factual information to define the health effects of exposure to individuals or populations to hazardous materials and situations"

The CDC and the NIH provided the basic definition for risk in their *Biosafety in Microbiological and Biomedical Laboratories*: -"Risk" implies the probability that harm, injury, or disease will occur. In the environment of the research, microbiological, teaching, and biomedical laboratories, the assessment of risk focuses first and foremost on the prevention of laboratory associated infections and the likelihood that the agent can be used as a weapon and the consequences of bioattack with the agent. The risk assessment helps to assign the BSL, PPE required, laboratory and facilities design, equipment that can be used, procedures and practices that can be implemented and that reduce, to a minimum, the personnel and the environmental risk of exposure to an agent. The risk evaluation should be made by the person with the best knowledge of the microorganism (*M. tuberculosis*) and the available containment measures. The risk assessment can be quantitative in the presence of known hazards or qualitative when the data will be incomplete or unknown.

The CDC and NIH recommend that the laboratory director or principal investigator, in close collaboration with the institutional biosafety committee, be responsible for assessing risk in order to set the BSL for the work.

The risk assessments should be conducted periodically and the analysis should include: new variables; updated information and procedures related to *M. tuberculosis*; management of the TB; MDR TB or XDR TB, and new international regulations applicable to the malicious use of the bacillus or bacillus-infected substances.

The CDC and NIH include the following important factors in a risk assessment:

1. The pathogenicity of the infectious or suspected infectious agent, in this case *M. tuberculosis*, including disease incidence and severity (morbidity and mortality). **Remark**: The more severe the potentially acquired disease, the higher the risk. With respect to *M. tuberculosis*, one has to consider the types of resistance (TB, MDR TB, and XDR TB).
2. The route of transmission (parenteral, airborne or ingestion). **Remark:** The greater the aerosol potential, the higher the risk (for *M. tuberculosis* the mode of transmission **is** usually airborne).
3. Agent stability: aerosol infectivity and the agent´s ability to survive over time in the environment. Factors such as desiccation, exposure to sunlight or ultraviolet light, or exposure to chemical disinfectants must be considered.
4. The infectious dose of *M. tuberculosis*.
5. The concentration (number of infectious organisms per unit volume).
6. The origin of the potentially infectious materials.
7. The availability of data from animal studies, in the absence of human data.
8. The established availability of an effective prophylaxis or therapeutic interventions.
9. Medical surveillance.
10. Evaluation of the experience and skill level of at-risk personnel.

Sandia National Laboratories International Biological Threat Reduction department worked with biosafety, infectious disease, and risk experts to develop a systematic and standardized methodology for biological safety risk assessments. This standardized methodology will enhance biosafety risk assessments by allowing them to be both repeatable and quantifiable. This methodology is not intended as an all-hazards assessment, but is focused on the risks associated with biological materials being handled in a laboratory setting. Sandia National Laboratories defined criteria related to:

- Agent factors which impact the biosafety risk to humans,
- Agent factors which impact the biosafety risk to animals,
- Procedures used for the activity being assessed, procedures and processes involving animals used for the procedure being assessed.

A "scoring system" was developed for each criterion, with zero defined as the absence of the element defined by the criterion and four defined as the highest possible value for the element (for some elements the highest possible value is the worst case and for others the highest possible value is the best case). For example:

Is this agent known to cause infection via inhalation in humans (to cause infection via droplets or droplet nuclei that have entered the upper or lower respiratory tract) in a laboratory setting?

4=Preferred route

2= A possible route

1=Unknown

0=Not a route

Taking the via inhalation in humans scenario for an agent which cannot cause infection via inhalation the score will be zero; for an agent which via inhalation as *M. tuberculosis* is the preferred route of infection the score will be four.

The biosafety risk assessment model has been coded into a software package which runs on Microsoft'sc .Net Framework. The software, titled "BioRAMSoftware.exe" (Version 1.0 dated September 2010), was planned to be released open source and discussions have started to freely license the software to organizations. The BioRAMSoftware allows visitors to provide the scores for all the criteria in a simple tool by answering a set of questions. The BioRAMSoftware calculates the risk scores using the algorithms and weights defined in the model and methodology. The BioRAMSoftware also allows visitors to modify the wording of questions and the definitions of the scoring scales to better reflect a unique laboratory situation or language differences. The software then produces a numeric and graphical document with the relative risk rankings for the visitors and a chart identifying the impact each question had on the final results. This feature is useful in understanding and communicating the risks, as well as providing guidance on risk management or mitigation efforts. Also, visitors can view and, if needed, modify the weights. The methodology outlined is consistent with internationally accepted risk assessment schemes and also parallels international biosafety risk assessment guidance.

Biosafety RAM includes generalized definitions of how to conduct a biosafety risk assessment:

Evaluate the biological agents that exist at the facility.

Evaluate the facility processes and procedures.

Evaluate the existing biorisk mitigation measures.

You can establish the procedures and concrete situations based upon your institution's particular environment, geographical conditions, and risk assessment. The BioRAMSoftw is available on: http://www.sandia.gov/

The selection should include all situations and procedures that represent a risk for employees, the community, the natural environment, and animals. Biosafety and biocontainment measures should then be implemented based upon each institution's particular situation. A risk assessment should be initiated that defines the specific problem. The method of risk assessment should be simple; easy to apply and interpret; and should permit a quantitative classification of risk on a scale ranging from very low, low, moderate, high, and very high risk.

A risk assessment should include the characteristics of *M. tuberculosis* that are described in the safety data sheet. The intrinsic properties and the laboratory techniques that are likely to generate infectious aerosols should be evaluated based upon each particular situation. For example, in a research laboratory one should establish the difference between the characteristics of bacteria's under study; the H37Ra (ATCC 25177) used in some experiments is classified as a RG 2 pathogen, while the H37Rv (ATCC 2618) strain is designated as RG 3 pathogen. The information collected in the risk assessment may confirm changes in the pathogenicity of the specific microorganism and, therefore, the risk assessment may be altered enough to require an increase in the BSL and PPE for its containment. For example, bacteria which have developed resistance to multiple therapeutic drugs, such as *M. tuberculosis* MDR or XDR are considered to be a higher risk due to the lack of treatment alternatives and are to be handled with more stringent precautions. This bacteria is RG 3, but the extra precautions required for safe work with *M. tuberculosis* MDR would not be expected to take it to a higher containment level than BSL 3.

The laboratory diagnosis of TB should determine the percentage of positivity of pathogenic mycobacteria of clinical specimens submitted for the *M. tuberculosis* test; reported studies estimate that only 1% is positive; however, this data will obviously vary according to region and the number of samples that each laboratory processes. Additionally, the following factors are of crucial relevance in the risk assessment:

- *M. tuberculosis* can be isolated from virtually any type of human or animal specimens.
- The infectious dose in humans is very low and some samples processed in a diagnostic laboratory, such as the sputum of an infected patient, can contain several millions of bacilli per milliliter.
- The infection predominantly occurs by inhalation of airborne bacilli and the manipulation of liquid clinical specimens that likely involves generation of infectious aerosols, although percutaneous injury or infection by secondary transmission through the use of contaminated PPE or laboratory surfaces may also result in infection (Miller 1987, and Muller 1988).

Studies of air transmission of TB conducted during the first half of the last century by Wells (Wells 1955), led to the framing of the concept of the "droplet nucleus." The great majority of laboratory technicians generate droplets of liquid or aerosols and each droplet may contain one or more bacillus. The aerosols that are produced can be classified according their size:

Droplet nuclei: with a size ranging from 1 to 10 µm in diameter and a velocity of propagation of 0.2 to 18 cm/minute or 0.1 to 1 µm in diameter and a velocity of propagation of 0.005 to 0.2 cm/minute.

Dust: with a size ranging from 10 to 100 µm in diameter and a velocity of propagation of 18 to 1800 cm/minute.

Droplet: with a size ranging from 100 to 400 µm in diameter and a velocity of propagation of 1800 to 15200 cm/minute. These particles containing *M. tuberculosis* can remain airborne from minutes to hours.

Larger droplets would not dry and could rapidly contaminate laboratory equipment and surfaces, and fingers or gloves, resulting in a secondary contamination of mouth and nasal cavities. The droplets settle very slowly and dry, and they are transformed into droplet nuclei. These droplet nuclei float in the air of a room and are spread by very small air currents; when inhaled they can settle in alveolar spaces and infect the employee.

Remark: among the laboratory techniques used for the identification and characterization of *M. tuberculosis,* the following ones are likely to increase the risk of contamination or to generate infectious aerosols producing droplet nuclei, such as: centrifugations, pipetting, mechanical homogenizing, sonication, heating, boiling, work with bacteriological loops, preparation and manipulation of frozen sections, handling of containers with clinical specimens, acid-fast staining, manipulation of solid and liquid cultures, flow cytometry, and animal studies.

The risk assessment should also be conducted in hospitals, healthcare units, respiratory isolation areas, ambulatory assistance spaces, and for the TB or non- TB patients transiting through the institution.

3. Biosafety

Biosafety currently involves a large, interdisciplinary group of professionals gathered with the unique objective of guaranteeing that the risk of contracting infection for employees of the institution, and animals, is reduced to a minimum, and that the environment is protected. Currently, however, many of the decisions implemented to reduce biorisk, and contain infectious agents, are also employed by the community-at-large as part of anti-pandemic programs. These activities are dynamic and are strengthened by recent scientific and industrial advances. Changes in the biological characteristics of microorganisms, and the pace of modern life, have generated host-parasite relations that facilitate the transmission of illnesses that are devastating for humanity. Thanks to the groups engaged in interdisciplinary, scientific work, many of these unusual relationships have been disclosed. General and basic recommendations, of a compulsory nature, to ensure biosecurity in the manipulation and containment of *M. tuberculosis*, are discussed below.

WHO classifies microorganisms within four RGs according to infectious characteristics, availability of treatment, preventive measures, and the possibility of containing dissemination (WHO 2004):

RG 1: no or low individual and community risk

RG 2: moderate individual risk, low community risk

RG 3: high individual risk, low community risk

RG 4: high individual and community risk

Current classifications, similar to those created by WHO, have been developed by other institutions, such as: Standars Australia/New Zealand 2002, Canadian Laboratory Biosafety Guidelines (Laboratory Centre for Disease Control 1996), European Economic Community Directive (Comission of the European Communities 2000), NIH Recombinant DNA guidelines, and CDC/NIH guidelines (NIH 2002).

M. tuberculosis is located within these classifications as a microorganism RG3; therefore, its management requires the implementation of PPE consistent with its biological characteristics; a level of security in facilities and laboratory equipment that will minimize the risk of infection and maximize the capability of containment; and measures focused on preventing the intentional, malicious use of this microorganism by the institution's staff or outside parties.

The WHO's *Laboratory Biosafety Manual*, 3rd ed., 2004, which addresses the general principles of biosecurity, establishes the recommended BSLs for the management of microorganisms according to their RG, offers examples of laboratory practices that should be frequently conducted, and the requisite safety equipment. The BSL designations are based on a combination of the containment facilities; design features, equipment, construction, practices and operational procedures required for working with agents belonging to the various RGs. The laboratory facilities are designated as:

- BSL 1 – basic laboratory: for microorganisms in RG 1; an example of a facility would be a basic teaching laboratory; requirements include a good microbiological technique, open bench work, and an autoclave for sterilization of material. The use of PPE is recommended in all procedures; however, safety equipment such as a biological safety cabinet (BSC) is not required.
- BSL 2 - basic laboratory: for microorganisms in RG 2; examples of laboratories are primary health services, primary level hospitals, diagnostic, teaching and public health. Require an implementation of good microbiological technique plus PPE in all procedures; biohazard signs, open benches or ventilation (inward air flow or mechanical via building system) plus BSC for the potential aerosols and autoclave. Various procedures related to the identification of *M. tuberculosis* through clinical samples are conducted at this BSL; therefore, specific PPE measures are obligatory in order to minimize the risk of infection. The following are some accepted procedures for the identification of *M. tuberculosis* through clinical samples:
- Making smear microscopy and diagnostic activities including primary culture of clinical specimens potentially infected by bacilli of *M. tuberculosis*. (Welch 1993)
- Extraction of DNA, RNA, proteins, cell compounds, and molecular methodologies, following the inactivation, death, and lysis of the microorganism; and, having previously determined that the experimental protocol for the extraction and separation of the bacterial components is completely secure in the particular laboratory conditions in which it is conducted (Burgos 2004, Castro 2009 and Warren 2006).
- BSL 3 – laboratory with containment conditions for microorganisms in RG3; examples of laboratories are special diagnostic, production facilities, national tuberculosis reference laboratory and research laboratories; all of the conditions that apply for BSL 2 are included, plus specific PPE, controlled access with double-door entry, isolation laboratory, room sealable for decontamination, directional air flow, ventilation (inward air flow, mechanical via building system and filtered air exhaust), safety equipment as BSC class II or III and autoclave, preferably double –ended. Positive, viable samples of *M. tuberculosis*, *M. tuberculosis* MDR, and *M. tuberculosis* XDR should be handled at this BSL (Sessler 1983), including the following activities:
- Handling solid and liquid positive culture
- Secondary cultures for diagnostic or research activities
- DNA or RNA extraction (initial step of each protocol)
- Biochemical test for *M. tuberculosis* identification
- Bacterial suspension preparation
- Detection drugs resistance
- Centrifugations
- Pipetting
- Mechanical homogenizing

- Sonication, heating or boiling
- Work with bacteriological loops
- Preparation and manipulation of frozen sections (biopsies)
- Animal studies
- Infected clinical specimens and others

BSL 4 – laboratory with maximum containment: for microorganisms in RG 4; this is the maximum containment-BSL and includes all of the requirements of BSL 3 plus airlock entry, airlock with shower, effluent treatment, BSC class III, shower exit, and special waste disposal.

Remark: although some of the precautions may appear to be unnecessary for some organisms, and no clinical or hospital laboratory has complete control over the specimens it receives, the staff may occasionally and unexpectedly be exposed to organisms in higher RGs; therefore, each employee is responsible for his/her own safety; this implies the obligatory and continuous use of PPE, and biosecurity and biocontainment measures, equipment and facilities while in areas of biological risk.

General considerations to guarantee biosecurity in each of the established levels are provided in the recommendations issued by WHO, CDC, NIH (American Thoracic Society 1983, Kent 1985, and CDC 1999 WHO 2004). Compliance with these measures should be part of a culture of biosecurity and professional responsibility. We consider it important to stress some of the following, specific measures for the handling of potentially contaminated material, or material infected with *M. tuberculosis*, in accordance with the requisite level of biosecurity:

BSL 2:

- The international biohazard sign should be displayed on the doors of rooms where the clinical specimens for the search of *M. tuberculosis* are being processed.
- The laboratory personnel have specific training in handling agents such as *M. tuberculosis* and are directed by a competent scientist.
- Access to the laboratory is limited when work is being conducted.
- Extreme precautions are taken with contaminated sharp items.
- The procedure in which infectious aerosols or splashes may be created are conducted in CBS (remember that the risk of aerosols possibly infected with *M. tuberculosis* in a clinical sample such as sputum, or a biopsy, vary according to the number of cases in a region and the number of samples processed by a laboratory; therefore, procedures including making smear microscopy should be conducted in a color booth with biological containment and specific filters for the retention of chemical vapors emitted during the coloration process) and additionally, films and smears for microscopy should be handled with forceps, stored appropriately, and sterilized before disposal.
- Persons wash their hands after they handle viable materials, after removing gloves, and before leaving the laboratory.
- Eating, drinking, smoking, handling contact lenses, and applying cosmetics are not permitted in the work areas.
- All procedures are performed carefully to minimize the creation of splashes or aerosols.

- The work surfaces are decontaminated on completion of work or at the end of the day and after any spill or splash of viable material with disinfectants that are effective against *M. tuberculosis*.
- The wastes are decontaminated before disposal by an approved decontamination against *M. tuberculosis*.
- An insect and rodent control program is in effect.

Recommendations for special procedures:

- Access to the laboratory is restricted by the laboratory director when the work with *M. tuberculosis* includes possibly infectious substances. **Remark:** persons who are at increased risk of acquiring infection, or for whom infection may have serious consequences, are not permitted in the laboratory. Every person, upon initiating employment, should have a medical exam and laboratory tests in order to confirm that he/she is not at risk. Each institution should establish requirements to guarantee that all staff members are clinically suited for this type of work; this process should be conducted in coordination with occupational health professionals, health insurers, and experts in risk assessment and biosafety. In some countries, such as Colombia, vaccination with BCG is indicated; in those nations that have imposed this requirement, the employer should request the appropriate certificate to document the vaccination.
- A degree of precaution must always be taken with any contaminated sharp items, including needles and syringes, slides, pipettes, capillary tubes and scalpels. These items should be used only when absolutely necessary and should be discarded in appropriate containers for subsequent decontamination, thereby preventing the formation of aerosols.
- Spills and accidents that result in over-exposure to substances possibly infected with *M. tuberculosis* are immediately reported to the chief. Medical evaluation and surveillance, and prophylaxis or treatment, should be provided based upon the severity of the accident and estimated risk of the procedure that was being conducted. Each institution should implement protocols for biorisk containment in order to maintain biosecurity; all personnel (housekeeping, professional, administrative, students, and others authorized to enter work areas) should be familiar with these policies. All laboratory areas should include a containment kit that facilitates the rapid implementation of corrective measures following an accident, including an appropriate disinfectant for laboratory surfaces and equipment, PPE, absorbent paper, tweezers for removal of glass particles, and signs to restrict access to the area where the accident occurred. The accident response should conclude with an analysis of causes and implementation of corrective measures.

BSL 3:

All general guidelines governing standard microbiological practices are applicable, in addition to the measures included in BSLs 1 and 2.

- The two person rule should apply, whereby no individual ever works alone in the laboratory.
- All procedures involving the *M. tuberculosis* manipulation are conducted within BSC.

- The laboratory has special engineering design features; however, in the case of those laboratories that do not possess all of these features, good ventilation, illumination, and disinfection of surfaces should be employed in order to guarantee good biosafety. Access to the laboratory is restricted, utilize standard microbiological practices. The decision to implement this modification of BSL 3 recommendations should be made only by the laboratory director.
- The laboratory doors are kept closed when experiments are in progress.
- The laboratory personnel receive the appropriate immunizations with BCG Vaccine or test for the infection surveillance with *M. tuberculosis,* TST or IGRAs.
- The biosafety manual specific to the laboratory is prepared or adopted by the laboratory director and biosafety precautions are incorporated into standard operating procedures.
- The laboratory and support personnel receive specific training about the potential hazards associated with *M. tuberculosis.*
- The laboratory director is responsible for ensuring that before working with *M. tuberculosis,* all workers demonstrate proficiency in standard microbiological practices and experience in handling *M. tuberculosis.*

The CDC and NIH, besides providing orientation about standard microbiological practices and special practices for each BSL, also describe the safety equipment or primary barriers and the laboratory facilities or secondary barriers (CDC 2000). In the following section we reproduce some of these recommendations and include information pertaining to the handling of *M. tuberculosis*:

Safety equipment or primary barriers for BSL 2

- All procedures should be conducted in BSC class II; the selection of BSC should be based upon the actual conditions of each laboratory as reflected in the risk assessment; all BSC's should include at least one HEPA (high efficiency particulated air) filter with at least 99.97% efficiency in retaining particles of 0.3 micrometers, protecting both the operator and the environment; various types may also provide greater protection for the product.

BSC class II type A1:

- Re-circulates 70% and removes 30% to the interior of the laboratory
- Minimum inflow 75 fpm
- Gas jets, volatile toxic chemicals, and radionucleotides cannot be used
- Includes a front aperture and guillotine-type window

BSC class II type A2:

- Re-circulates 70% and removes 30% to the interior of the laboratory
- Minimum inflow 100 fpm
- Gas jets, volatile toxic chemicals, and radionucleotides cannot be used
- Includes a front aperture and guillotine-type window
- Installation of a tube can allow 30% of the air to be ventilated to the exterior of the lab; traces of radionucleotides and small quantities of volatile, toxic liquids can be used

The two types of BSC class II can be used in BSLs 1, 2, and 3 (National Sanitation Foundation International -NSF- 2002).

- The centrifugation of specimens should be done in closed containers, i.e., centrifuge safety cups; these containers are opened only in BSC class II.
- Protective elements such as goggles, mask, and face shield, should be used in order to prevent splashes or sprays of material possibly contaminated with *M. tuberculosis* or other infectious substances. These measures should be used continuously while working, preferably when BSC protection is not available.
- Clothing appropriate for the laboratory should be used, such as impermeable uniforms, gowns that close at the back, caps, shoe protectors, and other items that the institution may consider to be necessary. Laboratory clothing should be used only in the laboratory and is not permitted in other areas such as cafeterias, bathrooms, libraries, on public transportation, offices, etc.

Remark: "all protective clothing is either disposed of in the laboratory or laundered by the institution; it should never be taken home by personnel."

- When working with contaminated material, on contaminated surfaces or equipment, it is recommended that two pairs of gloves be used. Every laboratory should establish a protocol for the disinfection of gloves and hand washing upon completing work.

The laboratory facilities or secondary barriers for BSL 2:

- Laboratory installations should be isolated from public areas, when possible
- Hand-washing and eyewash should be available
- Laboratory facilities, furniture and chairs, should be easy to clean and disinfect; avoid the use of carpets and rugs.
- The laboratory should not be accessible to unauthorized persons.

Safety equipment or primary barriers for BSL 3

- All PPE specific for the manipulation of *M. tuberculosis* should be used, including: caps, shoe protectors, impermeable clothing, and gowns that close in the back. These elements should be disinfected prior to leaving BSL 3 for the laundry or to be discarded.
- Frequent change of gloves and hand washing is recommended. Disposable gloves are not reused. Respiratory and face protection are used when handling or monitoring infected animals.
- In the case of *M. tuberculosis*, infected material is handled in BSC class II; the possibility of using BSC class II type B should be considered based upon the characteristics and risk assessment of each laboratory.

BSC class II type B1:

Re-circulates 40% and removes 60% to the exterior of the laboratory
Minimum inflow 100 fpm
Permits traces of radionucleotides and small quantities of volatile, toxic chemicals; the use of gas burners is not recommended.

BSC class II type B2:

Re-circulates 0% and removes 100% to the exterior of the laboratory

Minimum inflow 100 fpm

Recommended for the handling of radionucleotides and volatile, toxic chemicals; the use of gas burners is not recommended.

Remark: each laboratory should develop its own protocols for the use and disinfection of BSC, according to the instructions of the manufacturer, frequency of use, and risk assessment. The decision to use a BSC class III should be based upon the risk assessment of each laboratory.

Some PPE serve an important function, especially given the current, particular situation concerning *M. tuberculosis*. The short-term prospects of obtaining a vaccine or new, alternative methods of treatment are remote, and the evolving strain of *M. tuberculosis* that is resistant to various, contemporary therapies dictate effective methods of personal protection. Presently, individual respiratory protection is the most recommended measure, and not only for laboratory staff; these devices should also be used by hospital personnel (physicians, nurses, respiratory therapists, and administrative personnel who attend patients, among others); additionally, it is necessary to remark upon the differences between respirators and surgical masks (American National Standard Institute 1992, CDC 1994). The surgical masks provide protection against pathogens present in droplets emitted by coughing; protection is limited to the nose and mouth as the mask does not completely cover the face; therefore, masks do not provide protection against infection contained in droplet nuclei. These masks are now recommended for use by TB patients as they move throughout the hospital or when they are within confined spaces. Respirators, on the other hand, are designed to provide protection against pathogenic microorganisms contained in droplet nuclei; these can include respirators for the retention of particulates or the purification of air. Respirators that purify air function with batteries that power a ventilator providing filtered air to the user; this protective item can be disinfected, allows the change of HEPA filters, and guarantees a level of 100% purification of air. A particulate respirator can be reusable and employ filters that are easily replaced; the equipment can be disinfected and permits installation of a new filter. These respirators do not prevent transmission when used by infected persons. Disposable face respirators are made of filtered material that impedes the passage of large and small particles contained in the air; some include a valve for expelling air. The National Institute of Occupational Safety and Health –NIOSH- 2003 and 2004) has approved nine types of respirators for the retention of particulates. Differences include capacity to filter air, and resistance of the filter to oil (partially or strongly resistant). See table 2. Any of these can be used when handling *M. tuberculosis*.

General characteristics of respirators		
Class of respirators	**Resistance to oils**	**% of retention**
R 95	Resistant	95
R 99	Resistant	99
R 100	Resistant	99.97
P 95	Partial	95
P 99	Partial	99
P 100	Partial	99.97
N 95	No	95
N 99	No	99
N 100	No	99.97

Table 2. General characteristics of respirator.

Correct training in the use and care of these items is indispensable in order to guarantee their protective function; the respirators should be properly adjusted to the face; the perception of odors or the presence of air leaks is an indication that the respirator is not functioning properly. **Remark:** These elements are for individual use and should be discarded when alterations, stains, porosity, or humidity are present.

The laboratory facilities or secondary barriers for BSL 3:

-   All doors and windows should remain closed.
-   A double-door system should be in place that does not allow both doors to be open at the same time (an alarm should sound if this occurs).
-   A special ventilation system with HEPA filters and negative pressure should be installed.
-   All procedures should be conducted in BSC.
-   Autoclaves, preferably double-ended, should be on-site, in the laboratory room.
-   A constant supply of electricity, water, disposal, and gas should be guaranteed; filters and other necessary items should be available in order to ensure the containment of *M. tuberculosis* and other pathogens.
-   All necessary equipment should be available in order to conduct all processes and avoid the entrance and exit of material that should be contained.
-   All procedures that occur at this BLS should be documented and approved by the laboratory director and the institution's biosafety committee, who should then monitor compliance with the policies.
-   Illumination should be adequate and should avoid reflections on cabinet windows and on other materials that would impair the vision of the operator.
-   Installations and integrated systems at this BSL should be monitored and inspected periodically.
-   Work areas should include decontamination systems and an adequate waste-disposal program (a company should be employed that specializes in this area).
-   Equipment should be located in such a manner that facilitates disinfection below and between the items.
-   Equipment and work surfaces should be resistant to the action of disinfectants.
-   Professionals are now available who specialize in the planning, construction, and maintenance of laboratories at BSL 3; they should be consulted and evaluated by the biosafety committee of each institution.

3.1 Biosafety and hospital control

Hospital patient care areas, waiting rooms, healthcare units, respiratory isolation areas, and TB patients transiting through the institution, are just some examples of areas that require PPE for workers personnel and the requisite BSL in order to minimize the risk of exposure (CDC 1996). The implementation of biosafety and biocontainment measures in the hospital should begin with the creation of a TB control committee responsible for risk assessment (CDC 2003). The committee should be responsible for the following functions:

-   Comprised of professionals who are expert in the area of biological changes of *M. tuberculosis* and its forms of resistance.

- The risk area should be identified
- Provide preventive measures and guidelines for patient isolation; identify, intervene and monitor the transmission risk areas
- Develop protocols for the management of patients, accidents in areas of risk, anti-pandemic plans, and for other situations that may arise
- supervise the compliance with protocols and guidelines

The areas that comprise the greatest risk of transmission in a hospital, and over which the TB control committee should focus its attention, are: ambulatory waiting rooms; radiology room; broncoscopy and sputum induction rooms; respiratory isolation rooms; ventilator assistance areas; emergency room; autopsy room; and microbiology or micobacteria laboratories. A detailed analysis indicates that these areas comprise almost 70% of the services provided by a general hospital; therefore, the activities of the TB control committee should be continuous and rigorous.

One of the effective measures used to diminish the transmission of MDR TB and XDR TB in the community is the placement of the patient in a respiratory isolation room; the room should have HEPA filters for the recirculation of air with a minimum replacement of six air changes per hour. The room should have negative pressure, guarantee the privacy of the patient, permit effective disinfection measures, and preferably contain an anteroom in order to minimize escape risk.

The TB control committee should delegate authority to a designated professional to decide which ambulatory or hospitalized patients should be located within the isolation area. The patient should receive clear instructions regarding behavior while in the respiratory isolation area (Garner 1996). For example, the patient should cover his/her mouth and nose when coughing in the room; upon leaving the room, the patient should cover his/her mouth and nose with a surgical mask. Healthcare personnel should avoid, to the maximum extent possible, entering the isolation area (Chen 1994). A small number of professionals should care for the patient and, when doing so, utilize a special mask such as N95, or respirators.

Remark: the TB control committee should monitor areas where patients gather, and should prepare guidelines to ensure that patients with suspected respiratory illness, pediatric patients, infectious persons, and geriatric patients are not in the same waiting room.

The TB control committee should also develop guidelines for ambulatory care areas that provide for adequate ventilation, illumination, and periodic disinfection with effective chemical agents against the pathogens most frequently encountered in this area. Air conditioners and ventilators are permitted only when used in conjunction with HEPA air filtration systems (American Institute of Architects 2001). The assistance room should include a ventilator that maintains a barrier between the physician and patient. Air flow should be directed toward the air that enters through doors and windows. See figure 2.

3.2 Biosafety in the teaching laboratory

The teaching laboratories are usually found in academic institutions to provide a venue for instructing students on how sciences are conducted and for training in specific applications. This laboratory in all discipline is unique in at least one important aspect. As a general rule and particularly at introductory levels, teaching laboratories tend to be densely populated

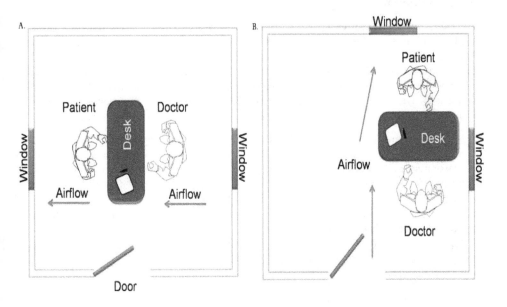

Fig. 2. Basic biosafety recommendations at the healthcare units.
On http://www.who.int/docstore/gtb/publications/healthcare/index.htm the WHO has
proposed practical and low cost interventions to reduce nosocomial transmission.

with large numbers of individuals with limited experience in hazard of a science laboratory
and certain number of then may be immunocompromised. Please answer the question ¿Are
teaching laboratories less safe than others laboratories? The correct answer is no, because in
this space de student must to learn the specific topics for risk assessment, biosafety and
biocontainment. Is a responsibility of educational institutions to teach about of biosafety
with the international and national guidelines and the use of PPE. (WHO 1992, CDC 1999,
2002, and 2005, Food and Drug Administration 2004).

3.3 Biosafety in the pharmaceutical industry

The microorganisms used in pharmaceutical companies are extremely diverse,
encompassing bacteria, viruses, fungi, helminthes and protozoa. The pharmaceutical
companies that use pathogenic microorganisms to produce or testing drugs, and vaccine
must establish a broad range of biosafety practice to ensure the safety of their workers
and their product. During the scale up, the biosafety practices employed should be in
harmony with the international guidelines to ensure that the manufacturing process and
product may be used and sold internationally. The biosafety in the pharmaceutical
encompasses both laboratory scale practices and requires a well organized and
implemented program of risk assessment, risk management, program evaluation and
modification (Advisory Committee on Dangerous Pathogens 1998). More information:
CDC 1997 and http://pharmacos.eudra.org/F2/eudralex/vol-4/pdfs-en/anx02en200408.pdf

4. Biocontainment

The biocontainment measures are very important, they arise from an adequate handling that an institution must do of their risk assessment, biological level, procedures, biosecurity measures, PPE, standards and protocols in order to prevent malicious use. The implementation and strict adherence of standard microbiological practices, it is currently considered the best measure of biocontainment for *M. tuberculosis* and other infectious substances is. The adoption of a biosafety culture together with a good laboratory practice and facilities design is a guarantee to preserve the environment and control risk.

The design of laboratories, as well as the supportive health and engineering staff faces great challenges like: to guarantee the maintenance of long-term infrastructure, to build efficiently at a reasonable cost and conscious planning of energy and water, localization of these laboratories (If the possibility is offered, this should be discussed with the regional development plans in each region). The biocontainment culture in an institution should anticipate the management of unexpected situations and for this; the institution must have contingency plans and emergency procedures.

4.1 The contingency plan must include

Operative procedures for the risk assessment, identification of high risk areas, to identify as much specific as possible to the population at risk and their characteristics, emergency transportation for the personnel exposed and prioritize this work when an incident occur, inventory of resources, suppliers commitment with availability of treatments, availability of PPE and properly trained personnel in the proper use and final disposal. Precise actions and simulations to verify the effectiveness of the evacuation plan and estimate the possibility of natural disaster like earthquakes powerful, storms and flooding, depending on the geographic region. (Lindell 1996 and, Young 2004)

Emergency procedures should include practical protocols, effective and achievable depending on the resources of the institution, these biocontainment protocols should include all possible events or accidents according with common activities like: ingestion or inhalation of potentially infectious material, broken containers and infectious spilled substances, breakage of tubes in centrifuges, puncture wounds, cuts and abrasions.

The police and fire departments should be involved in the development of emergency and contingency plans for fire or natural disasters, but they need to take a special training. Since, it is impossible to prevent all incidents of this nature, some precautions must be followed. These are some examples of what can be done to minimize the possibility of releasing pathogenic organism into the environment as the result of a natural disaster: post notices on all incubators, refrigerators, freezers and other storage facilities and contents listing persons to be notified in case of incident, secure store in culture collections, damage resistant cabinets or containers, cabinets or shelving provide for storing books, equipment, chemicals and others that close securely with doors, do not store heavy boxes and equipment above bench level.

5. Disinfection and sterilization

Understanding the importance of decontamination, cleaning, sterilization and disinfection is vital for implementing a laboratory biosafety plan. The descending order of resistance to

Disinfection					
Reagent	Concentration	Time exposure	Action	Funtion	Dificulties
Phenol	0.4 - 5%	10 minutes	Protein denaturation	Efficient disinfectants	Irritant, toxic, corrosive
Formal-dehyde	5%	10 minutes	Protein alkylation	Efficient disinfectants	Cutaneous irritant, respiratory irritant, eye irritant
Glutaral-dehyde	1 - 2%	20 - 30 minutes	Membrane disruption	Efficient disinfectants, or decontaminating surfaces	Toxic, cutaneous irritant, eye irritant
Sodium hypochlorite	0.2 - 5%, 5000 ppm, 1g/L	1 - 2 minutes	Enzymatic inhactivation	Efficient disinfectants	Toxic, corrosive, cutaneous irritant, respiratory irritant, eye irritant
Ethyl alcohol	70%, 96%	2 minutes	Protein action, membrane disruption	Surface disinfectant, mycobacterial disinfectants	Eye irritant
Hydrogen peroxide	3 - 10%	5 minutes	Free radicals, lipid and proteins action	Disinfectants	Corrosive, respiratory irritant
Iodophore	2 - 10 %, 75 ppm		Iodination and oxidation of proteins	Disinfectants	Cutaneous irritant, respiratory irritant, eye irritant, corrosive
Mix 1 : Iodine + ionophores, or ethyl alcohol	variable	variable	Iodination and oxidation of proteins	Efficient disinfectants	Cutaneous irritant, respiratory irritant, eye irritant, corrosive
Mix 2: paraformal dehyde + glutaraldeh yde or formalin solutions.	2- 5%	10 - 30 minutes	Protein alkylation, membrane disruption	Inactivation	Toxic, cutaneous irritant, respiratory irritant, eye irritant

Table 3. Summarizes the properties of some liquid germicides that are recommended again *M. tuberculosis.*

germicidal chemicals is: bacterial spores, Mycobacteria (especially *M. tuberculosis*), small viruses (Non lipid), fungi, vegetative bacteria, and medium size viruses (lipid) (Favero 1998, and 2001, and CDC 2003). Each laboratory must evaluate the efficacy of germicides. See table 3 (Kunz 1982, Best 1988, 1990, Rubin 1991, Rutala 1991, Sattar 1995, Schwebach 2001, and Blackwood 2005). Is essential that manufacturer's recommended use dilutions are followed.

Sterilization: susceptible to moist heat sterilization at 121°C for 15 minutes at 121 pounds of pressure.

6. Packing and shipping biological materials

The care and responsibility that one assumes when transporting infected material that contains live *M. tuberculosis* serve to guarantee the biosecurity of this important process. The transportation of infected material can occur within the same hospital (from the patient's room to the laboratory) or to an outside location (other institutions, cities, or countries). The transport of material infected with *M. tuberculosis* to areas within a hospital or laboratory should be made using resistant containers that can be easily disinfected; the container should have a hermetic seal capable of containing infectious substances during accidents, or until such time as the substances can be handled in a BSC. Currently, various organizations have prepared guidelines that should be used in order to reduce the risk of infection to personnel and the environment.

Current regulations governing the transport of hazardous items include obligatory actions that apply to the three parties involved in the process: the recipient (should receive import authorization and provide the appropriate documentation); the transporter or operator (should use a verification list, accept or reject the items to be transported, provide training, adequate documentation and instructions) and the shipper who should comply with packaging norms (should classify, identify and package the infected material, place markings and labels, document and have emergency plans in place).

The majority of the guidelines established for the transport of hazardous materials have been issued by the following agencies:

-   International Civil Aviation Organization (ICAO), a specialized United Nations (UN) agency with the regulations entitled "Safe Transport of Dangerous Goods by Air"
-   The IATA with regulations entitled "IATA Dangerous Goods Regulations
-   The U.S. Department of Transportation (DOT) with regulations entitled "United States Hazardous Material Uniform Safety Act."

These regulations are similar with respect to the following guidelines: classification and naming of diagnostic specimens and infectious substances; marking and labeling packaging material; training and certification of personnel; practical suggestions for classifying diagnostic specimens and infectious substances; resources for additional information and documentation; and instructions for completing a shipper's declaration for dangerous goods. This can change significantly as a result of investigations or sudden pandemics which may necessitate new measures and regulations.

IATA requirements and DOT regulations provide minimum requirements for packing and shipping diagnostic specimens and infectious substances. These provisions include:

- Classification and naming of the substances to be shipped: select the appropriate IATA packing instructions; in the case of category A material, submit the necessary information to complete the shipper's declaration. The substance or material should be classified in one of the nine IATA specified classes (1-explosivos, 2- gases, 3- flammable liquids, 4- flammable solids, 5- oxidizing substances and organic peroxides, 6- toxic and infectious substances, division 6.1: toxic substances, division 6.2 infectious substances, 7- radioactive materials, 8- corrosives and 9-miscellaneous dangerous goods) (IATA 2006).

- The classification 6.2 must be divided into one of nine IATA specific groups such as: - category A infectious substances, -category B infectious substances, –exempt human or animal specimens, -exempt substances, -patient specimens, -genetically modified organisms, -biological products, - infected animals, -medical waste.

The category A substances are specifically designated as pathogens which can be dangerous to both individual and public health. Category A pathogens and substances likely to contain category A pathogens must be assigned UN number UN2814 for infectious substances that affect humans or UN2900 for infectious substances affecting animals.

- The selection of package and packing the shipment correctly: after having classified the infectious substance, the shipper must officially name the Category A or B material; the substances must then be assigned one of the more than 3,000 IATA specified, and internationally recognized, UN numbers accompanied by the proper shipping name as provided by IATA regulations. This list provides information about 14 items, identified in alphabetical order from A to N, for each of the proper shipping names; this data is required in order to complete the shipper's declaration.

The PI describes the minimum standards for the safe transport of various biological materials. Shippers are legally obligated to comply with the regulations. Materials must be packaged properly in order to ensure the safety of all personnel who handle the package before, during, and after shipment. Clinical laboratories transporting category A infectious substances should use PI 602; for category B infectious materials, PI 650 should be used.

The PI 602 used for the packaging of infectious material should comply with the following requirements: leakproof and pressure-resistant for the first and second containers; absorbent between the first and second containers; list of contents between the second container and outer package; rigid outer packaging; positively sealed first container; name, address, and telephone number of responsible person on outer package or air waybill; shipper declaration for dangerous goods; outer packaging marking and labels; and strict manufacturing specifications. See table 4:

- The outer package should include appropriate markings and labels: labeling is the act of placing informational labels or stickers onto the surface of an outer package. The shipper is responsible for the proper marking and labeling of the outer shipping container. The labels and markings include:

Column	Information	2814	
A	United Nations number of the proper shipping name/description	2814	
B	Proper shipping name/description	Infectious Substance, Affecting Humans (Liquid)	Infectious Substance, Affecting Humans (Solid)
C	Class or division of dangerous good	6.2	6.2
D	NA		
E	Hazard label required on the outer package	Infectious substance	Infectious substance
F	NA		
G	NA		
H	NA		
I	PI to use for passenger and cargo aircraft	602	602
J	Maximum allowable amounts to be shipped in passenger and cargo aircraft	50 ml	50 g
K	PI to use for cargo aircraft only	602	602
L	Maximum allowable amounts to be shipped in cargo aircraft only	4 liters	4 kg
M	Applicable special provisions and exceptions	A81 A140	A81 A140
N	Emergency response code	11Y	11Y

Table 4. Shipping requirements for infection substances (*M. tuberculosis*).

- Name and direction of the shipper, name, address and telephone number of the responsible party, as provided by IATA regulations. The diamond-shaped infectious substances label should be used when shipping contaminated material, accompanied by a label which shows the proper shipping name, UN number, and quantity of the substances; the package orientation label must also be included and placed on opposite sides of the entire package. Additional markings may be included as required. The "cargo aircraft only" label indicates that the package may be shipped only in cargo, and not on passenger, aircraft; this label is used if the infectious substance is over 50 ml but less than 4 liters per the outer package being shipped. The "overpack" markings indicate that an overpack is used and that inner packages comply with the regulations. Packaging that meets UN specifications is marked by a "UN" inside of a circle and a series of letters and numbers which indicate the type of package, class of goods the package is designed to carry, the manufacturer, authorizing agency, and manufacturing date. The designation "Class 6.2" indicates that the container is approved for shipping infectious substances.(see figure 3)

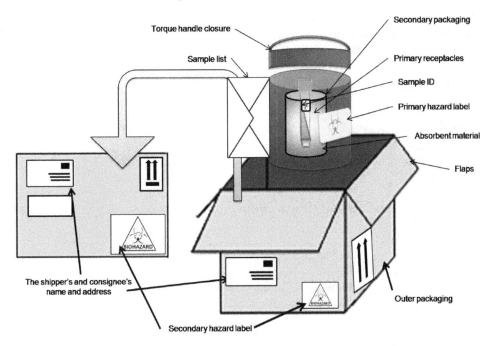

Fig. 3. Biomedical packaging for infectious substances, marking and labeling packages established by agencies governing transportation of dangerous goods.

- The relevant document: the preparation and delivery of a shipper's declaration is necessary in order to formalize a legal contract; this document is required for category A substances; however, it is not required for category B material. These documents should be completed in their entirety.
- Training for personnel: competent authorities such as the CDC offer training in the transport of infectious substances to laboratory personnel, members of biosecurity committees, and professionals in different areas.(IATA 2006, U.S. Department of Transportation 2004, and 2006, and WHO 2004, and 2005) Additional information concerning these regulations is available at http://www.iata.org or http://www.who.int/crs/resourceces/publications/biosafety/WWHO_CDS-EPR-2007_2/en/index.html

7. Conclusion

Is buying biosafety and biocontainment the best option?

The growing number of professionals infected by *M. tuberculosis*, many of whom have died due to this without knowing for certain the source of infection or exposure (whether the community or their workplace), and the dramatic figures of deaths caused by TB around the world among people infected or not with HIV confront us with a question to which we have no answer: Did the person get infected in a hospital waiting room, in an international flight? When did it happen? We don't know, and that is why it is so important to enhance community awareness on these issues.

Risk assessment and the adoption of biosecurity and biocontainment measures with the participation of academic institutions, scientists, designers and community at large represent paying the right price and obtaining the expected impact.

8. Self evaluation

Self evaluation:

1. What is *M. tuberculosis*?
    a.   Fungi
    b.   Bacteria
    c.   Virus
    d.   Other
2. Which is *M. tuberculosis* mode of transmission?
    a.   Airborne
    b.   Sexual contact
    c.   Vertical transmission.
3. How is *M. tuberculosis* spread person to person?
    a.   Inhalation of infectious aerosol or infected droplets
    b.   Water
    c.   Foods
    d.   Clothes
4. What is a N95?
    a.   Respirator
    b.   Surgical mask
    c.   HEPA filter
5. Is the infectious dose of *M. tuberculosis* less than 1000 bacilli by inhalation route in humans?
    a.   Yes
    b.   No
    c.   Is unknown
6. What are the tests for TB infection?
    a.   PPD or IGRAs
    b.   BCG
    c.   PPE

7. What is the meaning of microorganisms RG 3
   a. no or low individual and community risk
   b. high individual and community risk
   c. high individual risk, low community risk
   d. moderate individual risk, low community risk
8. What IATA category is *M. tuberculosis*?
   a. Category A
   b. Category B
   c. Category PI
9. The sterilization conditions for *M. tuberculosis* included?
   a. 121°C for 15 minutes at 121 pounds of pressure
   b. 121°C for 90 minutes at 140 pounds of pressure
   c. 15°C for 15 minutes at 121 pounds of pressure
   d. Unknown

9. References

Advisory Committee on Dangerous Pathogens. 1998. The Large Scale Contained Use of Biological Agents. Her Majesty's Stationery Office, London, England.

American Institute of Architects, Committee on Architecture for Health.2001. Guidelines for Construction and Equipment of Hospital and Medical Facilities. American Institute of Architects Press, Washington, D.C.

American National Standard Institute. 1992. American National Standard for Respirator Protection (ANSI Z88.2). American National Standards Institute, New York, N.Y.

American Thoracic Society. 1983. Levels of laboratory services for mycobacteria diseases. Am. Rev. Dis. 128:213.

Best M, Sattar S.A., Springthorpe V.S., Kennedy M.E. 1988. Comparative mycobactericidal efficacy of chemical disinfectans in suspension and carrier test. Appl Environ Microbiol. 54:2856-8.

Best M, Sattar S.A., Springthorpe V.S., Kennedy M.E. 1990. Efficacies of selected disinfectants against *Mycobacterium tuberculosis*. J Clin Microbiol 28:2234-9.

Blackwood K.s., Burdz T.V., Turenne C.Y., Sharma M.K., Kabani A.M. Wolfe J.N. 2005. Viability testing of material derived from *Mycobacterium tuberculosis* prior to removal from a containment Level-III Laboratory as part of a laboratory risk Assessment program. *BMC Infectious Diseases*, 5, (4): 1-7.

Boa, E., J. Lynch, and D.R. Liliquist. 2000. Risk Assessment Resource. American Industrial Hygiene Association, Fairfax, Va.

Burgos M.V., Mendez J.C., Ribón W. 2004. Molecular epidemiology of tuberculosis: methodology and applications. Biomédica. 24(Supl.):188-201

Castro C., González., Rozo J., Puerto G., Ribón W. 2009. Biosafety evaluation of the DNA extraction protocol for *Mycobacterium tuberculosis* complex species, as implemented at the Instituto Nacional de Salud, Colombia. Biomédica. 29:561-6

Centers for Disease Control and Prevention and National Institutes of Health. 1999. Biosafety in Microbiological and Biomedical laboratories, 4th ed. U.S. Government Printing Office, Washington, D.C. Centers for Disease Control and Prevention and

National Institutes of Health. 2006. Biosafety in Microbiology and Biomedical laboratories, 5th ed. U.S. Government Printing Office, Washington, D.C.

Centers for Disease Control and Prevention and the Healthcare Infection Control Advisory Committee. 2003. Guidelines for environmental infection control in health care facilities: recommendation of CDC and the Healthcare Infection Control Advisory Committee.

Centers for disease Control and Prevention. 1994. Guidelines for preventing the transmission of *Mycobacterium tuberculosis* in health-care facilities, 1994. Mor. Mortal. Wkly. Rep. 43(RR-13):1-132.

Centers for Disease Control and Prevention. 1996. Guideline for isolation precautions in hospitals. Am. J. Infect. Control 42:24-45.

Centers for Disease Control and Prevention. 1997. Goals Working safely with *Mycobacterium tuberculosis* in clinical, public health, and research laboratories.

Centers for Disease Control and Prevention. 2002. Guideline for hand hygiene in health-care settings. Morb. Mortal. Wkly. Rep. 51(RR-16):1-44.

Centers for Disease Control and Prevention. 2005. Possession, Use, and Transfer of Select Agents and Toxins. 42 CFR parts 72 and 73. U.S. Department of Health and Human Services. Fed. Regist. 70:13293-13325.

Centers for Diseases Control and Prevention and National Institutes of Health. 2000. Primary Containment for Biohazards: Selection, Installation and Use of Biological Safety Cabinets, 2nd ed. J. R. Richmond and R.W. McKinney (ed.) U.S. Government Printing Office, Washington, D.C.

Chen, S.-K., D. Vesley, L.M. Brosseau, and J.H. Vincent. 1994. Evaluation of single-use mask and respirators for protection of health care workers against mycobacterial aerosols. Am. J. Infect. Control. 22:65-74.

Commission of the European Communities. 2000. Directive 2000/54/EC of the European Parliament and of the Council of 18 September 2000 on the protection of workers from risks related to exposure to biological agents at work (seventhindividual directive within the meaning of Article 16 (1) of Directive 89/391/EEC). Official journal of the European Communities, L262/21-45,17.10.2000.

Cousins D.V., Bastida R., Cataldi A., Redrobe S., Dow s., Duignan P., Murray A., Dupont C., Ahmed N., Collins d. M. butler W.R., Dawson D., Rodriguez D., Loureiro J., Romano M.I., Alito A., Zumarraga M., Bernardelli A. 2003. Tuberculosis in seals caused by a novel member of the *Mycobacterium tuberculosis* complex: *Mycobacterium pinnipeddi* sp. Nov. Int Syst Evol Microbiol, 53,1305-1314.

Favero, M. 1998. Developing indicators for sterilization, p.119-132. In W.A. Rutala (ed.), Disinfection, Sterilization and Antisepsis in Health Cara. Association for Professionals in Infection Control and Epidemiology, Inc., Champlain, N.Y.

Favero, M. 2001. Sterility assurance: concepts for patient safety, p.110-119. In W.A. Rutala (ed.), Disinfection, Sterilization and antisepsis: Principles and Practices in Healthcare Facilities. Association for Professionals in Infection Control and Epidemiology, Inc., Washintong, D.C.

Favero, M., and W. Bond. 2001. Chemical disinfection of medical surgical material, p. 881-917.In S.S. Block (ed.) Disinfection, Sterilization, and Preservation, 5th ed. Lippincott, Williams and Wilkins, Philadelphia, Pa.

Food and Drug Administration. 2004. 21 CFR Part 211. Current Good Manufacturing Practices for finished pharmaceuticals. U.S. Code of Federal Regulations.

Garner, J.S., and the Hospital Infection Control Practices Advisory Committee. 1996. CDC guideline for isolation precautions in hospitals. Am. J. Infect. Control 24:24-52.

Garner, J.S., and the Hospital Infection Control Practices Advisory Committee. 1996. CDC guideline for isolation precautions in hospitals. Am. J. Infect. Control 24:24-52.

Ghosh J., Larsson P., Singh B., Pettersson B., Islam N., Sarkar S., Dasgupta S., and Kirsebom L. 2009. Sporulation in mycobacteria. PNAS 106: 10781–10.

Grange J.M. Tuberculosis. In: Topley and Wilson Principles of Bacteriology, Virology and Immunology, 9th ed. Year book, 1990. vol.3,p.94-121.

Hankenson, F. C., N.A. Johnson, B.J. Weigler, and R.F. Di Giacomo.2003.Overview: Zoonoses of occupational health importance in contemporary laboratory animal research. Comp. Med. 53:570-601.

Harrintong J.M., Shannon H.S. Incidence of tuberculosis, hepatitis, brucellosis and shigellosis in British Medical Laboratory workers. Br Med J 1976;1:759-62.

International Air Transport Association. 2006. IATA Dangerous Goods Regulations, 47th ed. International Air Transport Association, Montreal, Canada.

International Air Transport Association. 2006. Infectious Substances Shipping Guidelines, 7th ed. Ref. N°9052-07. International Air Transport Association, Montreal, Quebec, Canada.

Kent, P. T., and G. P. Kubica. 1985. Public Health Mycobacteriology. A guide for the level III Laboratory. Centers for Disease Control, Atlanta, Ga.

Krauss, H., A. Weber, M. Appel, B. Enders, H.D. Isenberg, H.G. Schiefer, W. Slenczka, A. von Graevenitz, and Zahner. 2003. Zoonoses: Infectious Diseases Transmissible from Animals to humans, 3rd ed. ASM Press, Washintong, D.C.

Kunz R., Gunderman KC. The survival of *Mycobacterium tuberculosis* on surfaces at different relative humidities. Zent Bakt Hyg 1982; 176. 105-115.

Laboratory Center for Diseases Control, Health Protection Branch, Health Canada. 1996. Laboratory Biosafety guidelines, 2nd ed. Ministry of Supply and Services, Ottawa, Ontario, Canada.

Lietman, T., and S. Blower.1999. Tuberculosis vaccines. Science 286:1300-1301.

Lindell, M. K., and R. W. Perry. 1996. Addressing gaps in environmental emergency planning hazardous materials releases during earthquakes. J. Environ. Planning Manag. 39:529-545.

Miller C.D. Songer J.R., Sullivan J.F. 1987. A twenty-five year review of laboratory acquired human infections at the National Animal Disease Center. Am Ind hyg assoc J, 48,271-275.

Muller H.E. 1988 Laboratory-acquired mycobacterial infection. Lancet, 2:331.

National Institute of Health. 2002. NIH guidelines for research involving recombinant DNA molecules (NIH guidelines). Fed. Regist. 59:34496 (July 5, 1994) as amended. (http:www4.od.nih.gov/oba/rac/guidelines/guidelines_html).

National Institutes of Health. 2002. NIH Guidelines for Research Involving Recombinant DNA Molecules (NIH Guidelines), 59 FR 34496 (July 5, 1994), as amended.

National Researgh Council. 1997. Occupational Health and Safety in the Care and Use of Research Animals. National Academy Press, Washintong, D.C.

National Researgh Council. 2003. Occupational Health and Safety in the Care and Use of Nonhuman Primates. National Academy Press, Washintong, D.C.

NSF International. 2002. Class II (Laminar Flow) Biosafety cabinetry. NSF/ANSI standard 49-2002. NSF International, Ann Arbor, Mich.

Occupational Safe and Health Administration (OSHA). 2003. Occupational exposure to tuberculosis. Notice. Fed. Regist. 68:75767-75775.

Occupational Safe and Health Administration (OSHA). 2003. Personal Protective Equipment. Publication 3151-12R. OSHA Publications Office, Washington, D.C.

Occupational Safety and Health Administration. 1996. CPL 2.106 Enforcement Procedures and Scheduling for Occupational Exposure to tuberculosis. Occupational Safety and Health Administration, Washington, D.C.

Occupational Safety and Health Administration. 1997. Occupational Exposure to tuberculosis; proposed rule. Fed. Regist. 62:54159-54309

Occupational Safety and health Administration. 30 July 2004. Standard Interpretations-Tuberculosis and Respiratory Protection. R. Davis Layne, Deputy Assistant secretary.

Pike R.M.1978. Past and present hazards of working with infectious agent. Arch. Pathol. Lab. Med. 102:333-36.

Pike, R.M. 1976. Laboratory-associated infections: summary and analysis of 3921 cases. Health Lab. Sci.13:105-114.

Pike.R.M. 1979. Laboratory-associated infections: incidence, fatalities, causes, and prevention. Annu. Rev. microbial. 33:41- 66.

Reid DD. Incidence of tuberculosis among workers in medical laboratories. Br Med J 1957;2:10-4.

Riley, R. 1961. Airborne pulmonary tuberculosis. Bacteriol. Rev. 25:243-248.

Riley, R.L. 1957. Aerial dissemination of pulmonary tuberculosis. Am. Rev. Tuberc. 76:931-941.

Rozo J., and Ribón W.2010. Molecular tools for *Mycobacterium tuberculosis* genotyping. Rev. salud pública. 12 (3): 510-521.

Rubin J. Mycobacterial disinfection and control. In: Seymour S. Block Lea and Febiger editors. Disinfection, sterilization and preservation, 4th edition, Year book, 1991.377-83.

Rutala W. A., Cole E.C., Wannamaker N.S. Weber D.J. 1991. Inactivation of *Mycobacterium tuberculosis* and *Mycobacterium bovis* by 14 hospitals disinfectans. Am J Med 91:267-271S.

Sattar S.A., Best M., Springthorpe V.S., Sanani G.1995. Mycobacterial testing of disinfectants: an update. Hosp Inf, 30 suppl. 372-382.

Schwebach J.R., Jacobs W.R. Jr, Casadevall A. 2001. Sterilization of *Mycobacterium tuberculosis* Erdman samples by antimicrobial fixation in biosafety level 3 laboratory. J Clin Microbiol, 39, 769-771.

Sessler, S.M., and R.M. Hoover. 1983. Laboratory Fume Hood Noise, Heating Piping and Air Conditioning. Penton/PC Reinhold, Cleveland, Ohio.

Standars Australia/Standars New Zealand. 2002. Safety in Laboratories. Part 3: Microbiological Aspects and Containment Facilities. Australia/New Zealand Standard AS/NZS2243.3:2002. Standards Australia International Ltd., Sydney, Australia.

Traag B., Driks A., Stragier P., Bitter W., Broussard G., Hatfull G., Chu F., Adams K., Ramakrishnan L., and Losick R.2010. Do mycobacteria produce endospores? PNAS 12:878–881

U.S. Department of transportation, Pipeline and Hazardous Materials Safety Administration. 2006. Hazardous materials: infectious substances; harmonization with the United Nations recommendations; proposed rule. Fed. Regist. 71:32244-32263.

U.S. Department of transportation, Research and Special Programs Administration. 2004. Harmonization with the United Nations recommendations. International Maritime Dangerous Goods Code, and International Civil Aviation Organizations Technical Instructions; final rule. Fed Regist. 69:76043-76187.

Verhagen, L. Van den Hof, S. Mycobacterial Factors Relevant for Transmission of Tuberculosis. Journal of Infectious Diseases Advance Access published March 4, 2011.

Warren R. Koch M., Engelke E., Myburgh R., van pittus N., Victor T., and van Helden P. 2006. Safe *Mycobacterium tuberculosis* DNA extraction method that does not compromise integrity. *Journal of Clinical Microbiology*, 44: 254-256.

Wayne L.G. Mycobacterial speciation. In Kubica G.P. Wayne LG. editors. The Mycobacteria. A sourcebook. New York: Marcel-Dekker: Year book, 1984. 26-65.

Welch, D. F., A. P. Guruswamy, S. J. Sides, C. J. Shaw, and M. J. R. Gilchrist. 1993. Timely culture for mycobacteria which utilizes a microcolony method. J. Clin. Microbiol. 31:2178-2184.

Wells, W. 1934. On air-borne infection. II. Droplets and droplet nuclei. Am. J. Hyg. 20:611-18.

Wells, W. F. 1955. Airborne contagion and Air Hygiene. Harvard University Press, Cambridge, Mass.

Wheelis, M.2002. Biological warfare at the 1346 Siegui of Caffa. Emerg. Infect. Dis. 8:971-975.

World Health Organization. 1992. Expert Committee on Specifications for Pharmaceutical Preparations, Thirty-Second Report. World Health Organization, New York, N.Y.

World Health Organization. 2004. Laboratory Biosafety Manual.3rd ed. World Health Organization, Geneva, Switzerland.

World Health Organization. 2004. Transport of infectious substances. Background to the amendments adopted in the 13th revision of the United Nations Model Regulations guiding the transport of infectious substances.

World Health Organizations. 2005. Guidance on Regulations for the Transport of Infectious Substances. World Health Organization, Geneva, Switzerland.

Young, S., L. Balluz, and J. Malilay. 2004. Natural and technologic hazardous material releases during and after natural disasters: a review: Sci. Total Environ.322:3-20.

10

Management of TB in HIV Subjects, the Experience in Thailand

Attapon Cheepsattayakorn

Thai Board of Preventive Medicine (Public Health Science)
10th Zonal Tuberculosis and Chest Disease Centre, Chiang Mai,
10th Office of Disease Prevention and Control,
Department of Disease Control,
Ministry of Public Health,
Thailand

1. Introduction

Currently, tuberculosis (TB) remains a major public health threats of humankind. It has been occurred since antiquity and is the second communicable-disease cause of death after the human immunodeficiency virus (HIV)/ acquired immunodeficiency syndrome (AIDS). Of the mycobacterial diseases, TB is by far the most important because of its most virulence. Most of the disease and nearly all of the deaths occurs in the developing countries. Co-infection with HIV/AIDS and TB represents a public health crisis worldwide. An estimated 2 billion people worldwide carry latent infection and more than 8 million persons develop active TB each year. Approximately, 3 million people per year die from TB (WHO, 2010). Various comorbidities, especially the immunocompromised statuses will accelerate the TB sickness and deaths. The prevalence of primary drug- (Jiang et al., 2011) and multidrug-resistant (MDR) (Wells, 2010) pulmonary TB among the immunocompromised populations is globally increased. In Thailand, total-estimated TB cases is more than 140,000, now ranking 18 of the 22 high-burden countries of the world (WHO, 2010). The clinical features of active TB are very highly variable, depend on the immune status of the host and the site and extent of disease. New diagnostic, therapeutic, preventive and control strategies for TB are heavily investigated throughout the world. How we can rapidly diagnose TB within few hours and how we can shorten the treatment regimens to weeks or days. World elimination of TB is expected to occur in 2050 when the incidence is 1 patient per 1 million populations per year (WHO, 2010).

2. Epidemiology

While HIV/AIDS has continued to pose greater threats to the public health system worldwide which is a major risk of double increasing within the first year after *Mycobacterium tuberculosis* exposure and 10% per year for developing TB (Barnes et al., 1991, as cited in Silva et al., 2010 & Sonnenberg et al., 2001, as cited in Nachega & Maartens, 2009). Now it is clear that non-communicable comorbidities such as diabetes mellitus, especially type 2 (Goldhaber-Fiebert et al., 2011), malignancies, chronic renal failure, immunosuppressive drug uses as well as biological modifiers such as rituximab and infliximab are undoubtedly adding to the multiple burdens the people suffer. A previous study in The Philippines demonstrated 37.4% of central nervous system TB among patients with systemic lupus erythematosus (SLE) (Vargas et al., 2009). Multiple immune system abnormalities contribute to high prevalence of TB with SLE (Prabu & Agrawal, 2010). Fatal tuberculous myositis at the left thigh was also reported in a 55-old-male patient with primary Sjögren's syndrome (Huang et al., 2010). TB patients with diabetes type 2 have lower antimicrobial peptides gene expression that contribute to enhance the TB-reactivation risk (Gonzalez-Curiel et al., 2011). A recent study conducted in India showed the ranks of risk factors for developing of TB disease as the following: diabetes (30.9%), smoking (16.9%), alcoholism (12.6%), HIV/AIDS (10.6%), malignancies (5.8%), chronic hepatic diseases (3.9%), history of TB contact (3.4%), chronic corticosteroid therapy (2.9%), chronic renal diseases and malnourishment (1.5%) (Gupta et al., 2011). No evidence was found that TB increases the risk of diabetes (Young et al., 2010). There has been a recent evidence of increased risk of lung malignancies among pulmonary TB patients and may increase further with coexisting chronic obstructive pulmonary disease (COPD) (Yu et al., 2011). A annual TB report of the fiscal year 2009 demonstrated that TB patients in northern Thailand who had COPD, HIV/AIDS, hypertension and diabetes mellitus ranked 1 to 4 of the specific causes of death (10th Zonal Tuberculosis and Chest Disease Centre, Chiang Mai, Thailand and the 10th Office of Disease Prevention and Control, Chiang Mai, Thailand, 2009 Tuberculosis annual report). A study in Brazil revealed that among the non-HIV-infected immunocompromised patients with TB, the only factor statistically related to mortality was the need for mechanical ventilation (Silva et al., 2010). In 2009, a total of 300,000 HIV-positive TB patients were enrolled on co-trimoxazole preventive therapy, and almost 140,000 were enrolled on antiretroviral therapy. In 2006 northern Thailand survey, only 69.6% and 63.1% of the HIV- infected/AIDS patients received co-trimoxazole prophylaxis therapy and antiretroviral therapy, respectively (10th Zonal Tuberculosis and Chest Disease Centre, Chiang Mai, Thailand and the 10th Office of Disease Prevention and Control, Chiang Mai, Thailand, 2006 Tuberculosis annual report). Almost 80,000 persons living with HIV were provided with isoniazid preventive therapy. This represents less than 1% of estimated number of HIV- infected persons worldwide. The 2015 targets are HIV testing of 100% of TB patients, enrolment of 100% of HIV-infected TB patients on antiretroviral therapy and co-trimoxazole preventive therapy while in 2009 revealed only 26%, 75% and 37%, respectively (WHO, 2010).

In northern Thailand, TB is the most common opportunistic infection among HIV-infected/AIDS individuals (38.9%) (Cheepsattayakorn et al., 2009). The highest prevalence of TB co-infected with HIV/AIDS in northern Thailand appeared in 1999 which was 48.8% of the total registered TB cases in the same year compared to 12.2% of the country (10th Zonal Tuberculosis and Chest Disease Centre, Chiang Mai, Thailand and the 10th Office of Disease Prevention and Control, Chiang Mai, Thailand, 2005 Tuberculosis annual report, Figure 1). In 2004 northern Thailand survey revealed that the extrapulmonary site of TB among HIV-infected/AIDS cases was accounted for 18.7% of the total TB cases, especially TB of the jugular lymph nodes (Cheepsattayakorn & Cheepsattayakorn, 2009). A recent study of extrapulmonary TB in a Caucasian population demonstrated that the proportion of extrapulmaonry TB has been increased while the overall incidence of TB has been reduced (Garcia-Rodriguez et al., 2011). This could be explained by an increase of life expectancy. There is no statistically significant difference between the development of pulmonary and extrapulmonary TB among diabetic persons (Young et al,. 2010). A recent study in the United States and Mexico revealed high diabetes prevalence among newly-diagnosed TB cases which was 39% in Texas and 36% in Mexico, respectively (Restrepo et al., 2011). A recent study on TB among end-stage renal disease (ESRD) patients in Taiwan showed that the independent risk factors for TB infection in ESRD are male gender, old age, chronic obstructive pulmonary disease (COPD), and silicosis (Li et al., 2011). A survey between 2001-2007 in northern Thailand showed the highest incidence of TB among the populations with more than 64 years of age (10th Zonal Tuberculosis and Chest Disease Centre, Chiang Mai, Thailand and the 10th Office of Disease Prevention and Control, Chiang Mai, Thailand, 2007 Tuberculosis annual report, Figure 2).

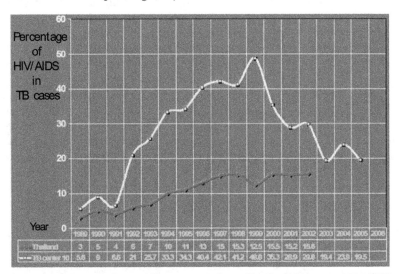

Fig. 1. TB/HIV/AIDS sentinel surveillance in northern Thailand between 1989-2005.

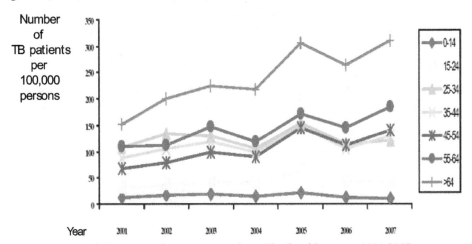

Fig. 2. Incidence of TB patients by ages in northern Thailand between 2001-2007.

3.Tuberculosis investigations in immunocompromised patients

3.1 Acid-Fast Bacilli (AFB) smear and culture

The finding of AFB on stained specimens is the only reliable and affordable rapid diagnostic method of TB which has lower yield (40%-70%) compared to the mycobacterial culture (75-90%) (Nachega & Maartens, 2009).

3.2 Interferon-gamma release assays

Since 2001, development of interferon-gamma release assays (IGRAs) for the detection of TB infection has been initiated in addition to the tuberculin skin test (TST). It detects sensitization to *Mycobacterium tuberculosis* by measuring interferon-gamma release in response to *Mycobacterium tuberculosis* complex antigens (Converse et al., 1997, Rothel et al., 1990 & Streeton et al., 1998, as cited in Mazulek et al., 2010 & Walsh et al., 2011). QuantiFERON-TB test (QFT) (Cellestis Limited, Carnegie, Victoria, Australia) was the first assay approved by the Food and Drug Administration (FDA) in 2001 (FDA, 2010 & Mazurek & Villarino, 2003, as cited in Mazulek et al., 2010). The QuantiFERON-TB Gold test (GFT-G) (Cellestis Limited, Carnegie, Victoria, Australia) was the second IGRA approved by FDA in 2005 (FDA, 2010 & Mazulek et al., 2005, as cited in Mazulek et al., 2010). The United States Centers for Disease Control and Prevention (CDC) published guidelines for using QFT and QFT-G in 2003 and 2005, respectively (Mazurek & Villarino, 2003, Mazulek et al., 2005, as cited in Mazulek et al., 2010). The CDC recommended that a positive interferon-gamma release test should be confirmed with a TST (Mazurek & Villarino, 2003, as cited in Hopewell, 2005). A recent study compared the sensitivity of QFT- G to enzyme-linked immunospot (ELISPOT) among pulmonary TB including HIV - negative immunocompromised patients and demonstrated the superiority of ELISPOT over QFT-G at the low lymphocyte count conditions, not depending on gender, age, and nutritional status (Komiya et al., 2010).

Many studies have been shown that these new assays are useful for diagnosis of active TB in both immunocompromised patients and immunocompetent ones such as HIV/AIDS, diabetes mellitus, systemic immunosuppressant administration, malignant diseases and chronic renal failure (Ito et al., 2011, Nachega & Maartens, 2009, Tan et al., 2010 & Walsh et al., 2011). The sensitivity of the interferon-gamma release assays are not compromised by serum glucose levels in TB patients with diabetes (Walsh et al., 2011) including other immunocompromised TB patients (Ito et al., 2011). A study demonstrated that, unlike the tuberculin skin test, the sensitivity of these assays are less interfered by moderately advanced HIV status (Rangaka et al., 2007, as cited in Nachega & Maartens, 2009). The QFT-G assay has higher detection rate of the latent TB infection than the TST. It may has lower sensitivity among the immunocompromised persons but requires shorter turnaround time than the TST (Baboolal et al., 2010). A previous study of QuantiFERON-TB Gold In-Tube (QFT-GIT) showed 33.4% of indeterminate results among HIV-infected/AIDS patients with CD4-T cell count below 200 cells/μL and the TST has higher degree of agreement than QFT-GIT in patients with immune-mediated inflammatory diseases. This study results indicated that the performance of QFT-GIT varied between different types of immunocompromised patients (Sauzullo et al., 2010). The CDC do not recommend the blood interferon-gamma release assay for pregnant women, individuals with HIV/AIDS, individuals with increased risk of TB, screening children younger than 17 years old, contacts with an infectious case of TB, or individuals being evaluated for suspected TB (Mazurek & Villarino, 2003, as cited in Hopewell, 2005).

3.3 Imaging

Several chest roengenographic pictures plays a critical role in the diagnosis of TB in HIV-infected/AIDS patients, however, the degree of immunosuppression is a core determinant of the roentgenographic appearance. Most notably the presence of bilateral hilar lymphadenopathy is highly suggestive of TB, but is not diagnostic (Nachega & Maartens, 2009, Figure 3). When a CD4+ T-cell count is higher than 200 cells/μL, the pulmonary infiltrates are characteristic adult picture with cavitation and upper lobe predominance. But when a CD4+ T-cell count is below 200 cells/μL, the pulmonary infiltrates shift toward atypical patterns for adults: hilar or mediastinal adenopathy, and mid- ,lower-zone or military infiltrates (Nachega & Maartens, 2009, Figure 4). Pleural effusion can occur with any CD4+ T-cell count (Havlir & Barnes, 1999, as cited in Nachega & Maartens, 2009, Post et al., 1995, Long et al., 1991, as cited in Nachega & Maartens, 2009, Perlman et al., 1997, Wendel & Sterling, 2002, as cited in Nachega & Maartens, 2009, Figure 5). There is no statistically significant pulmonary shadowing among old patients with TB (Toure' et al., 2010).

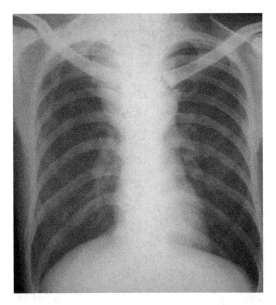

Fig. 3. Chest roentgenogram from the initial presentation of a 34-year-old Thai male with HIV-infection/AIDS who attended the tenth Zonal Tuberculosis and Chest Disease Centre, Chiang Mai, Thailand showing bilateral hilar adenopathy. The sputum smears for AFB and cultures revealed positive results. Diagnosis of pulmonary TB was made.

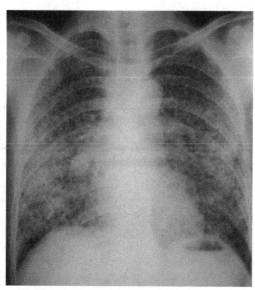

Fig. 4. Chest roentgenogram from initial presentation of a 44-year-old Thai female with chronic smoking who attended the tenth Zonal Tuberculosis and Chest Disease Centre, Chiang Mai, Thailand showing military infiltrates. Her three consecutive sputum smears for AFB and cultures revealed negative results. After completeness of anti-TB chemotherapy her chest roentgenogram completely resoluted.

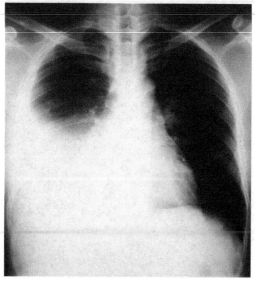

Fig. 5. Chest roentgenogram from initial presentation of another 34-year-old Thai male with HIV-infection/AIDS who attended the tenth Zonal Tuberculosis and Chest Disease Centre, Chiang Mai, Thailand showing a right massive pleural effusion. His pleural biopsy revealed tuberculous pleurisy.

A recent study of TB patients with diabetes conducted in India revealed that lower lung field involvement was predominant (84%) as compared to upper lung field. Cavitation was predominantly confined to the lower lung field (80%) while nodular lesions were found in 36% and exudative lesions were found in 22% (Patel et al.,2011). A previous report in 2000 also demonstrated a higher lower-lung field involvement (Perez-Guzman et al., 2000, as cited in Patel et al.,2011). Some investigators have demonstrated no major differences of the roentgenographic pictures (Bacakoglu et al., 2001, as cited in Patel et al.,2011) while other previous studies have reported more common multiple cavities among diabetic patients (Sen et al., 2009, as cited in Patel et al.,2011). There are not clear reasons for atypical images in TB patients with diabetes.

Alveolar infiltration which indicates tuberculous pneumonia mostly occurs in the upper lung fields is frequently found in HIV-infected/AIDS (20%) and diabetes (15%) patients (Moreira et al., 2011).

Other imaging techniques may be helpful depending on localization of the clinical manifestations. Magnetic resonance imaging (MRI) or computed tomography (CT) scans are specifically detection of TB of the central nervous system (Figure 6 A & B) while ultrasonography can detect intraperitoneal TB such as splenic microabscesses, mesenteric lymphadenopathy and hepatic tuberculous granulomas. CT of the chest is superior to chest roentgenogram to demonstrate latent TB infiltrate in patient with hepatic transplantation (Lyu et al., 2011).

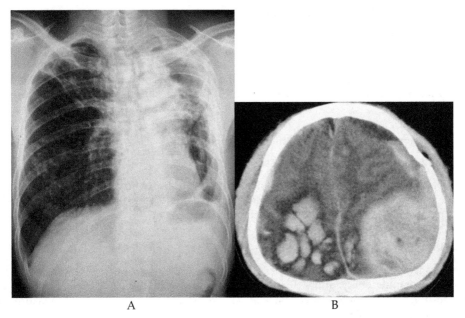

A   B

Fig. 6. A: Chest roentgenogram from initial presentation of a 46-year-old Thai male with HIV-infection/AIDS who attended the tenth Zonal Tuberculosis and Chest Disease Centre, Chiang Mai, Thailand showing bilaterally diffuse reticulo-nodular infiltrates with left pleural effusion. His three consecutive sputum smears for AFB and cultures revealed positive results. B: Computed tomography of the brain from initial presentation of the same patient in Figure 6 A showing multiple tuberculous granulomas with various sizes throughout both parietal lobes.

3.4 Tuberculin skin test

The tuberculin skin test is now the standard technique to detect the latent TB infection. The sensitivity and specificity of the TST in immunocompromised persons with TB infection are very low. A study on latent TB infection during renal replacement therapy in India demonstrated that TST was insensitive and nonspecific to detect latent TB infection (Bhowmik et al., 2010). The TST in HIV-infected/AIDS patients is more likely to be negative due to the declines of the CD4+ T-cell count (Markowitz et al., 1993, as cited in Nachega & Maartens, 2009). More than 5 mm. induration on the Mantoux test in HIV-infected/AIDS patients is a positive result but this has been challenged by a previous study with sensitivity of 64.3% at a cutoff value of 10 mm. and of 71.2% at a cutoff value of 5 mm. and after adjustment for tuberculosis-specific anergy, the sensitivity was 67.6% and 74.5%, respectively (Cobelens et al., 2006, as cited in Nachega & Maartens, 2009). The sensitivity and specificity of TST for diagnosis of latent TB infection in patients on renal replacement therapy were only 20% and 9%, respectively, showed in a previous study (Agarwal et al., 2010). The only benefit and effectiveness of the positive-result TST is TB preventive therapy (Woldehanna & Volmink, 2004, as cited in Nachega & Maartens, 2009).

3.5 Tissue aspiration, excision and biopsy

Aspiration of lymph node with macroscopic tuberculous caseation demonstrates positive results 40.8% of cases (Bem et al., 1993, as cited in Nachega & Maartens, 2009, Pithie & Chicksen, 1992, as cited in Nachega & Maartens, 2009). Patients with negative-result aspiration should be performed needle-core biopsy or excisional biopsy. First needle-core biopsy made a definite diagnosis in 85% of cases (Wilson et al., 2005, as cited in Nachega & Maartens, 2009).

3.6 Mycobacterial molecular identification modalities

3.6.1 Amplicor Polymerase Chain Reaction (PCR)

A previous study in Kenya showed that the sensitivity and specificity of this technique were 93% and 94%, respectively and did not affected by the HIV status (Kivihya-Ndugga et al., 2004, as cited in Cheepsattayakorn & Cheepsattayakorn, 2006).

3.6.2 IS6110-PCR

The sensitivity of this technique was 100% in smear-positive, 81.8% in smear- negative, 66.7% in extrapulmonary, and 42.9% in blood specimens of HIV-infected/AIDS patients as demonstrated in a study (Schijman et al., 2004, as cited in Cheepsattayakorn & Cheepsattayakorn, 2006).

3.6.3 Nested PCR

This technique was studied in urine specimens of the HIV-infected/AIDS participants and revealed the sensitivity of 40.5% in smear-positive, 66.7% in smear-negative, and 57.1% in extrapulmonary cases. The overall specificity was 98.2%. This study results were different in the non-HIV-infected/AIDS and HIV-infected/AIDS patients (Torrea et al., 2005, as cited in Cheepsattayakorn & Cheepsattayakorn, 2006).

3.6.4 GeneXpert MTB/RIF test

This test is based on nucleic acid amplification and detection of an *Mycobacterium tuberculosis*-specific region of the *rpoB* gene, use real-time PCR with molecular beacons. It also detects mutation associated with rifampicin resistance. It is fully automated system which integrates sputum processing, deoxy-ribonucleic acid extraction, and amplification to diagnose TB. Its results are available within 90 minutes. It is minimized biosafety and contamination because of its closed system (Lockman, 2011). A clinical study conducted in Azerbaijan, India, Peru and South Africa showed the sensitivity of this test for only one sputum specimen examination was 92.2% for all positive-culture, 98.2% for positive AFB smear and positive culture, and 72.5% for negative AFB smear and positive culture cases with a specificity of 99.2%. When 3 specimens were tested the sensitivity was 97.6%, 99.8%, and 90.2% with a specificity of 98.1%, respectively (Boehme et al., 2010, as cited in Lockman, 2011). This test would increase case finding by 30% (replacing or adding to the conventional sputum AFB smear) and MDR case finding by 3-fold (replacing sputum culture and conventional drug-susceptibility testing) (Boehme et al., 2011, as cited in Lockman, 2011). The WHO stated in 2010 that this test should be used as the initial diagnostic test in persons suspected of being HIV/AIDS-associated TB or MDR-TB and it may be used as a follow-on test in smear-negative specimens where HIV/AIDS and/or MDR are of lesser concern (WHO, 2010, as cited in Lockman, 2011). Thailand will soon start using 4 GeneXpert MTB/RIF units in collaboration with the United States CDC.

4. Diagnosis of pulmonary tuberculosis (Sociedade Brasileira de Pneumologia e Tisiologia, 2004 & WHO, 2010)

The diagnosis of pulmonary TB is based on meeting one or more the following criteria: 3.1 detection by two positive sputum smear examinations 3.2 detection by one positive sputum smear examination and positive sputum culture 3.3 detection by one positive sputum smear examination and roentgenographic pictures consistent TB positive sputum culture or 3.4 clinical manifestations, epidemiological findings and roentgenographic pictures consistent TB, together with a favorable response to anti-TB drugs.

5. Antituberculous chemotherapy

There have been substantial studies from both prospective and retrospective demonstrated that standard 6-month rifampicin and isoniazid-contained regimens supplemented by pyrazinamide and ethambutol are effective for cure in treating HIV-seropositive patients with TB (Hopewell & Chaisson, 2000). The WHO recommends standard regimen (2HRZE/4HR, H=isoniazid, R=rifampicin, Z=pyrazinamide, E=ethambutol) for new TB patients with seropositive-HIV and all TB patients living in HIV-prevalent settings should receive daily antituberculous therapy at least during the intensive phase (Khan et al., 2010, as cited in WHO, 2010). Co-trimoxazole preventive therapy should be started as soon as possible and prescribed throughout antituberculous therapy (International Standards for

Tuberculosis Care (ISTC), 2009, as cited in WHO, 2010) which substantially reduces mortality among these patients (Harries et al., 2009, as cited in WHO, 2010 & WHO, 2006). The standard 6-month regimen is currently recommended for treating TB of any site, excepts of the central nervous system, which is recommended 2HRZE/7HR or 2HRZE/10HR (Nachega & Maartens, 2009). Recurrent rates of pulmonary TB among patients with and without HIV/AIDS have varied among various studies, mostly of 5% or less (Kassim et al., 1995, as cited in Nachega & Maartens, 2009, Chaisson et al., 1996, as cited in Nachega & Maartens, 2009, el-Sadr et al.,1998, as cited in Nachega & Maartens, 2009, Connolly et al.,1999, as cited in Nachega & Maartens, 2009 & Sterling et al., 1999, as cited in Nachega & Maartens, 2009). The recurrent rates of TB among HIV-infected/AIDS patients were associated with the duration of rifampicin-based regimens which rifampicin durations of 2-3, 5-6, and more than 7 months were associated with rates of 4, 2, and 1.4 cases per 100 person-years, respectively (Korenromp et al., 2003, as cited in Nachega & Maartens, 2009). WHO and the International Union Against Tuberculosis and Lung Disease (IUATLD) recommends a standardized 6-month rifampicin-based regimen with directly observed treatment for highly TB/HIV-endemic, low- income countries for at least the first 2 months for all positive-sputum smear cases (Korenromp et al., 2003, as cited in Nachega & Maartens, 2009). The IUATLD recommends an 8-month regimen (2HRZE/6HE) for negative-smear HIV-infected/AIDS cases but this regimen is related to high relapse rates (Korenromp et al., 2003, as cited in Nachega & Maartens, 2009). A study in Zaire among HIV-infected/AIDS-related TB patients demonstrated that additional 3 months in the continuation phase (2HRZE/7HR) of the standardized 6- month short-course regimen (2HRZE/4HR) resulted in 1% versus 8% of relapse rates, respectively but the survival rates were no different in patients given extended regimen (Perriens et al., 1995, as cited in Hopewell & Chaisson, 2000). Other studies revealed relapse rates of TB with various treatment regimens among HIV-infected/AIDS patients between 2%-7% (Kassim et al., 1995, as cited in Hopewell & Chaisson, 2000, Chaisson et al., 1996, as cited in Hopewell & Chaisson, 2000, el-Sadr et al., 1998, as cited in Hopewell & Chaisson, 2000). The United States CDC , the American Thoracic Society (ATS) and the Infectious Disease Society of America (IDSA) recommend the extension of the continuation phase from 6 to 9 months of the standardized 6-month rifampicin-based regimen for patients with positive cultures and cavitary TB, regardless of the HIV status (Chaisson & Nachega, 2010). Acquired- rifampicin resistance has been occurred among HIV-infected with advanced immune suppression treated with twice weekly rifampicin-based or rifabutin-based regimens (Chaisson & Nachega, 2010). The continuation phase of isoniazid plus rifapentine once weekly is contraindicated in HIV-infected/AIDS patients because of acquired resistance to rifamycins and unacceptably high rate of relapse (Chaisson & Nachega, 2010). Patients with CD4-T cell count < 100 cells/μL should receive daily or three-times weekly regimens (Chaisson & Nachega, 2010). WHO recommends the same regimens for extrapulmonary and pulmonary TB excepts longer treatment for TB of bone or joint and TB of meninges (WHO, 2010). Progress against TB is being made on several fronts. Several new drugs are being studied for TB therapy, including nitroimidazopyrans (e.g., PA-824), quinolone (moxifloxacin & gatifloxacin), oxazolidinones (e.g., PNU-100480, linezolid), macrolides (e.g., clarithromycin, azithromycin), ring-substituted imidazoles, and diamines (e.g., SQ109). Finally, new TB vaccines is being directed toward developing and should be ready for human testing within a few years.

6. Empirical antituberculous therapy

Empirical therapy will often initiated pending culture results in areas where mycobacterial culture is available, especially in areas of high proportion of sputum smear-negative cases and relatively rapid disease progression of HIV-related TB. Three consecutive-negative smear results, a compatible chest roentgenogram, and no response to a 2-week trial of antibiotics for pneumonitis is the common case definition for negative-smear pulmonary TB used in resource-poor settings (WHO, 2010, Figure 7). This case definition has been modified by WHO to include consideration of acutely-ill patients (especially with Pneumocystis pneumonia). If there has been a clinical response with negative-culture results, the empirical therapy should be continued. A previous study of case definitions in South Africa demonstrated high positive predictive value for a modified case definition of negative-smear pulmonary TB and case definitions of extrapulmonary TB and found that improvement of symptoms, Karnosky performance score, and serum C-reactive protein level were very sensitive to evaluation of the empirical therapy, excepted improvement of body weight and hemoglobin level (Wilson et al., 2006, as cited in Nachega & Maartens, 2009). The specificity of case definitions cannot be 100% so patients who have no response to empirical therapy within 2-8 weeks need to be investigated for alternative diagnoses discontinuation of their empirical therapy (Nachega & Maartens, 2009). In developing countries, the national TB control programs and the international agencies discourage the clinical trials of antituberculous therapy.

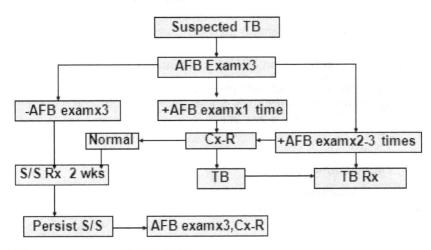

Fig. 7. TB case management (WHO, 2010)

7. Antiretroviral therapy

TB patients with advanced HIV disease/AIDS indicates antiretroviral therapy (ART) which improves survival (Harries et al., 2009, as cited in WHO, 2010), reduces TB disease rates by 60% at a population level, by up to 90% at personal level and reduces TB recurrence rates by 50% (Lawn & Churchyard, 2009, as cited in WHO, 2010 & Golub et al., 2008, as cited in WHO, 2010). Patients co-administered ART and antituberculous therapy may increase risk of adverse drug reactions, especially hepatitis (McIlleron et al., 2007, as cited in Nachega & Maartens, 2009). Around 25%-40% of these patients develop the so-called immune reconstitute inflammatory syndrome (IRIS) which paradoxically deteriorate TB disease (Lawn et al., 2005, as cited in Nachega & Maartens, 2009). Factors related to an increased risk of TB-IRIS include rapidly decreasing viral loads, lower CD4+ T-cell count and more shorter intervals between starting of antituberculous therapy and ART (Lawn et al., 2005, as cited in Nachega & Maartens, 2009). These worsening clinical manifestations should be excluded notably poor compliance to antituberculous therapy, systemic drug hypersensitivity reactions, MDR-TB, and new opportunistic infections. The most common manifestation of TB-IRIS is enlarging lymphadenopathy with caseous necrosis. The optimal timing of starting ART in relation to starting antituberculous therapy is unclear but TB treatment should always be initiated first, and waits at least until the patient is tolerating the antituberculous therapy before initiating ART as soon as possible and within the first 8 weeks of initiating antituberculous therapy (Nachega & Maartens, 2009 & WHO, 2010). All active-TB patients living with HIV should be initiated ART irrespective of CD4+ T-cell count (WHO, 2009, as cited in WHO, 2010). In 2010 Thailand's guidelines, starting ART when CD4 T-cell count is below 350 cells/µL. Patients who are already receiving an ART regimen, ART should be continued (Nachega & Maartens, 2009). WHO recommends the first-line ART regimens contain two nucleoside reverse transcriptase inhibitors (NRTIs-zidovudine (AZT) or tenofovir disproxil fumarate (TDF) plus lamivudine (3TC) or emtricitabine (FTC)) plus one non-nucleoside reverse transcriptase inhibitors (NNRTI-efavirenz (EFV) or nevirapine (NVP)) (WHO, 2010). In Thailand, the available regimens are stavudine plus lamivudine plus efavifenz or stavudine plus lamivudine plus nevirapine or stavudine plus lamivudine plus indinavir or ritonavir (Cheepsattayakorn & Cheepsattayakorn, 2009).

8. Adjunctive glucocorticoids in TB patients with HIV-infection/AIDS

There is lacking of evidence base for adjunctive glucocorticoids among these patients. There is likely to be a mortality benefit when used in HIV-infected/AIDS patients with tuberculous meningitis and pericarditis, but more larger studies are needed (Nachega & Maartens, 2009).

9. Adjuvant immunotherapy

A previous study demonstrated that immunization with killed *Mycobacterium vaccae* had ability to modify immune response to TB, but failed to showed clinical benefit in HIV-infected/AIDS patients (Mwinga et al., 2002, as cited in Nachega & Maartens, 2009).

10. Monitoring during antituberculous therapy

Sputum-smear examinations at the completion of the intensive phase of treatment course is a conditional, rather than a strong WHO recommendation (WHO, 2010). The evidence of a positive smear at this stage has a very poor ability to predict relapse or pretreatment isoniazid resistance (WHO, 2010). A positive-sputum smear at the end of the intensive phase among new patients should trigger sputum-smear examinations at the end of the third month and if it is positive, sputum culture and antituberculous-drug susceptibility testing should be done (WHO, 2010). There is no longer recommends to extend the intensive phase for patients have a positive-sputum smear at the end of the second month of treatment course (WHO, 2010).

11. Antituberculous therapy in non-HIV-infected immunocompromised patients

Regimens used in these patients are the same as used in HIV-infected/AIDS patients except regimens used in military TB, TB of bone or joint, and meninges which are more longer than 6 months, usually at least 8 months (WHO, 2010).

12. Treatment of latent TB infection

The IUATLD conducted a study in Eastern Europe and revealed that 3 months of isoniazid therapy reduced the TB incidence by 20%, 66% for 6 months, and 75% for 12 months (Chaisson & Nachega, 2010). This study also resulted in 92% reduction in TB risk for patients completing 12 months of isoniazid compared to 69% decrease for patients completing the standard-6 month regimen. A recent study in Alaskan populations revealed that the optimal duration of isoniazid therapy was 9 months therefore, the new ATS/CDC recommendation is 9 months of isoniazid as the preferred regimen, and the alternative regimen is 6 months (Chaisson & Nachega, 2010). A previous study in northern Thailand showed that 78% of HIV-infected/AIDS patients did not have TB disease at the end of 24 months after completion of 9 months of isoniazid therapy (Cheepsattayakorn, 1998, as cited in Cheepsattayakorn & Cheepsattayakorn, 2009).

13. Bacille Calmette-Gue'rin (BCG) vaccination

The protective benefit of BCG for active TB disease and death is about 50% (Chaisson & Nachega, 2010). It decrease hematogenous dissemination of primary TB infection and so reduces the incidence of military TB and childhood tuberculous meningitis (Chaisson & Nachega, 2010). BCG should not be given to immunocompromised individuals, including those with HIV-infection/AIDS, or to pregnant women (Hopewell, 2005).

14. Further research areas

It demonstrates that the WHO's DOTS strategy for case finding and effectively treating cases is not sufficient to eliminate TB, particularly in countries with HIV epidemics. Neither combination ART nor treatment of latent TB infection has a significant impact on community TB incidence. The most effective measures are reduced HIV incidence and improved TB case finding and treatment success rates. A better understanding of natural immunity to TB and its pathogenesis may contribute to the development of a new more effective vaccine. The genome sequencing of *Mycobacterium tuberculosis* promises to produce a new generation of TB control research.

15. References

Agarwal SK, Gupta S, Bhow D & Mahajan S. (2010). Tuberculin skin test for the diagnosis of latent tuberculosis during renal replacement therapy in an endemic area: a single center study. *Indian J Nephrol,* Vol. 20, No. 3, (July 2010), pp. 132-136, ISSN: 0971-4065.

Baboolal S, Ramoutar D & Akpaka PE. (2010). Comparison of the QuantiFERON®-TB assay and tuberculin skin test to detect latent tuberculosis infection among target groups in Trinidad & Tabago. *Rev Panam Salud Publica,* Vol. 28, No. 1, (July 2010), ISSN: 1020-4989, doi: 10.1590/S1020- 4982010000700006

Bacakoglu F, Basoglu OK, Cok G, Sayiner A & Ates M. (2001). Pulmonary tuberculosis in patients with diabetes mellitus. *Respiration,* Vol. 68, No. 6 , (November-December 2001), pp. 595-600, ISSN: 0993-9490.

Barnes PF, Bloch AB, Davidson PT & Snider DE Jr. (1991). Tuberculosis in patients with human immunodeficiency virus infection. *N Eng J Med,* Vol. 324, No. 23, (June 1991), pp. 1644- 1650, ISSN: 0028-4793.

Bem C, Patil PS, Elliot AM, Namaambo KM, Bharucha H & Porter JD. (2010). The value of wide-needle aspiration in diagnosis of tuberculous lymphadenitis in Africa. *AIDS,* Vol. 7, No. 9, (September 2010), pp. 1221-1225, ISSN: 0269-9370.

Bhowmik D, Agarwal SK, Gupta S & Mahajan S. (2010). Tuberculin skin test for diagnosis of latent tuberculosis during renal replacement therapy in an endemic area: a single center study. *Indian J Nephrol,* Vol. 20, No. 3, (October 2010), pp. 132-136, ISSN: 0971-4065.

Boehme CC, Nabeta P, Hillemann D, Nicol MP, Shenai S, Krapp F, Allen J, Tahirli R, Blakemore R, Rustomjee R, Milovic A, Jones M, O'Brien SM, Persing DH, Ruesch-Gerdes S, Gotuzzo E, Rodrigues C, Alland D & Perkins MD. (2010). Rapid molecular detection of tuberculosis and rifampicin resistance. *N Eng J Med,* Vol. 363, No. 11, (September 2010), pp. 1005-1015, ISSN: 0028- 4793.

Boehme CC, Nicol MP, Nabeta P, Michael JS, Gotuzzo E, Tahirli R, Gler MT, Blakemore R, Worodria W, Gray C, Huang L, Caceres T, Mehdiyey R, Raymond L, Whitelaw A, Sagadevan K, Alexander H, Albert H, Cobelens F, Cox H, Alland D & Perkins MD. (2011). Feasibility, diagnostic accuracy, and effectiveness of decentralized use of the xpert MTB/RIF test for diagnosis of tuberculosis and multidrug resistance: a multicentric implementation study. *Lancet,* Vol. 377, No. 9776, (April 2011), pp. 1495-1505, ISSN: 0099-5355.

Chaisson RE, Clermont HC, Holt E, Holt EA, Cantave M, Johnson MP, Atkinson J, David H, Boulos R, Quinn TC & Halsey NA. (1996). Six-month supervised intermittent tuberculosis therapy in Haitian patients with and without HIV infection. *Am J Respir Crit Care Med,* Vol. 154, No. 4 Pt 1 (October 1996), pp. 1034-1038, ISSN: 1073-449X.

Chaisson RE & Nachega JB. (2010). Tuberculosis. In: *Oxford textbook of Medicine.* Warrell DA, Cox TM, Firth JD & Ogg GS., pp. (810-831), Oxford University Press, 978-0-1992-0485-4, Oxford.

Cheepsattayakorn A. (1998). Isoniazid prophylactic therapy in HIV-infected individuals. *Thai Journal of Tuberculosis and Chest Diseases,* Vol. 19, No. 3, (July-September 1998), pp. 149-157, ISSN: 0125-5029.

Cheepsattayakorn A & Cheepsattayakorn R. (2006). Rapid diagnosis of pulmonary tuberculosis by polymerase chain reaction and other advanced molecular diagnostic technologies in comparison to conventional bacteriological methods. *Thai Journal of Tuberculosis Chest Diseases and Critical Care,* Vol. 27, No. 3, (July-September 2006), pp. 191- 216, ISSN: 0125-5029.

Cheepsattayakorn A & Cheepsattayakorn R. (2009). The outcome of tuberculosis control in special high-risk populations in northern Thailand: an observational study. *Journal of Health Systems Research,* Vol. 3, No. 4, (October-December 2009), pp. 558-566, ISSN: 0858-9437.

Cobelens FG, Egwaga SM, van Ginkel T, Muwinge H, Matee MI & Borgdorff MW. (2006). Tuberculin skin testing in patients with HIV infection: limited benefit of reduced cutoff values. *Clin Infect Dis,* Vol. 43, No. 5, (September 2006), pp. 634-639, ISSN: 1058-4838.

Connolly C, Reid A, Davies G, Sturm W, McAdam KP & Wilkinson D. (1999). Relapse and mortality among HIV-infected and uninfected patients with tuberculosis successfully treated with twice weekly directly observed therapy in rural South Africa. *AIDS,* Vol. 13, No. 12, (August 1999), pp. 1543-1547, ISSN: 0269-9370.

Converse PJ, Jones SL, Astemborski J, Vlahov D & Graham NM. (1997). Comparison of a Tuberculin-interferon-gamma assay with the tuberculin skin test in high-risk adults: effect of human immunodeficiency virus infection. *J Infect Dis,* Vol. 176, No. 1, (July 1997), pp. 144- 150, ISSN: 0022-1899.

el-Sadr WM, Perlman DC, Matts JP, Nelson ET, Cohn DL, Salomon N, Olibrice M, Medard F, Chirgwin KD, Mildvan D, Jones BE, Telzak EE, Klein O, Heifets L & Hafner R. (1998). Evaluation of an intensive intermittent-induction regimen and duration of short-course treatment for human immunodeficiency virus-related pulmonary tuberculosis. Terry Beirn Community Programs for Clinical Research on AIDS (CPCRA) and AIDS Clinical Trials Group (ACTG). *Clin Infect Dis,* Vol. 26, No. 5, (May 1998), pp. 1148-1158, ISSN: 1058-4838.

Food and Drug Administration. (2010). QuantiFERON-TB-P010033. June 16, 2010, Available from:
http://www.fda.gov/MedicalDevices/ProductandMedicalProcedures/DeviceAp provals- ApprovedDevices/ucmo84025.htm

Food and Drug Administration. (2010). QuantiFERON-TB Gold-P010033/S006. June 16, 2010, Available from:
http://www.fda.gov/MedicalDevices/ProductandMedicalProcedures/DeviceAp provals- ApprovedDevices/ucmo84025.htm

Garcia-Rodriguez JF, Alvarez-Diaz H, Lorenzo-Garcia MV, Marino-Callejo A, Ferna'ndez-Rial A & Sesma-Sa'nchez P. (2011). Extrapulmonary tuberculosis: epidemiology and risk factors. *Enferm Infecc Microbiol Clin,* (May 2011), ISSN: 0213-005X, [Epub ahead of print].

Goldhaber-Fiebert JD, Jeon CY, Cohen T & Murray MB. (2011). Diabetes mellitus and tuberculosis in countries with high tuberculosis burdens: individual risk and social determinants. *Int J Epidemiol,* Vol. 40, No. 2, (April 2011), pp. 417-428, ISSN: 0300-5771.

Golub JE, Astemborski J, Ahmed M, Cronin W, Mehta SH, Kirk GD, Vlahov D & Chaisson RE. (2008). Long-term effectiveness of diagnosing and treating latent tuberculosis infection in a cohort of HIV-infected and at risk injection drug users. *J Acquir Immune Defic Syndr,* Vol. 49, No. 5, (December 2008), pp. 532-537, ISSN: 1525-4135.

Gonzalez-Curiel I, Castaneda-Delgado J, Lopez-Lopez N, Araujo Z, Hernandez-Pando R, Gandara- Jasso B, Macias-Segura N, Enciso-Moreno A & Rivas-Santiago B. (2011). Differential expression of antimicrobial peptides in active and latent tuberculosis and its relationship with diabetes mellitus. *Hum Immunol,* Vol. 72, No. 8, (August 2011), pp. 656-662, ISSN: 0198-8859.

Gupta S, Shenoy VP, Mukhopadhyay C, Bairy I & Muralidharan S. (2011). Role of risk factors and socio-economic status in pulmonary tuberculosis: a search for the root cause in patients in a tertiary care hospital, South India. *Trop Med Int Health*, Vol. 16, No. 1, (January 2011), pp. 74-78, ISSN: 1360-2276.

Harries AD, Zachariah R, Lawn SD. (2009). Providing HIV care for co-infected tuberculosis patients: a perspective from sub-Saharan Africa. *Int J Tuberc Lung Dis*, Vol. 13, No. 1, (January 2009), pp. 6-16, ISSN: 1027-3719.

Havlir DV & Barnes PF. (1999). Tuberculosis in patients with human immunodeficiency virus infection. *N Eng J Med*, Vol. 340, (February 1999), pp. 367-373, ISSN: 0028-4793.

Hopewell PC. (2005). Tuberculosis and other mycobacterial diseases. In: *Murray and Nadel's textbook of respiratory medicine*, Mason RJ, Murray JF, Broaddus VC & Nadel JA, pp. 979-1043, Elsevier Saunders, Inc, ISSN: 0-7216-0327-0, Philadelphia.

Hopewell PC & Chaisson RE. (2000). Tuberculosis and human immunodeficiency virus infection. In: *Tuberculosis: a comprehensive international approach*, Reichman LB & Hershfield ES, pp. 525-552, Marcel Dekker, Inc, ISSN: 0-8247-8121-X, New York.

Huang CC, Liu MF, Lee NY, Chang CM, Lee HC, Wu CJ & Ko WC. (2010). Fatal tuberculous myositis in a immunocompromised adult with primary Sjögren's syndrome. *J Formos Med Assoc*, Vol. 109, No. 9, (September 2010), pp. 680-683, ISSN: 0929-6646.

International Standards for Tuberculosis Care (ISTC). (2009). *The Hague, Tuberculosis Coalition for Technical Assistance (2nd ed)*, World Health Organization, Geneva.

Ito I, Tada K, Ootera H, Sakurai T & Iwasaki H. (2011). Analysis of usefulness of a whole blood interferon-gamma assay (QuantiFERON TB-2G) for diagnosing active tuberculosis in immunocompromised patients. *Kekkaku*, Vol. 86, No. 2, (February 2011), pp. 45-50, ISSN: 0022-9776.

Jiang JR, Yen SY & Wang JY. (2011). Increased prevalence of primary drug-resistant pulmonary tuberculosis in immunocompromised patients. *Respirology*, Vol. 16, No. 2, (February 2011), pp. 308-313, ISSN: 1323-7799.

Kassim S, Sassan-Morokro M, Ackah A, Abouya LY, Digbeu H, Yesso G, Coulibaly IM, Coulibaly D, Whitaker PJ & Doorly R. (1995). Two year follow-up of persons with HIV-1-associated and HIV-2-associated pulmonary tuberculosis treated with short-course chemotherapy in West Africa. *AIDS*, Vol. 9, No. 10, (October 1995), pp. 1185-1191, ISSN: 0269-9370.

Khan FA, Minion J, Pai M, Royce S, Burman W, Harries AD & Menzies D. (2010). Treatment of active tuberculosis in HIV co-infected patients: a systematic review and meta-analysis. *Clin Infect Dis*, Vol. 50, No. 9, (May 2010), pp. 1288-1299, ISSN: 1058-4838.

Kivihya-Ndugga L, van Cleeff M, Juma E, Kimwomi J, Githui W, Oskam L, Schuitema A, van Soolinger D, Nganga L, Kibuga D, Odhiambo J & Klatser P. (2004). Comparison of PCR with the routine procedure for diagnosis of tuberculosis in a population with high prevalence of tuberculosis and human immunodeficiency virus. *J Clin Microbiol*, Vol. 42, No. 3, (March 2004), pp. 1012-1015, ISSN: 0095-1137.

Komiya K, Ariga H, Nagai H, Teramoto S, Kurashima A, Shoji S & Nakajima Y. (2010). Impact of peripheral lymphocyte count on the sensitivity of 2 interferon-gamma release assays, QFT- G and ELISPOT, in patients with pulmonary tuberculosis. *Intern Med*, Vol. 49, No. 17, (September 2010), pp. 1849-1855, ISSN: 0918-2918, doi: 10.2169/internalmedicine.49.3659

Korenromp EL, Scano F, Williams BG, Dye C & Nunn P. (2003). Effects of human immunodeficiency virus infection on recurrence of tuberculosis after rifampicin-based treatment: an analytical review. *Clin Infect Dis*, Vol. 37, No. 1, (July 2003), pp. 101-112, ISSN: 1058- 4838.

Lawn SD, Bekker L-G & Miller RF. (2005). Immune reconstitution disease associated with Mycobacterial infections in HIV-infected individuals receiving antiretrovirals. *Lancet Infect Dis*, Vol. 5, No. 6, (June 2005), pp. 361-373, ISSN: 1473-3099.

Lawn SD & Churchyard G. (2009). Epidemiology of HIV-associated tuberculosis. *Curr Opin HIV AIDS*, Vol. 4, No. 4, (July 2009), pp. 325-333, ISSN: 1746-630X.

Li SY, Chen TJ, Chung KW, Tsai LW, Yang WC, Chen JY & Chen TW. (2011). Mycobacterium tuberculosis infection of end-stage renal disease patients in Taiwan: a national longitudinal study. *Clin Microbiol Infect*, (January 2011), 1469-0691, Jan 24. doi: 10.1111/j.1469- 0691.2011.03473.x [Epub ahead of print].

Lockman S. (June 6, 2011). A new era: molecular tuberculosis diagnosis. Title, In: *Search Medscape News*, June 29, 2011, Available from:
http://www.medscape.com/viewarticle/745030?src=nl_topic

Long R, Scalcini M, Manfreda J, Carre' G, Philippe E, Hershfield E, Sekla L & Stackiw W. (1991). Impact of human immunodeficiency virus type 1 on tuberculosis in rural Haiti. *Am Rev Respir Dis*, Vol. 143, No. 1, (January 1991), pp. 69-73, ISSN: 1073-449X.

Lyu J, Lee SG, Hwang S, Lee SO, Cho OH, Chae EJ, Lee SD, Kim WS, Kim DS & Shim TS. (2011). Chest CT is more likely to show latent tuberculosis foci than simple chest radiography in liver transplantation candidates. *Liver Transpl*, Vol. 17, No. 8, (August 2011), pp. 963-968, ISSN: 1527- 6465, doi: 10.1002/lt.22319

Markowitz N, Hansen NI, Wilcosky TC, Hopewell PC, Glassroth J, Kvale PA, Mangura BT, Osmond D, Wallace JM, Rosen MJ & Reichman LB. (1993). Tuberculin and anergy testing in HIV-seropositive and HIV-seronegative persons. Pulmonary Complications of HIV Infection Study Group. *Ann Intern Med*, Vol. 119, No. 3, (August 1993), pp. 185-193, ISSN: 0003-4819.

Mazulek GH, Jereb J, LoBue P, Iademarco MF, Metchock B & Vernon A. (2005). Guidelines for using the QuantiFERON-TB Gold test for detecting Mycobacterium tuberculosis infection, United States. *MMWR*, Vol. 54, No. RR15, (December 2005), pp. 49-55, ISSN: 1057-5987.

Mazulek GH, Jereb J, Vernon A, LoBue P, Goldberg S & Castro K. (2010). Updated guidelines for using interferon-gamma release assays to detect Mycobacterium tuberculosis infection--- United States, 2010. *MMWR*, Vol. 59, No. RR05, (June 2010), pp. 1-25, ISSN: 1057-5987.

Mazurek GH & Villarino ME. (2003). Guidelines for using the QuantiFERON-TB test for diagnosing latent Mycobacterium tuberculosis infection. *MMWR*, Vol. 52, No. RR02, (January 2003), pp. 15-18, ISSN: 1057-5987.

McIlleron H, Meintjes G, Burman WJ & Maartens G. (2007). Complications of antiretroviral therapy in patients with tuberculosis-drug interactions, toxicity and immune reconstitute inflammatory syndrome. *J Infect Dis*, Vol. 196 (Suppl 1), (August 2007), pp. S63-75, ISSN: 0022- 1899.

Moreira J, Fochesatto JB, Moreira AL, Pereira M, Porto N & Hochhegger B. (2011). Tuberculous pneumonia: a study of 59 microbiologically confirmed cases. *J Bras Pneumol*, Vol. 37, No. 2, (April 2011), pp. 232-237, ISSN: 1806-3713.

Mwinga A, Nunn A, Ngwira B, Chintu C, Warndorff D, Fine P, Darbyshire J & Zumla AI; LUSKAR collaboration. (2002). Mycobacterium vaccae (SRL 172) immunotherapy as an adjunct to Standard antituberculosis treatment in HIV-infected adults with pulmonary tuberculosis: a randomized placebo-controlled trials. *Lancet*, Vol. 360, No. 9339, (October 2002), pp. 1050-1055, ISSN: 0099-5355.

Nachega JB & Maartens G. (2009). Clinical aspects of tuberculosis in HIV-infected adults, In: *Tuberculosis: a comprehensive clinical reference*, Schaaf HS & Zumla AI, pp. 524-531, Suanders Elsevier, ISSN: 978-1-4160-3988-4, London.

Patel AK, Rami KC & Ghanchi FD. (2011). Radiological presentation of patients of pulmonary tuberculosis with diabetes mellitus. *Lung India*, Vol. 28, No. 1, (January-March 2011), pp. 70, ISSN: 0970-2113.

Perez-Guzman C, Torres-Cruz A, Villarreal-Velarde H & Vargas MH. (2000). Progressive age- related changes in pulmonary tuberculosis images and the effect of diabetes. *Am J Respir Crit Care Med*, Vol. 162, No. 5, (November 2000), pp. 1738-1740, ISSN: 1073-449X.

Perlman DC, el-Sadr W, Nelson ET, Matts JP, Telzak EE, Salomon N, Chirgwin K & Hafner R. (1997). Variation of radiographic patterns in pulmonary tuberculosis by degree of human immunodeficiency virus-related immunosuppression. The Terry Beirn Community Programs for Clinical Research on AIDS (CPCRA). The AIDS Clinical Trials Group (ACTG). *Clin Infect Dis*, Vol. 25, No. 2, (August 1997), pp. 242-246, ISSN: 1058-4838.

Perriens JH, St. Louis ME, Mukadi YB, Brown C, Prignot J, Pouthier F, Portaels F, Willame JC, Mandala JK, Kaboto M, Ryder RW, Roscigno G & Piot P. (1995). Pulmonary tuberculosis in HIV-infected patients in Zaire: a controlled trial of treatment for either 6 or 12 months. *N Eng J Med*, Vol. 332, No. 12, (March 1995), pp. 779-784, ISSN: 0028-4793.

Pithie AD & Chicksen B. (1992). Fine-needle extrathoracic lymph-node aspiration in HIV-associated sputum-negative tuberculosis. *Lancet*, Vol. 340, No. 8834-8835, (n.d. 1992), pp. 1504- 1505, ISSN: 0099-5355.

Post FA, Wood R & Pillay GP. (1995). Pulmonary tuberculosis in HIV infection: radiographic appearance is related to CD4+ T-lymphocyte count. *Tuber Lung Dis*, Vol. 76, No. 6, (December 1995), pp. 518-521, ISSN: 0962-8479.

Prabu VNN & Agrawal S. (2010). Systemic lupus erythematosus and tuberculosis: a review of complex interactions of complicated diseases. *J Postgrad Med*, Vol. 56, No. 3, (August 2010), pp. 244-250, ISSN: 0022-3859, doi: 10.4103/0022-3859.68653

Rangaka MX, Wilkinson KA, Seldon R, Van Cutsem G, Meintjes GA, Morroni C, Mouton P, Diwakar L, Connell TG, Maartens G & Wilkinson RJ. (2007). Effect of HIV-1 infection on T cell based and skin test detection of tuberculosis infection. *Am J Respir Crit Care Med*, Vol. 175, No. 5, (March 2007), pp. 514-520, ISSN: 1073-449X.

Restrepo BI, Camerlin AJ, Rahbar MH, Wang W, Restrepo MA, Zarate I, Mora-Guzma'n F, Crespo-Solis JG, Briggs J, McCormick JB & Fisher-Hoch SP. (2011). Cross-sectional assessment reveals high diabetes prevalence among newly-diagnosed tuberculosis cases. *Bull World Health Organ*, Vol. 89, No. 5, (May 2011), pp. 352-359, ISSN: 0042-9686.

Rothel JS, Jones SL, Corner LA, Cox JC & Wood PR. (1990). A sandwich enzyme immunoassay for bovine interferon-gamma and its use for detection of tuberculosis in cattle. *Aust Vet J*, Vol. 67, No. 4, (April 1990), pp. 134-137, ISSN: 0005-0423.

Sauzullo I, Mengoni F, Scrivo R, Valesini G, Potenza C, Skroza N, Marocco R, Lichtner M, Vullo V & Mastroianni CM. (2010). Evaluation of QuantiFERON-TB Gold In-Tube in human immunodeficiency virus infection and in patients candidates for anti-tumor necrosis factor- alpha treatment. *Int J Tuberc Lung Dis*, Vol. 14, No. 7, (July 2010), pp. 834-840, ISSN: 1027-3719.

Schijman AG, Losso MH, Montoto M, Saez CB, Smayevsky J & Benetucci JA. (2004). Prospective evaluation of in-house polymerase chain reaction for diagnosis of mycobacterial diseases in patients with HIV infection and lung infiltrates. *Int J Tuberc Lung Dis*, Vol. 8, No. 1, (January 2004), pp. 106-113, ISSN: 1027-3719.

Sen T, Joshi SR & Udwadia ZF. (2009). Tuberculosis and diabetes mellitus: Merging epidemics. *J Assoc Physicians India*, Vol. 57, (May 2009), pp. 399-404, 0004-5772.

Silva DR, Menegotto DM, Schulz LF, Gazzana MB & Dalcin PdeTR. (2010). Clinical characteristics and evolution of non-HIV-infected immunicompromised patients with an in- hospital diagnosis of tuberculosis. *J Bras Pneumol*, Vol. 36, No. 4, (August 2010), pp. 475-484, ISSN: 1806-3713.

Sociedade Brasileira de Pneumologia e Tisiologia. (2004). 11 Consenso Brasileiro de Tuberculose-Diretrizes Brasileiras para Tuberculose. *J Bras Pneumol*, Vol. 30 (Puppl 1), (n.d. 2004), pp. S4-S56, ISSN: 1806-3713.

Sonnelberg P, Murray J, Glynn JR, Shearer S, Kambashi B & Godfrey-Faussett P. (2001). HIV-1 and recurrence, relapse, and reinfection of tuberculosis after cure: a cohort study in South African mineworkers. *Lancet*, Vol. 358, No. 9294, (November 2001), pp. 1687-1693, ISSN: 0099-5355.

Sterling TR, Alwood K, Gachuhi R, Coggin W, Blazes D, Bishai WR & Chaisson RE. (1999). Relapse rates after short-course (6-month) treatment of tuberculosis in HIV-infected and uninfected persons. *AIDS*, Vol. 13, No. 14, (October 1999), pp. 1899-1904, ISSN: 0269-9370.

Streeton JA, Desem N & Jones SL. (1998). Sensitivity and specificity of a gamma-interferon blood test for tuberculosis infection. *Int J Tuberc Lung Dis*, Vol. 2, No. 6, (June 1998), pp. 443-450, ISSN: 1027-3719.

Tan CK, Lai CC, Chen HW, Liao CH, Chou CH, Huang YT, Yang WS, Yu CJ & Hsueh PR. (2010). Enzyme-Linked immunospot assay for interferon-gamma to support the diagnosis of tuberculosis in diabetic patients. *Scand J Infect Dis*, Vol. 42, No. 10, (October 2010), pp. 752- 756, ISSN: 0036-5548.

Tenth Zonal Tuberculosis and Chest Disease Centre, Tenth Office of Disease Prevention and Control, Chiang Mai, Thailand. (2005). *Tuberculosis annual report*, Tenth Zonal Tuberculosis and Chest Disease Centre, Tenth Office of Disease Prevention and Control, Chiang Mai, Thailand.

Tenth Zonal Tuberculosis and Chest Disease Centre, Tenth Office of Disease Prevention and Control, Chiang Mai, Thailand. (2006). *Tuberculosis annual report*, Tenth Zonal Tuberculosis and Chest Disease Centre, Tenth Office of Disease Prevention and Control, Chiang Mai, Thailand.

Tenth Zonal Tuberculosis and Chest Disease Centre, Tenth Office of Disease Prevention and Control, Chiang Mai, Thailand. (2007). *Tuberculosis annual report*, Tenth Zonal Tuberculosis and Chest Disease Centre, Tenth Office of Disease Prevention and Control, Chiang Mai, Thailand.

Tenth Zonal Tuberculosis and Chest Disease Centre, Tenth Office of Disease Prevention and Control, Chiang Mai, Thailand. (2009). *Tuberculosis annual report*, Tenth Zonal Tuberculosis and Chest Disease Centre, Tenth Office of Disease Prevention and Control, Chiang Mai, Thailand. Toure' NO, Dia Kane Y, Diatta A, Ba Diop S, Niang A, Ndiaye EM, Thiam K, Mbaye FB, Badiane M & Hane AA. (2010). Tuberculosis in elderly persons. *Rev Mal Respir*, Vol. 27, No. 9, (November 2010), pp. 1062-1068, ISSN: 0761-8425.

Torrea G, Van de Perre P, Ouedraogo M, Zougba A, Sawadogo A, Dingtoumda B, Diallo B, Defer MC, Sombie' I, Zanetti S & Sechi LA. (2005). PCR-based detection of the Mycobacterium tuberculosis complex in urine of HIV-infected and uninfected pulmonary and extrapulmonary tuberculosis patients in Burkina Faso. *J Med Microbiol*, Vol. 54, No. Pt 1, (January 2005), pp. 39-44, ISSN: 0022-2615.

Vargas PJ, King G & Navarra SV. (2009). Central nervous system infections in Filipino patients with systemic lupus erythematosus. *Int J Rheum Dis*, Vol. 12, No. 3, (September 2009), pp. 234-238, ISSN: 1756-1841.

Walsh MC, Camerlin AJ, Miles R, Pino P, Martinez P, Mora-Guzma'n F, Crespo-Solis JG, Fisher- Hoch SP, McCormick JB & Restrepo BI. (2011). The sensitivity of interferon-gamma release assays is not compromised in tuberculosis patients with diabetes. *Int J Tuberc Lung Dis*, Vol. 15, No. 2, (February 2011), pp. 179-184, ISSN: 1027-3719.

Wells CD. (2010). Global impact of multidrug-resistant pulmonary tuberculosis among HIV-infected and other immunocompromised hosts: epidemiology, diagnosis, and strategies for management. *Curr Infect Dis Rep*, Vol. 12, No. 3, (May 2010), pp. 192-197, ISSN: 1523-3847.

Wendel KA & Sterling TR. (2002). Tuberculosis and HIV. *AIDS Clin Care*, Vol. 14, No. 2, (February 2002), pp. 9-15, ISSN: 1043-1543.

Wilson D, Nachega J, Chaisson R & Maartens G. (2005). Diagnostic yield of peripheral lymph node needle-core biopsies in HIV-infected adults with suspected smear-negative tuberculosis. *Int J Tuberc Lung Dis*, Vol. 9, No. 2, (February 2005), pp. 220-222, ISSN: 1027-3719.

Wilson D, Nachega J, Morroni C, Chaisson RE & Maartens G. (2006). Diagnosing smear-negative tuberculosis using case definitions and treatment response in HIV-infected adults. *Int J Tuberc Lung Dis*, Vol. 10, No. 1, (January 2006), pp. 31-38, ISSN: 1027-3719.

Woldehanna S & Volmink J. (2004). Treatment of latent tuberculosis infection in HIV infected persons. *Cochrane Database Syst Rev*, No. 1, (n.d. 2004): CD000171, ISSN: 1469-493X.

World Health Organization. (2010). *Global tuberculosis control: WHO report 2010*, World Health Organization, ISSN: 978 92 4 156406 9, Geneva.

World Health Organization. (2006). *Guidelines on co-trimoxazole prophylaxis for HIV-related infections among children, adolescents and adults in resource-limited settings: recommendations for a public health* approach, ISSN: 97892 4 159470 7, Geneva.

World Health Organization. (2009). Key recommendations, In : *Rapid advice for antiretroviral therapy for HIV infection in adults and adolescents*, June 6, 2011, Available from: http://www.who.int/hiv/pub/arv/rapid_advice_art.pdf

World Health Organization. (2010). About WHO expert group and STAG-TB recommendations, In: *Roadmap for rolling out Xpert MTB/RIF for rapid diagnosis of tuberculosis and MDR-TB*, June 6, 2011, Available from: http://www.who.int/tb/laboratory/roadmap_xpert_mtb-rif.pdf

World Health Organization. (2010). *Treatment of tuberculosis: guidelines* (4th ed), World Health Organization, ISSN: 978 92 4 154783 3, Geneva.

Young F, Wotton CJ, Critchley JA, Unwin NC & Goldacre MJ. (2010). Increased risk of tuberculosis disease in people with diabetes mellitus: record-linkage study in a UK population. *J Epidemiol Community Health*, (November 2010), ISSN: 0143-005X, Nov 24. [Epub ahead of print].

Yu YH, Liao CC, Hsu WH, Chen HJ, Liao WC, Muo CH, Sung FC & Chen CY. (2011). Increased lung cancer risk among patients with pulmonary tuberculosis: a population cohort study. *J Thorac Oncol*, Vol. 6, No. 1, (January 2011), pp. 32-37, ISSN: 1556-0864.

Permissions

The contributors of this book come from diverse backgrounds, making this book a truly international effort. This book will bring forth new frontiers with its revolutionizing research information and detailed analysis of the nascent developments around the world.

We would like to thank Dr. Pere-Joan Cardona, for lending his expertise to make the book truly unique. He has played a crucial role in the development of this book. Without his invaluable contribution this book wouldn't have been possible. He has made vital efforts to compile up to date information on the varied aspects of this subject to make this book a valuable addition to the collection of many professionals and students.

This book was conceptualized with the vision of imparting up-to-date information and advanced data in this field. To ensure the same, a matchless editorial board was set up. Every individual on the board went through rigorous rounds of assessment to prove their worth. After which they invested a large part of their time researching and compiling the most relevant data for our readers. Conferences and sessions were held from time to time between the editorial board and the contributing authors to present the data in the most comprehensible form. The editorial team has worked tirelessly to provide valuable and valid information to help people across the globe.

Every chapter published in this book has been scrutinized by our experts. Their significance has been extensively debated. The topics covered herein carry significant findings which will fuel the growth of the discipline. They may even be implemented as practical applications or may be referred to as a beginning point for another development. Chapters in this book were first published by InTech; hereby published with permission under the Creative Commons Attribution License or equivalent.

The editorial board has been involved in producing this book since its inception. They have spent rigorous hours researching and exploring the diverse topics which have resulted in the successful publishing of this book. They have passed on their knowledge of decades through this book. To expedite this challenging task, the publisher supported the team at every step. A small team of assistant editors was also appointed to further simplify the editing procedure and attain best results for the readers.

Our editorial team has been hand-picked from every corner of the world. Their multi-ethnicity adds dynamic inputs to the discussions which result in innovative outcomes. These outcomes are then further discussed with the researchers and contributors who give their valuable feedback and opinion regarding the same. The feedback is then collaborated with the researches and they are edited in a comprehensive manner to aid the understanding of the subject.

Apart from the editorial board, the designing team has also invested a significant amount of their time in understanding the subject and creating the most relevant covers. They scrutinized every image to scout for the most suitable representation of the subject and create an appropriate cover for the book.

The publishing team has been involved in this book since its early stages. They were actively engaged in every process, be it collecting the data, connecting with the contributors or procuring relevant information. The team has been an ardent support to the editorial, designing and production team. Their endless efforts to recruit the best for this project, has resulted in the accomplishment of this book. They are a veteran in the field of academics and their pool of knowledge is as vast as their experience in printing. Their expertise and guidance has proved useful at every step. Their uncompromising quality standards have made this book an exceptional effort. Their encouragement from time to time has been an inspiration for everyone.

The publisher and the editorial board hope that this book will prove to be a valuable piece of knowledge for researchers, students, practitioners and scholars across the globe.

List of Contributors

Patrick Eberechi Akpaka and Shirematee Baboolal
Unit of Microbiology & Pathology, Department of Para Clinical Sciences, Faculty of Medical Sciences, The University of the West Indies, St. Augustine, Trinidad & Tobago

N. Esther Babady
Memorial Sloan-Kettering Cancer Center, New York, New York, USA

Nancy L. Wengenack
Mayo Clinic, Rochester, Minnesota, USA

Sahal Al-Hajoj
Biological and Medical Research Department, King Faisal Specialist Hospital and Research Centre, Kingdom of Saudi Arabia

Simeon I.B. Cadmus
Department of Veterinary Public Health and Preventive Medicine, University of Ibadan, Ibadan, Nigeria

Osman El Tayeb
Damien Foundation, Belgium

Dick van Soolingen
Departments of Pulmonary Diseases and Medical Microbiology, Radboud University of Nijmegen Medical Centre, Nijmegen, Netherlands
National Tuberculosis Reference Laboratory, National Institute for Public Health and the Environment (RIVM), Bilthoven, Netherlands

Faten Al-Zamel
King Saud University, Saudi Arabia

Claude Mambo Muvunyi
Department of Clinical Chemistry, Microbiology and Immunology, Ghent University Hospital, De Pintelaan, Ghent, Belgium
Department of Clinical Biology, Centre Hospitalier Universitaire-Butare, National University of Rwanda, Butare, Rwanda

Florence Masaisa
Department of Clinical Chemistry, Microbiology and Immunology, Ghent University Hospital, De Pintelaan, Ghent, Belgium
Department of Internal Medicine, Centre Hospitalier Universitaire-Butare, National University of Rwanda, Butare, Rwanda

Shamsher S. Kanwar
Department of Biotechnology, Himachal Pradesh University, Summer Hill, Shimla, India

Iacob Simona Alexandra and Banica Dorina
National Institute of Infectious Diseases "Matei Bals", Bucharest, Romania

Iacob Diana Gabriela and Panaitescu Eugenia
The University of Medicine and Pharmacy "Carol Davila" Bucharest, Romania

Radu Irina
The University of Bucharest, Romania

Cojocaru Manole
The "Titu Maiorescu" University, Romania

Wellman Ribón
Universidad Industrial de Santander, Bucaramanga, Colombia

Attapon Cheepsattayakorn
Thai Board of Preventive Medicine (Public Health Science), 10th Zonal Tuberculosis and Chest Disease Centre, Chiang Mai, 10th Office of Disease Prevention and Control, Department of Disease Control, Ministry of Public Health, Thailand

Printed in the USA
CPSIA information can be obtained
at www.ICGtesting.com
JSHW011430221024
72173JS00004B/746

9 781632 412041